Barbara O'N

Natural Holistic Remedies

Complete Collection

Over 1000 Herbal Remedies Based on Barbara O'Neill's Teachings for Sustained Wellness

By

Rebecca Wimborne

Disclaimer notice

Table of Contents

Introduction

In an era where quick fixes and symptom-focused treatments often dominate healthcare, a quiet revolution is brewing—a return to nature's wisdom and holistic healing. The profound teachings of Barbara O'Neill, a leading figure in natural health, inspire this comprehensive guide. Her integrative approach blends time-honored remedies with modern scientific understanding, offering a pathway to genuine wellness and vitality.

The genesis of this project lies in a personal journey towards finding sustainable, natural health solutions. The limitations of conventional medicine, which often targets symptoms without addressing underlying causes, prompted a deep dive into alternative approaches. Barbara O'Neill's holistic philosophies, emphasizing the body's innate ability to heal, provided the perfect foundation for this exploration.

At the heart of this guide is the principle that proper health is multifaceted, encompassing physical, emotional, and environmental well-being. This holistic perspective is woven throughout, emphasizing the interconnectedness of our choices and their cumulative impact on health. Readers are introduced to various natural healing modalities grounded in Barbara O'Neill's practical and compassionate approach.

One of the key themes explored is the importance of detoxification. In our modern world, exposure to toxins is nearly unavoidable. This guide provides clear, actionable steps to cleanse the body, highlighting the benefits of detox practices in restoring balance and enhancing vitality.

Nutrition plays a pivotal role in Barbara O'Neill's teachings. This guide offers detailed insights into how a balanced diet, rich in whole foods and devoid of harmful substances, can prevent illness and support overall well-being. It goes beyond essential dietary advice, delving into the healing properties of specific foods and how they can be used therapeutically.

Herbal remedies are another cornerstone of natural health, and this guide demystifies their use. Readers will discover how to harness the power of herbs to support the body's healing processes, alleviate symptoms, and enhance immunity. Practical advice on sourcing, preparing, and using these natural medicines is provided, making it easy for anyone to incorporate them into their daily routine.

The transformative power of essential oils is also explored. These potent plant extracts offer myriad benefits, from stress relief to immune support. This guide explains how to use essential oils safely and effectively, whether through aromatherapy, topical application, or other methods.

Chronic illness and pain are pervasive issues that often defy conventional treatment. This guide emphasizes the role of lifestyle modifications, dietary changes, and natural therapies in achieving lasting relief and improved quality of life, providing readers with a sense of reassurance and hope.

Emotional and mental health are integral to overall wellness. Techniques for stress reduction, mindfulness, and emotional support are discussed, offering readers tools to enhance their mental well-being.

In essence, this comprehensive guide is a call to action. It invites readers to embrace natural healing practices, make informed health choices, and cultivate a deeper connection with themselves and the natural world.

BOOK 1: Meet Barbara O'Neill

The Inspiring Journey of a Trailblazing Health Pioneer

Chapter 1: Biography and background

Barbara O'Neill, a leading figure in natural health and herbal medicine, has devoted her entire life to comprehending and advocating the benefits of holistic healing. Born into a family that cherished natural remedies, Barbara's journey into herbal medicine commenced at a tender age. Her upbringing, steeped in the rich natural healing traditions passed down through generations, ignited her enduring passion for herbal medicine.

Barbara's formal education took a different path initially. She pursued studies in conventional healthcare, believing that a strong foundation in medical science would complement her interests in natural remedies. She earned a degree in nursing, which provided her with valuable insights into the workings of the human body and the principles of medical treatment. Her experience in the healthcare system, however, exposed her to the limitations and side effects of conventional medicine. This realization reinforced her belief in the potential of natural remedies to offer safer, more holistic alternatives.

After completing her nursing degree, Barbara sought to deepen her knowledge of natural health. She embarked on extensive studies in nutrition, herbal medicine, and naturopathy. Her education included rigorous training and certifications from reputable institutions, where she learned from some of the leading experts in the field. This comprehensive education equipped her with a deep understanding of the therapeutic properties of herbs and the principles of natural healing.

Barbara's career as a health practitioner took flight when she established her wellness center. Here, she amalgamated her medical background with her expertise in natural remedies to offer holistic healthcare to her clients. Her approach was distinctive; she didn't just alleviate symptoms but concentrated on identifying and tackling the root causes of health issues. This holistic perspective resonated with many people who were in search of alternatives to conventional treatments.

Over the years, Barbara's practice grew, and she became a sought-after speaker and educator. She conducted workshops, seminars, and lectures worldwide, sharing her knowledge and insights with laypeople and healthcare professionals. Her ability to explain complex concepts in simple, understandable terms made her a popular and effective teacher. She also authored numerous articles and books on natural health, establishing her as a leading voice.

Barbara's impact extends beyond her personal practice and educational efforts. She has been instrumental in advocating for recognizing and integrating natural remedies within mainstream healthcare. Her work has helped to bridge the gap between conventional medicine and natural health practices, promoting a more inclusive and comprehensive approach to wellness.

Despite her professional success, Barbara remains deeply committed to personal growth and continuous learning. She regularly updates her knowledge by attending conferences, conducting research, and collaborating with other experts in the field. This commitment to lifelong education ensures that her teachings and practices remain current and evidence-based.

Throughout her career, Barbara has maintained a strong focus on empowering individuals to take charge of their own health. She believes that education is the key to health and wellness, and she strives to provide people with the knowledge and tools they need to make informed decisions about their health. Her approach is compassionate and practical, emphasizing the importance of a balanced lifestyle, proper nutrition, and the therapeutic use of herbs, empowering her audience to take control of their health.

In her personal life, Barbara practices what she preaches. She leads a healthy, balanced lifestyle, incorporating the principles of natural health into her daily routine. Her personal experiences with natural remedies and holistic living serve as a testament to the efficacy of her approach and inspire those around her.

Barbara O'Neill's journey from a young girl fascinated by the healing power of nature to a respected authority in natural health is a testament to her dedication, knowledge, and passion. Her work continues to inspire and educate people worldwide, helping them achieve better health and well-being through the power of nature. As she looks to the future, Barbara remains committed to advancing the field of herbal medicine and promoting a holistic approach to health that honors the wisdom of nature.

Chapter 2: His journey into herbal remedies

Barbara O'Neill's journey into herbal remedies is a fascinating story of passion, education, and dedication to holistic health. This journey can be divided into three main phases: her early influences and inspirations, her formal education and training, and her practical application and professional growth.

2.1 Early Influences and Inspirations

Barbara's interest in herbal remedies began in her childhood. Growing up in a family that valued natural health practices, she was exposed to the healing power of herbs and plants from a young age. Her parents and grandparents often used herbal teas, poultices, and natural concoctions to treat common ailments. This early exposure instilled in her a deep appreciation for nature's pharmacy and a curiosity about how these remedies worked.

During her teenage years, Barbara began to explore herbal remedies more deeply. She spent hours reading books on herbal medicine, learning about the different plants and their medicinal properties. She started a small herb garden, experimenting with growing and using various herbs. This hands-on experience allowed her to see firsthand the benefits of natural remedies. Her success in treating minor health issues with her homemade remedies strengthened her belief in the power of herbs and fueled her desire to learn more.

2.2 Formal Education and Training

As Barbara grew older, she decided to pursue a career in healthcare. She believed that a strong foundation in medical science would complement her interest in herbal medicine and enable her to provide comprehensive care. She enrolled in a nursing program, where she gained valuable knowledge about human anatomy, physiology, and the principles of conventional medicine. Her nursing education provided her with a deep understanding of the human body and the disease processes, which would later prove invaluable in her practice of herbal medicine.

However, Barbara soon realized that conventional medicine had its limitations. She saw patients who were suffering from chronic conditions that medications could only manage, not cure. She also witnessed the side effects and complications that often accompany pharmaceutical treatments. These experiences reinforced her belief in the importance of natural and preventative healthcare.

Determined to integrate her medical knowledge with her passion for natural remedies, Barbara sought further education in herbal medicine. She enrolled in nutrition, naturopathy, and herbal medicine courses from reputable institutions. She studied under renowned herbalists and natural health practitioners, learning about the therapeutic properties of plants, the principles of holistic health, and the art of formulating herbal remedies. This rigorous training provided her with a solid foundation in herbal medicine and equipped her with the skills needed to practice it professionally.

2.3 Practical Application and Professional Growth

With her comprehensive education and training, Barbara was ready to put her knowledge into practice. She opened her wellness center, combining her nursing background with her expertise in herbal medicine to provide holistic healthcare to her clients. Her approach was unique and holistic; she didn't just focus on treating symptoms but aimed to identify and address the root causes of health issues.

In her practice, Barbara used a variety of herbal remedies to treat a wide range of conditions. She formulated personalized treatment plans for her clients, incorporating herbal teas, tinctures, salves, and dietary recommendations. Her treatments were based on thoroughly understanding each client's health history, lifestyle, and needs. This personalized approach not only provided effective relief but also empowered her clients to take charge of their health.

Barbara's success in her practice quickly gained her a reputation as a skilled and compassionate practitioner. She became a sought-after speaker and educator, conducting workshops and seminars to share her knowledge and experience. Her ability to explain complex concepts in simple, understandable terms made her a popular teacher. She also authored numerous articles and books on herbal medicine, establishing her as a leading voice in the field.

Throughout her career, Barbara has remained committed to advancing the field of herbal medicine. She regularly updates her knowledge by attending conferences, conducting research, and collaborating with other experts. This commitment to continuous learning ensures that her practice remains current and evidence-based.

Barbara's journey into herbal remedies is marked by a deep passion for natural health, a dedication to education, and a commitment to holistic care. Her early influences and hands-on experiences laid the foundation for her interest in herbal medicine. Her formal education and rigorous training provided her with the knowledge and skills needed to practice it professionally. Her practical application and professional growth have allowed her to make a significant impact in the field of natural health, helping countless individuals achieve better health and well-being through the power of herbs.

Chapter: 3 Philosophy and basic principles of his approach

Barbara O'Neill's approach to health and wellness is deeply rooted in a holistic philosophy that views the body as an interconnected system. Her principles are derived from traditional wisdom and contemporary scientific understanding. This philosophy is based on the belief that proper health is achieved through balance and harmony within the body, mind, and spirit. Here, we will delve into the core elements of Barbara O'Neill's philosophy and principles, which include holistic health, natural remedies, prevention over cure, the importance of diet and lifestyle, and patient empowerment.

3.1 Holistic Health

At the heart of Barbara O'Neill's approach is holistic health. Holistic health recognizes that the body is not merely a collection of parts but an integrated whole with interconnected physical, mental, emotional, and spiritual aspects. Barbara emphasizes that to achieve optimal health, one must consider all these facets.

Body-Mind Connection: Barbara believes physical health cannot be separated from mental and emotional well-being. Stress, anxiety, and emotional trauma can manifest as physical ailments. Conversely, physical health issues can affect one's mental and emotional state. Therefore, her approach addresses the physical symptoms and the underlying emotional and psychological factors.

Spiritual Well-being: While not tied to any specific religion, Barbara acknowledges the role of spiritual health in overall well-being. This can involve a sense of purpose, connection to nature, meditation, or other practices that foster inner peace and fulfillment.

Environmental Factors: She also considers the impact of the environment on health. This includes exposure to toxins, quality of air and water, and even the electromagnetic fields surrounding us. Barbara advocates for creating a living environment that supports health, such as using natural cleaning products, ensuring good air quality, and minimizing exposure to harmful substances.

3.2 Natural Remedies

Barbara O'Neill is a strong proponent of natural remedies. She believes nature provides everything we need to maintain health and treat illness. Several principles guide her use of natural remedies:

Plant-based Healing: The cornerstone of her natural remedies is the use of herbs and plants. Plants contain a wide array of compounds that can have therapeutic effects. Barbara's extensive knowledge of herbal medicine allows her to recommend specific herbs for various conditions, ensuring they are used safely and effectively.

Minimizing Side Effects: One of the key advantages of natural remedies, according to Barbara, is their lower risk of side effects compared to synthetic drugs. While she acknowledges that natural does not always mean safe when used correctly, herbal and natural remedies often have a gentler impact on the body.

Supporting the Body's Natural Processes: Natural remedies support the body's healing processes rather than overriding them. For instance, instead of using pharmaceuticals to suppress symptoms, Barbara uses herbs and other natural treatments to enhance the body's ability to heal.

Holistic Formulations: She often creates holistic formulations that combine herbs and natural ingredients to address multiple aspects of a condition. These formulations are designed to be synergistic, where the combined effect is greater than the sum of the individual components.

3.3 Prevention Over Cure

A central tenet of Barbara O'Neill's philosophy is the emphasis on prevention rather than cure. She believes many health problems can be avoided through proactive measures that maintain and enhance health. This preventive approach involves several strategies:

Regular Detoxification: Barbara advocates for regular detoxification practices to eliminate toxins from the body. This can include dietary changes, specific herbs, and other natural methods to support the liver, kidneys, and other organs involved in detoxification.

Nutritional Support: Adequate nutrition is fundamental to preventing disease. Barbara stresses the importance of a diet rich in fruits, vegetables, whole grains, and other nutrient-dense foods. She often recommends dietary supplements to address specific deficiencies and support overall health.

Healthy Lifestyle Practices: Beyond diet, Barbara promotes a lifestyle that includes regular physical activity, adequate sleep, stress management, and other healthy habits. She believes these lifestyle factors are critical to preventing chronic diseases and maintaining long-term health.

Early Intervention: When signs of imbalance or illness appear, Barbara advocates for early intervention with natural remedies and lifestyle adjustments. Addressing issues promptly can prevent them from developing into more severe health problems.

3.4 Importance of Diet and Lifestyle

Barbara O'Neill places significant emphasis on the role of diet and lifestyle in achieving and maintaining health. She believes that what we eat and how we live have profound effects on our overall well-being. Her dietary and lifestyle principles include:

Whole Foods Diet: Barbara advocates for a diet based on whole, unprocessed foods. She emphasizes the importance of eating various fruits, vegetables, whole grains, nuts, and seeds. These foods provide essential nutrients that support the body's functions and promote health.

Avoiding Harmful Substances: She advises against consuming processed foods, refined sugars, artificial additives, and other substances that can harm the body. Barbara is particularly critical of the excessive intake of sugar and refined carbohydrates, which she links to numerous health problems.

Hydration: Adequate hydration is another key component of her dietary advice. Barbara encourages the consumption of pure water and herbal teas while limiting caffeinated and sugary beverages.

Regular Physical Activity: Physical activity is crucial for maintaining health. Barbara recommends regular exercise tailored to an individual's abilities and preferences. She highlights the benefits of aerobic and strength-training activities and the importance of incorporating movement into daily routines.

Stress Management: Recognizing the impact of stress on health, Barbara includes stress management techniques in her approach. This can involve mindfulness practices, meditation, yoga, and other activities that promote relaxation and mental well-being.

Sleep and Rest: Adequate sleep and rest are essential for the body to repair and rejuvenate. Barbara emphasizes the importance of good sleep hygiene and ensuring that individuals get enough restful sleep each night.

3.5 Patient Empowerment

A crucial element of Barbara O'Neill's philosophy is empowering individuals to take charge of their health. She believes that education and self-awareness are key to achieving and maintaining wellness, providing a sense of control and empowerment. Her principles of patient empowerment include:

Education and Knowledge: Barbara is passionate about educating her clients and the public about health and wellness. She provides information on how the body works, the impact of diet and lifestyle on health, and the use of natural remedies. Her goal is to equip individuals with the knowledge they need to make informed decisions about their health.

Personal Responsibility: She encourages individuals to take personal responsibility for their health, fostering a sense of accountability and proactivity. This means making conscious choices about diet, lifestyle, and healthcare practices. Barbara believes that individuals are their best health advocates and that empowerment comes from taking an active role in one's health.

Holistic Self-Care: Barbara promotes holistic self-care practices that individuals can incorporate into their daily lives. This includes not only diet and exercise but also practices like journaling, spending time in nature, and engaging in activities that bring joy and fulfillment.

Supportive Guidance: While she emphasizes self-care and personal responsibility, Barbara also recognizes the importance of supportive guidance. She works closely with her clients to develop personalized health plans, providing the support and encouragement needed to implement and sustain healthy changes. This emphasis on supportive guidance is designed to make everyone feel reassured and confident in their health journey, fostering a sense of security and confidence.

Community and Connection: Barbara believes in the power of community and connection in achieving health. She fosters a sense of community among her clients and encourages them to seek support from family, friends, and like-minded individuals. Social connections and a sense of belonging are important aspects of holistic health.

Adaptability and Personalization: Recognizing that each individual is unique, Barbara's approach is highly adaptable and personalized. She tailors her recommendations to fit the specific needs, preferences, and circumstances of each person. This personalized approach ensures that everyone feels understood and catered to, making the health strategies practical and effective for each individual.

Book 2: Introduction to Natural Healing

Unlocking the Secrets to Holistic Health, Wellness, and Sustainable Living for a Vibrant Life

Chapter 1: Understanding the Basics of Natural Healing

1.1 Definition and Principles of Natural Healing

Natural healing is an approach to health and wellness that prioritizes the body's intrinsic ability to heal itself using natural, non-invasive methods. This philosophy is deeply rooted in the belief that the body, mind, and spirit are interconnected and that true health encompasses all aspects of a person's life. Natural healing practices seek to address the root causes of illness rather than merely treating symptoms, promoting a holistic and sustainable approach to wellness.

At its core, natural healing emphasizes the use of natural remedies, including herbs, essential oils, proper nutrition, physical activity, and stress management techniques. These methods are chosen for their minimal side effects and their ability to support the body's natural processes. This approach stands in contrast to conventional medicine, which often relies on synthetic drugs and invasive procedures that can sometimes lead to adverse effects or only provide temporary relief.

Barbara O'Neill, a renowned naturopath and health educator, champions natural healing as a vital path to achieving optimal health. She advocates for a comprehensive understanding of the body's needs and encourages individuals to take an active role in their health journey. According to O'Neill, the principles of natural healing are grounded in several key concepts:

1. Holistic Approach: Natural healing views the body as an integrated whole rather than a collection of separate parts. It considers the physical, mental, emotional, and spiritual dimensions of health, acknowledging that imbalances in one area can affect the others. This holistic perspective ensures that all aspects of a person's well-being are addressed in the healing process.

2. Prevention Over Cure: Prevention is a cornerstone of natural healing. By maintaining a healthy lifestyle and making informed choices, individuals can prevent many illnesses before they develop. This proactive approach includes adopting a balanced diet, regular physical activity, adequate sleep, and effective stress management techniques. Prevention not only enhances quality of life but also reduces the need for medical interventions.

3. Empowerment Through Education: Barbara O'Neill believes in empowering individuals with knowledge about their health. Education is a crucial component of natural healing, as it enables people to make informed decisions about their well-being. Understanding how the body works and what it needs to thrive helps individuals take responsibility for their health and make choices that promote healing and prevention.

4. Use of Natural Remedies: Natural healing relies on the therapeutic properties of natural substances such as herbs, essential oils, and whole foods. These remedies are used to support the body's natural healing processes and restore balance. For example, herbs like echinacea and turmeric are known for their

immune-boosting and anti-inflammatory properties, respectively, while essential oils like lavender and peppermint offer relaxation and pain relief.

5. Support of the Body's Innate Healing Ability: Natural healing trusts in the body's inherent wisdom and capacity to heal itself. Practitioners aim to create an environment that supports these natural processes, whether through detoxification, proper nutrition, or stress reduction. This principle underscores the importance of not interfering unnecessarily with the body's attempts to restore health.

6. Lifestyle and Environmental Factors: Natural healing recognizes the significant impact of lifestyle and environment on health. Factors such as diet, exercise, sleep, and exposure to toxins all play critical roles in overall well-being. By addressing these elements, individuals can create a supportive environment that fosters healing and prevents disease.

In summary, natural healing is a comprehensive approach to health that focuses on nurturing the body's natural abilities and addressing the root causes of illness. Through a combination of education, prevention, natural remedies, and lifestyle adjustments, individuals can achieve and maintain optimal health. Barbara O'Neill's principles of natural healing serve as a guide for those seeking to embrace a holistic and empowering path to wellness.

1.2 Historical Background of Natural Healing Practices

The roots of natural healing practices extend deep into human history, long before the advent of modern medicine. Ancient civilizations recognized the healing potential of natural elements and developed extensive knowledge of plants, minerals, and other natural substances to treat ailments and maintain health. These early practices laid the foundation for contemporary natural healing methods, blending centuries of empirical wisdom with modern scientific understanding.

One of the earliest known systems of natural healing is Traditional Chinese Medicine (TCM), which dates back over 2,500 years. TCM is grounded in the concept of Qi, the vital life force that flows through the body. According to TCM, health is achieved by maintaining the balance and flow of Qi through practices like acupuncture, herbal medicine, dietary therapy, and Tai Chi. The Chinese pharmacopoeia includes thousands of herbs, each classified by their properties and therapeutic actions, illustrating a sophisticated understanding of plant-based healing.

Similarly, Ayurveda, the traditional medicine system of India, has been practiced for over 3,000 years. Ayurveda, meaning "science of life," emphasizes balance among the body, mind, and spirit. It categorizes individuals into three primary doshas (Vata, Pitta, and Kapha), each representing different physiological and psychological traits. Ayurvedic practitioners use a variety of natural treatments, including herbal medicine, dietary adjustments, yoga, and meditation, tailored to the individual's dosha to promote health and prevent disease.

In ancient Greece, Hippocrates, often referred to as the "Father of Medicine," advocated for natural healing methods in the 5th century BCE. He believed in the body's intrinsic ability to heal itself and emphasized the importance of diet, exercise, and environmental factors in maintaining health. His famous maxim, "Let food be thy medicine and medicine be thy food," underscores the enduring relevance of nutrition in natural healing. Hippocrates' holistic approach laid the groundwork for later developments in Western herbalism and naturopathy.

The Indigenous peoples of the Americas have also contributed significantly to natural healing practices. Native American healing traditions are deeply connected to nature and the spiritual world. These practices often involve the use of medicinal plants, rituals, and ceremonies to restore balance and harmony within the individual and the community. The extensive botanical knowledge of Indigenous healers has informed modern herbal medicine, highlighting the therapeutic potential of plants native to the Americas.

In Europe, during the Middle Ages and Renaissance, herbal medicine was widely practiced by monks, nuns, and lay healers. Monastic gardens were cultivated with medicinal plants, and texts such as the "Herbarium" by Apuleius Platonicus and the "Physica" by Hildegard of Bingen compiled extensive herbal knowledge. The Renaissance period saw the resurgence of ancient Greek and Roman medical texts, further enriching the European tradition of herbal medicine. Paracelsus, a Swiss physician and alchemist, introduced the concept of "like cures like," which influenced the development of homeopathy in the 18th century.

The 19th and early 20th centuries marked the formalization of natural healing practices into recognized medical disciplines. Naturopathy emerged in Europe and North America, integrating the principles of herbal medicine, nutrition, hydrotherapy, and lifestyle counseling. Figures such as Sebastian Kneipp, who popularized hydrotherapy, and Benedict Lust, who founded the first naturopathic medical school in the United States, played pivotal roles in establishing naturopathy as a holistic medical system.

Concurrently, the practice of homeopathy, developed by Samuel Hahnemann, gained popularity for its principle of "like cures like" and the use of highly diluted substances to stimulate the body's healing response. Homeopathy's emphasis on individualized treatment and minimal intervention resonated with the broader movement towards natural and holistic medicine.

The mid-20th century saw the rise of the modern holistic health movement, which sought to integrate natural healing practices with contemporary medical knowledge. Pioneers like Dr. John Christopher and Dr. Bernard Jensen promoted herbal medicine, nutrition, and detoxification as essential components of health care. The growing interest in alternative medicine led to the establishment of professional organizations, educational programs, and research institutions dedicated to natural healing.

Today, natural healing practices continue to evolve, informed by both ancient traditions and modern scientific discoveries. The integration of traditional knowledge with contemporary research has led to a deeper understanding of the mechanisms underlying natural remedies and their efficacy in promoting health and preventing disease. This historical continuum underscores the enduring relevance of natural healing and its potential to contribute to a more holistic and sustainable approach to health care.

The historical background of natural healing practices is a rich tapestry woven from the diverse traditions of ancient civilizations, indigenous cultures, and modern holistic pioneers. These practices, rooted in the wisdom of the past, continue to offer valuable insights and approaches to health and wellness in the contemporary world.

1.3 Comparison with Conventional Medicine

Natural healing and conventional medicine represent two distinct paradigms in health care, each with its own philosophy, methodologies, and areas of strength. Understanding the differences and complementary aspects of these approaches is essential for individuals seeking the best care for their health needs.

Conventional medicine, also known as allopathic or Western medicine, is characterized by its reliance on scientific research, pharmaceutical interventions, and advanced technological procedures. It excels in acute care, emergency situations, and conditions requiring surgical intervention. The approach is typically symptom-focused, aiming to diagnose and treat specific diseases or injuries through standardized methods. Conventional medicine operates within a reductionist framework, where diseases are often seen as isolated from the broader context of the patient's overall health.

In contrast, natural healing, often referred to as holistic or complementary and alternative medicine (CAM), emphasizes the body's innate ability to heal itself. This approach is based on the principles of holistic care, where the mind, body, and spirit are viewed as interconnected and essential to overall health. Natural healing employs a variety of non-invasive methods, including herbal remedies, nutrition, acupuncture, massage, and lifestyle changes, to support the body's natural healing processes and address the root causes of illness.

One of the primary distinctions between the two approaches is their perspective on disease and treatment. Conventional medicine tends to be disease-centered, focusing on identifying pathogens or physiological malfunctions and then eliminating or correcting them. Treatments often involve medications, surgeries, and other interventions that directly target the symptoms or the underlying cause of a specific condition. For example, antibiotics are used to combat bacterial infections, and surgeries are performed to remove tumors.

Natural healing, on the other hand, adopts a more patient-centered approach. It seeks to understand the individual's unique physical, emotional, and environmental context and how these factors contribute to their health. Rather than targeting specific symptoms in isolation, natural healing aims to restore balance and support the body's self-healing capabilities. For instance, an herbalist might use anti-inflammatory herbs, dietary changes, and stress reduction techniques to manage chronic inflammation, considering both the physical and emotional factors contributing to the condition.

Preventive care is another area where the two approaches differ significantly. Conventional medicine often emphasizes preventive care through screenings, vaccinations, and early detection of diseases. While these measures are crucial, they typically focus on identifying and mitigating risks rather than promoting overall wellness. Natural healing, however, places a stronger emphasis on lifestyle and dietary choices as primary preventive measures. Practitioners encourage habits that support long-term health, such as regular physical activity, balanced nutrition, adequate sleep, and stress management.

The methodologies used in these approaches also differ. Conventional medicine relies heavily on pharmacological treatments and high-tech diagnostic tools. While these have proven highly effective in many cases, they can also lead to side effects and complications. Additionally, the cost and accessibility of such treatments can be prohibitive for some individuals. Natural healing methods, such as herbal remedies, acupuncture, and nutritional counseling, tend to have fewer side effects and are often more accessible and affordable. However, the effectiveness of these treatments can vary, and they may not always provide the immediate results that some conventional treatments offer.

Integration of both approaches can provide a more comprehensive care strategy. Many health care providers and patients recognize the value of combining the strengths of conventional medicine with the holistic principles of natural healing. For instance, a patient undergoing surgery (a conventional approach) might also use herbal supplements and acupuncture to support recovery and manage pain (natural healing methods).

While conventional medicine excels in acute and emergency care, and in addressing specific diseases with targeted interventions, natural healing offers valuable approaches for chronic conditions, prevention, and overall wellness. By recognizing the strengths and limitations of both paradigms, individuals can make informed decisions about their health care, often finding that a combination of both conventional and natural methods provides the most effective and comprehensive path to wellness. This integrated approach, often termed integrative or complementary medicine, aims to harness the best of both worlds to support optimal health outcomes.

Chapter 2: Barbara O'Neill's Philosophy and Approach

2.1 Core Beliefs and Principles

Natural healing is built upon a foundation of core beliefs and principles that distinguish it from conventional medical approaches. These principles emphasize the body's inherent ability to heal, the importance of holistic care, and the necessity of addressing the root causes of illness rather than merely treating symptoms. The core beliefs and principles of natural healing can be encapsulated as follows:

The Body's Innate Healing Ability

At the heart of natural healing is the belief in the body's intrinsic ability to heal itself. This principle, often referred to as the "vis medicatrix naturae" or the healing power of nature, asserts that the body is naturally designed to maintain health and recover from illness. Natural healers focus on supporting and enhancing this self-healing capacity through non-invasive methods and lifestyle adjustments. Rather than suppressing symptoms, they aim to create conditions that facilitate the body's natural healing processes.

Holistic Approach to Health

Natural healing emphasizes a holistic approach, which means considering the whole person—body, mind, and spirit—in the context of their environment. This principle recognizes that physical health cannot be separated from emotional, mental, and spiritual well-being. Practitioners of natural healing strive to address all aspects of a person's life, understanding that imbalances in one area can affect overall health. This comprehensive approach ensures that treatment plans are personalized and tailored to the individual's unique needs and circumstances.

Prevention Over Cure

A cornerstone of natural healing is the emphasis on preventive care. The belief is that maintaining health through proactive measures is far more effective than treating diseases after they have developed. Preventive care in natural healing involves adopting a healthy lifestyle, which includes a balanced diet, regular exercise, sufficient sleep, stress management, and avoiding toxins. By focusing on prevention, individuals can reduce their risk of developing chronic diseases and improve their overall quality of life.

Treating the Root Cause

Natural healing is distinguished by its focus on identifying and treating the underlying causes of illness rather than just addressing symptoms. Symptoms are viewed as signals from the body indicating deeper imbalances or dysfunctions. Practitioners spend time understanding the patient's history, lifestyle, and environment to uncover these root causes. Treatments are then designed to correct these underlying issues, leading to more sustainable and long-lasting health improvements.

Individualized Treatment

Every person is unique, and natural healing respects this individuality. Treatments are customized based on the patient's specific needs, preferences, and circumstances. This personalized approach contrasts with the one-size-fits-all methodology that is often seen in conventional medicine. By considering genetic predispositions, lifestyle choices, and emotional state, practitioners can develop more effective and tailored treatment plans.

Use of Natural Remedies

Natural healing heavily relies on natural remedies, including herbs like chamomile for relaxation, essential oils such as lavender for stress relief, and whole foods like garlic for immune support. These remedies are chosen for their ability to support the body's natural functions and promote health without the side effects often associated with synthetic drugs. Herbal medicine, for example, uses plants with medicinal properties to treat various conditions, while nutrition therapy focuses on using food as medicine to support overall health.

Patient Empowerment and Education

Empowering patients through education is a fundamental principle of natural healing. Practitioners believe that informed patients are better equipped to make decisions about their health and take an active role in their healing journey. Education involves teaching patients about the principles of natural healing, the importance of lifestyle choices, and how to use natural remedies effectively. This knowledge fosters a sense of responsibility and autonomy in patients, encouraging them to take charge of their health.

Balance and Harmony

Natural healing advocates restoring and maintaining balance and harmony within the body and the environment. Whether nutritional, emotional, or environmental, imbalances are seen as the root of illness. Practices like meditation, yoga, and Tai Chi are often recommended to help achieve mental and emotional balance. Creating a healthy living environment by reducing exposure to toxins and embracing natural elements is vital for overall well-being, highlighting the importance of balance and harmony in your health journey.

Integration with Conventional Medicine

While natural healing emphasizes non-invasive and holistic methods, it does not reject conventional medicine outright. Instead, it seeks to integrate the best of both worlds. This integrative approach recognizes that conventional medicine excels in acute and emergency care, while natural healing offers valuable insights into chronic disease management and preventive care. By combining these approaches, practitioners aim to provide comprehensive and effective health care.

In summary, the core beliefs and principles of natural healing center on the body's innate ability to heal, a holistic view of health, the importance of prevention, addressing root causes, individualized treatment, the use of natural remedies, patient empowerment, balance and harmony, and integration with conventional medicine. These principles collectively form a comprehensive approach to health that emphasizes long-term well-being and the body's natural wisdom.

2.2 Holistic Health: Body, Mind, and Spirit Connection

Holistic health is an approach that seeks to treat and care for the whole person, recognizing the intricate connections between the body, mind, and spirit. This perspective goes beyond merely addressing physical symptoms; it involves understanding how mental, emotional, and spiritual factors contribute to overall well-being. The concept of holistic health is rooted in the belief that optimal health cannot be achieved by focusing solely on one aspect of a person's life but rather by acknowledging and nurturing the interconnectedness of all these elements.

2.2.1 Body: The Physical Foundation

The body is the tangible aspect of our being and the foundation for holistic health. Physical health involves maintaining the body's systems in optimal working order through proper nutrition, regular exercise, adequate rest, and preventive care. Natural healing practices strongly emphasize these aspects, advocating for a balanced diet rich in whole foods, regular physical activity to strengthen and sustain bodily functions, and sufficient sleep to repair and rejuvenate the body.

Nutrition plays a critical role in holistic health. Consuming various nutrient-dense foods supports bodily functions and provides the necessary vitamins, minerals, and antioxidants to prevent disease and promote healing. Regular exercise strengthens muscles, improves cardiovascular health, boosts the immune system, and enhances mental well-being by releasing endorphins. Adequate sleep is essential for overall health, as it allows the body to repair tissues, consolidate memories, and regulate hormones.

Moreover, natural remedies such as herbal supplements and essential oils are often used to support physical health. These remedies can help alleviate symptoms, enhance immune function, and promote overall vitality without the side effects commonly associated with synthetic drugs. By nurturing the body with these holistic practices, individuals can maintain physical health and prevent many common ailments.

2.2.2 Mind: The Mental and Emotional Sphere

Mental and emotional health is another crucial component of holistic well-being. The mind influences the body through complex interactions that affect hormone levels, immune function, and overall health. Stress, anxiety, and depression can manifest as physical symptoms such as headaches, digestive issues, and weakened immunity. Thus, addressing mental and emotional health is essential for achieving holistic health.

Stress management is a significant aspect of mental health within holistic healing. Techniques such as meditation, mindfulness, and deep-breathing exercises are commonly recommended to reduce stress and promote relaxation. These practices help calm the mind, lower cortisol levels and improve overall mood. Regular practice of mindfulness and meditation has been shown to enhance emotional resilience, increase self-awareness, and promote a sense of inner peace.

Emotional health also involves processing and expressing emotions in healthy ways. Practices such as journaling, counseling, and engaging in creative activities can help individuals understand and manage their emotions. Building strong social connections and maintaining supportive relationships are also vital for emotional well-being, as they provide a sense of belonging and reduce feelings of isolation.

2.2.3 Spirit: The Core of Being

The spiritual aspect of holistic health pertains to the deeper sense of purpose, meaning, and connection to something greater than oneself. Spiritual health does not necessarily involve religious beliefs but rather encompasses a broader sense of connection to the universe, nature, or a higher power. This connection can provide comfort, foster resilience, and enhance overall well-being.

Practices such as prayer, meditation, and spending time in nature can nurture spiritual health. These activities help individuals connect with their inner selves, find meaning in their experiences, and develop a sense of peace and contentment. For some, spiritual health may involve engaging in community service or activities that align with their values and beliefs, fostering a sense of purpose and fulfillment.

Integrating spiritual practices into daily life can provide a sense of balance and harmony, helping individuals navigate life's challenges with greater ease. Spiritual well-being can also promote a positive outlook on life, increase resilience in the face of adversity, and enhance overall happiness.

2.2.4 The Interconnection of Body, Mind, and Spirit

Holistic health recognizes that the body, mind, and spirit are deeply interconnected and that imbalance in one area can affect the others. For example, chronic physical pain can lead to emotional distress and spiritual disconnection, while unresolved emotional issues can manifest as physical symptoms. By addressing all three aspects, holistic health aims to create a harmonious state of well-being.

Natural healing practices often involve treatments that simultaneously address physical, mental, and spiritual health. Yoga, for instance, combines physical postures, breath control, and meditation to enhance physical strength, mental clarity, and spiritual awareness. Similarly, acupuncture can help alleviate physical pain, reduce stress, and restore energetic balance.

In holistic health, the practitioner takes a comprehensive view of the individual, considering lifestyle, environment, emotional state, and spiritual beliefs in the treatment plan. This approach ensures that care is personalized and aligned with the individual's unique needs and circumstances.

Holistic health is an integrative approach that emphasizes the interconnectedness of the body, mind, and spirit. By nurturing each aspect, individuals can achieve a balanced and harmonious state of well-being, leading to optimal health and a fulfilling life. This comprehensive perspective not only addresses symptoms but also fosters long-term health and resilience, providing a more sustainable and enriching path to wellness.

2.3 Importance of Lifestyle Changes in Natural Healing

Lifestyle changes are a cornerstone of natural healing, playing a crucial role in preventing illness, promoting wellness, and enhancing the body's ability to heal itself. Unlike conventional medicine, which often focuses on treating specific symptoms or diseases, natural healing emphasizes the significance of everyday choices and behaviors in maintaining and improving health. Adopting healthy lifestyle habits can lead to profound and lasting health benefits, transforming not only the physical body but also mental, emotional, and spiritual well-being.

2.3.1 The Role of Diet and Nutrition

One of the most impactful lifestyle changes in natural healing involves diet and nutrition. Proper nutrition is fundamental to health, as the nutrients in food are the building blocks of the body. A diet rich in whole, unprocessed foods—such as fruits, vegetables, whole grains, nuts, seeds, and lean proteins—provides essential vitamins, minerals, and antioxidants that support bodily functions and enhance immune defense. These foods help reduce inflammation, balance blood sugar levels, and provide the energy needed for daily activities and healing processes.

Conversely, diets high in processed foods, refined sugars, unhealthy fats, and artificial additives can lead to nutrient deficiencies, chronic inflammation, and a range of health problems such as obesity, diabetes, cardiovascular disease, and cancer. Natural healing advocates for a return to nutrient-dense, natural foods that nourish the body and support overall health. Tailoring dietary choices to individual needs, such as food sensitivities and metabolic types, can further optimize health outcomes.

2.3.2 Physical Activity and Exercise

Regular physical activity is another essential lifestyle change in natural healing. Exercise helps maintain a healthy weight, boosts cardiovascular health, strengthens muscles and bones, and improves flexibility and balance. It also plays a significant role in mental and emotional health by reducing stress, anxiety, and depression. Physical activity stimulates the release of endorphins, the body's natural mood elevators, promoting a sense of well-being and happiness.

Natural healing encourages finding enjoyable and sustainable forms of exercise, such as walking, swimming, cycling, yoga, or dancing. Incorporating movement into daily routines, like taking the stairs instead of the elevator or gardening, can also contribute to overall physical health. The key is consistency and making physical activity a regular part of life.

2.3.3 Stress Management and Mental Health

Effective stress management is crucial in natural healing, as chronic stress can have detrimental effects on both physical and mental health. Stress can weaken the immune system, increase inflammation, disrupt sleep, and contribute to the development of chronic diseases. Natural healing emphasizes techniques to manage and reduce stress, such as mindfulness, meditation, deep breathing exercises, and relaxation techniques.

Practices like yoga and tai chi combine physical movement with mindfulness and breath control, helping to alleviate stress and improve mental clarity. Engaging in hobbies, spending time in nature, and cultivating supportive relationships are important strategies for maintaining mental and emotional health. Prioritizing mental health through these practices can lead to improved resilience, better mood regulation, and enhanced overall well-being.

2.3.4 Sleep and Rest

Adequate sleep and rest are foundational to natural healing. Sleep is the body's time for repair and regeneration, essential for cognitive function, emotional balance, and physical health. Chronic sleep deprivation can impair immune function, increase the risk of chronic diseases, and negatively affect mood and cognitive performance.

Natural healing promotes good sleep hygiene practices, such as maintaining a regular sleep schedule, creating a restful sleep environment, and avoiding stimulants like caffeine and electronic devices before bedtime. Techniques such as relaxation exercises, herbal teas, and aromatherapy with essential oils like lavender can also support better sleep quality.

Chapter 3: Fundamental Natural Healing Techniques

3.1 Diet and Nutrition

Diet and nutrition are fundamental pillars of natural healing, crucial in maintaining health, preventing disease, and supporting the body's natural healing processes. A well-balanced, nutrient-rich diet provides the essential building blocks for the body's cells, tissues, and organs, ensuring optimal functioning and resilience against illnesses. Understanding the principles of a natural healing diet can empower individuals to make informed dietary choices that promote long-term health and vitality.

Whole Foods Over Processed Foods

The cornerstone of a natural healing diet is the emphasis on whole foods over processed foods. Whole foods are minimally processed and as close to their natural state as possible. These include fresh fruits, vegetables, whole grains, nuts, seeds, legumes, and lean proteins. Whole foods are rich in essential nutrients, including vitamins, minerals, antioxidants, and fiber, which support the body's functions and protect against diseases.

Processed foods, on the other hand, are often stripped of their natural nutrients and contain unhealthy additives such as artificial flavors, preservatives, and excessive sugar and salt. Regular consumption of processed foods is associated with numerous health issues, including obesity, diabetes, cardiovascular disease, and cancer. By prioritizing whole foods, individuals can reduce their intake of harmful substances and increase their consumption of beneficial nutrients.

Plant-Based Emphasis

A natural healing diet typically emphasizes plant-based foods. Fruits and vegetables are essential because they are high in vitamins, minerals, and antioxidants, which help to reduce inflammation and combat oxidative stress. The most nutrient-dense options are leafy greens, berries, cruciferous vegetables, and citrus fruits.

Legumes, nuts, and seeds are excellent plant-based proteins and healthy fats sources. They provide essential amino acids, omega-3 fatty acids, and fiber, which are essential for maintaining cardiovascular health, supporting brain function, and promoting digestive health. Whole grains such as quinoa, brown rice, and oats offer complex carbohydrates that provide sustained energy and support metabolic health.

Healthy Fats

Healthy fats are a crucial component of a natural healing diet. These fats in avocados, nuts, seeds, and fatty fish play a vital role in brain health, hormone production, and cellular function. Omega-3 fatty acids, in particular, have anti-inflammatory properties and are essential for heart health. Incorporating healthy fats while avoiding trans fats and excessive saturated fats found in processed and fried foods is important for overall health.

Hydration

Adequate hydration is essential for every aspect of health. Water is involved in virtually all bodily functions, including digestion, nutrient absorption, temperature regulation, and toxin elimination. Drinking plenty of water throughout the day helps keep the body hydrated, supports metabolic processes, and efficiently removes waste products.

In addition to water, herbal teas, and fresh vegetable juices can also contribute to hydration and provide additional nutrients and antioxidants. Avoiding sugary drinks, excessive caffeine, and alcohol is important as they can lead to dehydration and negatively impact health.

<u>Avoiding Toxins</u>

A key principle of natural healing is minimizing exposure to dietary toxins. This involves choosing organic foods, when possible, to reduce exposure to pesticides and genetically modified organisms (GMOs). It also means avoiding foods that contain artificial additives, preservatives, and colorings, which can have harmful effects on health.

Additionally, reducing the intake of sugar and refined carbohydrates is important. High sugar consumption is linked to various health issues, including obesity, diabetes, and cardiovascular disease. Instead, natural sweeteners like honey or maple syrup can be used in moderation.

<u>Personalized Nutrition</u>

Natural healing recognizes that there is no one-size-fits-all diet. Personalized nutrition involves tailoring dietary choices to an individual's specific needs, preferences, and health conditions. Factors such as age, gender, activity level, and genetic predispositions can influence nutritional requirements. Working with a nutritionist or a healthcare provider can help individuals create a personalized eating plan that supports their unique health goals and needs.

<u>Detoxification</u>

Diet plays a significant role in the body's natural detoxification processes. Certain foods can support the liver, kidneys, and other organs involved in detoxification. For example, cruciferous vegetables like broccoli and Brussels sprouts contain compounds that enhance liver detoxification enzymes. Foods high in fiber, such as fruits, vegetables, and whole grains, help to promote regular bowel movements and the elimination of toxins.

<u>Mindful Eating</u>

Mindful eating is an integral part of a natural healing diet. This involves paying attention to hunger and satiety cues, eating slowly, and savoring each bite. Mindful eating encourages a healthy relationship with food, reduces overeating, and enhances the enjoyment and appreciation of meals. It also helps individuals become more aware of how different foods affect their body and mind.

Diet and nutrition are central to natural healing, offering a powerful means to support overall health and well-being. By focusing on whole, nutrient-dense foods, staying hydrated, avoiding dietary toxins, and adopting personalized and mindful eating practices, individuals can harness the healing power of nutrition to achieve and maintain optimal health. These dietary principles provide the necessary nutrients for bodily functions and help prevent chronic diseases and promote longevity and vitality.

3.2 Whole Foods and Plant-Based Diet

A fundamental aspect of natural healing is emphasizing whole foods and adopting a plant-based diet. Whole foods are minimally processed and as close to their natural state as possible, providing a rich source of nutrients essential for optimal health. These include fresh fruits and vegetables, whole grains, nuts, seeds, and legumes. A plant-based diet, which prioritizes these foods, is associated with numerous health benefits, including reduced risk of chronic diseases, enhanced immune function, and improved overall well-being.

3.2.1 The Nutritional Superiority of Whole Foods

Whole foods are nutritionally superior to their processed counterparts. They are packed with vitamins, minerals, antioxidants, and fiber, all vital for maintaining bodily functions and preventing disease. For instance, fruits and vegetables are rich in vitamins A, C, and E, which have powerful antioxidant properties that help protect cells from damage caused by free radicals. Whole grains such as quinoa, brown rice, and oats provide essential B vitamins and complex carbohydrates that offer sustained energy and support metabolic health.

Processed foods, in contrast, often contain added sugars, unhealthy fats, and artificial additives while lacking the natural nutrients found in whole foods. Regular consumption of processed foods is linked to numerous health issues, including obesity, diabetes, cardiovascular disease, and certain cancers. Individuals can significantly improve their nutrient intake and reduce exposure to harmful substances by focusing on whole foods.

3.2.2 The Health Benefits of a Plant-Based Diet

A plant-based diet emphasizes the consumption of plant-derived foods while minimizing or eliminating animal products. This dietary approach has been shown to confer various health benefits. Plant-based diets are typically high in fiber, which aids in digestion, promotes satiety, and helps regulate blood sugar levels. They are also rich in phytonutrients—compounds found in plants with anti-inflammatory and antioxidant properties, such as flavonoids, carotenoids, and polyphenols.

Research has consistently shown that plant-based diets can reduce the risk of chronic diseases. For example, studies have found that individuals who follow plant-based diets have lower rates of heart disease, hypertension, type 2 diabetes, and certain types of cancer. This is primarily attributed to the high intake of fruits, vegetables, whole grains, nuts, and seeds, all rich in nutrients that support cardiovascular health, regulate blood pressure, and enhance immune function.

3.2.3 Environmental and Ethical Considerations

In addition to the health benefits, a plant-based diet is also more environmentally sustainable and ethically responsible. The production of plant-based foods generally requires fewer resources, such as water and land, and generates lower greenhouse gas emissions compared to animal agriculture. By choosing plant-based options, individuals can contribute to reducing their environmental footprint and promoting a more sustainable food system.

Moreover, a plant-based diet aligns with ethical considerations regarding animal welfare. It reduces the demand for factory farming, which is often associated with poor animal treatment and significant environmental degradation. Adopting a plant-based diet is a compassionate choice that reflects a commitment to ethical and sustainable living.

3.2.4 Practical Tips for Adopting a Whole Foods, Plant-Based Diet

Transitioning to a whole-food, plant-based diet can be both enjoyable and rewarding. Start by incorporating more fruits and vegetables into meals, aiming for a variety of colors to ensure a range of nutrients. Experiment with whole grains such as quinoa, farro, and brown rice, and include a variety of legumes like lentils, chickpeas, and black beans for protein. Nuts and seeds make excellent snacks and can be added to dishes for extra texture and nutrition.

Planning and preparation are key to success. Batch cooking and meal prepping can save time and ensure that healthy options are readily available. Exploring plant-based recipes and experimenting with herbs and spices can make meals exciting and flavorful. Additionally, being mindful of nutrient intake, particularly protein, iron, calcium, and vitamin B12, is essential for maintaining a balanced and healthful diet.

Embracing whole foods and a plant-based diet is a powerful step toward natural healing and well-being. This approach not only enhances physical health by providing essential nutrients and reducing disease risk, but also supports environmental sustainability and ethical living. By making informed and conscious dietary choices, individuals can take control of their health and contribute to a more sustainable future, harnessing the benefits of whole foods and plant-based eating to achieve long-term health and vitality.

3.3 Importance of Hydration

Hydration is a cornerstone of natural healing, vital in maintaining overall health and well-being. Adequate water intake is essential for many bodily functions, including temperature regulation, nutrient transportation, joint lubrication, and waste elimination. Despite its fundamental importance, hydration is often overlooked in discussions about health and wellness. Understanding the significance of proper hydration and its impact on the body can empower individuals to prioritize this crucial aspect of their health regimen.

The Role of Water in Bodily Functions

Water is involved in nearly every physiological process within the body. It is a major component of blood, transporting oxygen and nutrients to cells and removing waste products. Proper hydration ensures these processes occur efficiently, supporting cellular function and overall metabolic health. Additionally, water helps regulate body temperature through sweating and respiration. In hot conditions or during physical activity, adequate hydration is critical to prevent overheating and maintain homeostasis.

Joint health is another area where hydration is crucial. Water acts as a lubricant and cushion for joints, helping to protect them from damage and reduce the risk of conditions like arthritis. Similarly, it is essential for the proper functioning of the digestive system. Sufficient water intake aids in the digestion and absorption of nutrients, and it prevents constipation by softening stools and promoting regular bowel movements.

Hydration and Detoxification

One of water's most important roles is its contribution to the body's detoxification processes. The kidneys, which filter blood to remove toxins and waste products, rely heavily on adequate hydration to function effectively. Water helps dissolve waste substances and facilitates their excretion through urine. Without sufficient water, the kidneys cannot perform optimally, leading to a buildup of toxins that can negatively impact health.

Sweating is another natural detoxification pathway that depends on proper hydration. The body can expel various waste products through sweat, including heavy metals and metabolic byproducts. Drinking enough water ensures the sweat glands function effectively, supporting the body's natural detox mechanisms.

Hydration and Cognitive Function

The brain is particularly sensitive to changes in hydration status. Even mild dehydration can impair cognitive functions such as concentration, alertness, and short-term memory. Water is essential for maintaining the balance of electrolytes, which are critical for nerve signal transmission. Adequate hydration supports cognitive performance, mood stability, and overall mental clarity. Ensuring regular water intake can help maintain optimal brain function and improve mental well-being.

<u>Signs of Dehydration</u>

Recognizing the signs of dehydration is essential for maintaining health. Symptoms of dehydration can range from mild to severe and include dry mouth, fatigue, dizziness, dark-colored urine, and reduced urine output. In severe cases, dehydration can lead to confusion, rapid heartbeat, and even loss of consciousness. It is important to listen to the body's signals and respond promptly by increasing water intake when necessary.

<u>Practical Tips for Staying Hydrated</u>

Incorporating habits to ensure adequate hydration is a practical approach to natural healing. Aim to drink at least eight 8-ounce glasses of water a day, often referred to as the "8x8" rule, although individual needs may vary based on factors such as activity level, climate, and overall health. Carrying a reusable water bottle can be a constant reminder to drink water throughout the day. Setting regular reminders on the phone or using apps designed to track water intake can also be helpful.

In addition to plain water, other hydrating beverages, such as herbal teas and infused waters, can contribute to overall hydration. Eating water-rich foods like fruits and vegetables, such as cucumbers, oranges, and watermelon, can also help maintain hydration levels. It is important to moderate the consumption of diuretic beverages like coffee and alcohol, which can increase water loss and contribute to dehydration.

Hydration is a fundamental aspect of natural healing that supports various bodily functions and promotes overall health. By ensuring adequate water intake, individuals can enhance physical and cognitive performance, support detoxification processes, and maintain optimal cellular function. Prioritizing hydration is a simple yet powerful strategy to foster long-term health and well-being. Through mindful hydration practices, one can harness the healing power of water and achieve a balanced, vibrant life.

3.4 Detoxification Methods

Detoxification, a central tenet of natural healing, empowers individuals to take control of their health. It aims to eliminate toxins that accumulate in the body due to various environmental exposures, dietary choices, and metabolic processes. Effective detoxification methods can enhance the body's natural ability to cleanse itself, promoting overall health and preventing disease. Several holistic approaches to detoxification emphasize using natural remedies and lifestyle practices to support the body's innate detox pathways, primarily the liver, kidneys, lymphatic system, and skin.

1) Dietary Detoxification

Diet plays a pivotal role in the body's detoxification processes. Consuming a diet rich in detoxifying foods can help stimulate and support the organs responsible for eliminating toxins. Cruciferous vegetables, such as broccoli, cauliflower, and Brussels sprouts, are particularly beneficial as they contain compounds that boost the liver's detoxification enzymes. Leafy greens like kale and spinach are high in chlorophyll, which helps to remove toxins from the bloodstream.

Incorporating fiber-rich foods, such as fruits, vegetables, legumes, and whole grains, is crucial for detoxification. Fiber aids in the elimination of waste through the digestive tract, preventing the reabsorption of toxins. Additionally, staying hydrated by drinking plenty of water helps to flush out toxins through urine and supports kidney function.

2) Herbal Supplements

Herbal supplements can be powerful allies in the detoxification process. Milk thistle, for example, is well-known for its liver-protective properties and can help regenerate liver cells while boosting the organ's ability to filter toxins. Dandelion root is another effective herb that supports liver and kidney function by promoting bile production and acting as a diuretic to increase urine output.

Other beneficial herbs include burdock root, which helps to purify the blood and enhance lymphatic drainage, and turmeric, known for its anti-inflammatory and antioxidant properties that support overall detoxification. Using these herbs in teas, tinctures, or supplements can boost the body's natural detox processes.

3) Hydration and Detoxification

Adequate hydration is essential for effective detoxification. Water facilitates the elimination of waste products through urine and sweat and helps maintain lymph flow. This fluid carries toxins away from tissues and into the bloodstream for elimination. Drinking sufficient water daily, along with herbal teas and fresh vegetable juices, can significantly enhance the body's detoxification ability.

Lemon water is particularly beneficial as it provides vitamin C and antioxidants, which support liver function and stimulate digestive processes. Starting the day with warm lemon water can kickstart the body's detox mechanisms.

4) Physical Activity and Sweating

Physical activity, a natural way to promote detoxification, invigorates the body. Exercise increases circulation and promotes sweating, which helps to eliminate toxins through the skin. Activities like yoga, which combines movement with deep breathing, can enhance the body's detoxification processes by improving circulation and stimulating the lymphatic system.

Regular exercise also supports the health of vital detox organs, such as the liver and kidneys. Incorporating a variety of physical activities, including aerobic exercises, strength training, and stretching, can provide comprehensive support for the body's detox pathways.

5) Sauna and Steam Therapy

Using saunas and steam rooms can significantly aid in the detoxification process by promoting sweating. Sweating helps to expel toxins from the body through the skin, the body's largest detox organ. Infrared saunas, in particular, penetrate deeper into the skin, encouraging more profound detoxification at the cellular level.

Regular sauna use can improve circulation, relax muscles, and enhance overall detoxification. It's important to stay hydrated and replenish electrolytes when using saunas to support the body's detox efforts. Electrolytes, such as potassium and sodium, are essential for maintaining proper fluid balance and muscle function, and sweating in a sauna can deplete these important minerals.

6) Dry Brushing and Lymphatic Drainage

Dry brushing is a technique that involves brushing the skin with a natural bristle brush in a specific pattern to stimulate the lymphatic system. This practice helps to remove dead skin cells, improve circulation, and promote lymphatic drainage, which aids in the removal of toxins from the body.

Lymphatic drainage massage is another method to enhance lymph flow and detoxification. This gentle massage technique encourages the movement of lymph fluid, helping to clear toxins and support the immune system.

Detoxification methods are integral to natural healing, providing various ways to enhance the body's ability to eliminate toxins and maintain health. By incorporating dietary detoxification, herbal supplements, adequate hydration, physical activity, sauna therapy, and practices like dry brushing and lymphatic drainage, individuals can support their body's natural detox pathways. These holistic approaches not only promote the removal of harmful substances but also contribute to overall well-being, vitality, and disease prevention. Embracing these detoxification methods as part of a regular health regimen can lead to a cleaner, healthier, and more balanced body.

3.5 Benefits of Detoxification

Detoxification is a foundational practice in natural healing that offers a multitude of benefits for overall health and well-being. This holistic approach focuses on supporting the body's natural detoxification pathways to eliminate accumulated toxins and restore balance. By incorporating detoxification into a wellness regimen, individuals can experience improved physical vitality, mental clarity, and enhanced immune function. Understanding the specific benefits of detoxification empowers individuals to prioritize this essential practice for optimal health.

3.5.1 Enhanced Energy and Vitality

One of the primary benefits of detoxification is increased energy and vitality. Toxins from environmental pollutants, processed foods, and medications can burden the body's organs and impair cellular function. The body can operate more efficiently by eliminating these toxins through detoxification methods such as dietary changes, hydration, and sauna therapy. This boosts energy levels as metabolic processes improve, allowing individuals to feel more vibrant and alert.

3.5.2 Improved Digestive Health

Detoxification supports digestive health by promoting the elimination of waste and toxins from the digestive tract. A diet rich in fiber, found in fruits, vegetables, and whole grains, aids in regular bowel movements and prevents constipation. Herbal supplements like dandelion root and milk thistle can enhance liver and gallbladder function, facilitating the breakdown of fats and promoting bile production for efficient digestion. By reducing the burden on the digestive system, detoxification can alleviate symptoms such as bloating, gas, and indigestion, promoting overall gut health.

3.5.3 Strengthened Immune System

A well-functioning immune system is crucial for defending against infections and maintaining overall health. Detoxification supports immune function by reducing the load of toxins that can compromise immune response. When the body is burdened with toxins, the immune system may become overtaxed, making it less effective in fighting pathogens. By eliminating toxins through methods like hydration, herbal supplements, and sweat-inducing therapies, detoxification helps to strengthen the immune system and enhance its ability to protect against illness.

3.5.4 Clearer Skin and Youthful Appearance

The skin is a major organ of detoxification, playing a vital role in eliminating toxins through sweat. Individuals can promote clearer skin and a more youthful appearance by supporting detoxification practices such as sauna therapy, dry brushing, and hydration. Sweating helps unclog pores, remove impurities, and promote circulation, reducing acne breakouts and improving skin tone. Additionally, reducing toxin buildup internally can contribute to a brighter complexion and healthier skin overall.

3.5.5 Mental Clarity and Improved Cognitive Function

Toxins can also affect cognitive function and mental clarity. Heavy metals and environmental pollutants can accumulate in the brain, potentially impairing neurotransmitter function and cognitive performance. Detoxification methods that support liver and kidney function, such as herbal supplements and hydration, help to remove these toxins from the body and support brain health. Many individuals report improved concentration, memory, and overall mental acuity after incorporating detoxification practices into their routine.

3.5.6 Weight Management and Metabolic Health

Detoxification can aid in weight management and support metabolic health. Toxins stored in fat cells can interfere with hormone balance and metabolic processes, contributing to weight gain and difficulty losing weight. Individuals can promote a healthy metabolism and facilitate weight loss by reducing toxin exposure and supporting liver function through dietary changes and hydration. Detoxification also encourages the consumption of nutrient-dense foods and hydration, which can further support weight management efforts.

3.5.7 Enhanced Mood and Emotional Well-being

The link between physical health and emotional well-being is well-established. Detoxification practices that support overall health, such as hydration, exercise, and herbal supplements, can positively impact mood and emotional stability. By reducing the body's toxic load and supporting detoxification pathways, individuals may experience reduced feelings of stress, anxiety, and depression. Improving physical health through detoxification can contribute to a more balanced and resilient emotional state.

3.5.8 Long-term Disease Prevention

Detoxification is a proactive approach to health that can help prevent chronic diseases over the long term. By reducing exposure to toxins and supporting the body's natural detoxification mechanisms, individuals can lower their risk of developing conditions such as cardiovascular disease, diabetes, and certain cancers. Maintaining a clean internal environment through regular detoxification practices supports overall health and longevity, enabling individuals to enjoy a higher quality of life as they age.

Detoxification offers a comprehensive array of benefits that support holistic health and well-being. By implementing detoxification methods such as dietary changes, hydration, herbal supplements, and sweat-inducing therapies, individuals can enhance energy levels, improve digestive health, strengthen the immune system, promote clearer skin, boost mental clarity, support weight management, enhance mood, and reduce the risk of chronic diseases. These benefits underscore the importance of detoxification as a foundational practice in natural healing, empowering individuals to optimize their health and vitality through proactive self-care strategies. Integrating detoxification into a balanced lifestyle can lead to profound improvements in overall health, enabling individuals to thrive physically, mentally, and emotionally.

3.6 Simple Detox Practices

Incorporating simple detox practices into your daily routine can significantly enhance your body's natural ability to cleanse and rejuvenate. These practices focus on supporting the organs of detoxification—such as the liver, kidneys, and skin—and promoting overall health and vitality. By adopting these accessible and effective techniques, individuals can experience numerous benefits, including increased energy, improved digestion, clearer skin, and enhanced immune function. Here are some straightforward detox practices that you can incorporate into your daily life:

Hydration

Proper hydration is essential for effective detoxification. Water helps flush toxins from the body through urine and supports kidney function. Start your day with a glass of warm lemon water to stimulate digestion and promote detoxification. Aim to drink at least eight 8-ounce glasses of water (the "8x8" rule) throughout the day to stay adequately hydrated. You can also enjoy herbal teas, such as dandelion or ginger tea, which have detoxifying properties and support liver health.

Nutrient-Dense Diet

Eating a diet rich in nutrient-dense, whole foods is fundamental to supporting detoxification. Focus on incorporating plenty of fruits and vegetables high in antioxidants, vitamins, and minerals that support cellular function and protect against oxidative stress. Include leafy greens, cruciferous vegetables (like broccoli and Brussels sprouts), berries, and citrus fruits in your meals. Choose organic options when possible to reduce exposure to pesticides and toxins.

Avoid processed foods, refined sugars, and trans fats, which can burden the liver and contribute to inflammation. Instead, opt for whole grains like quinoa and brown rice, lean proteins such as beans and legumes, and healthy fats like avocados, nuts, and seeds. Fiber-rich foods, such as flaxseeds and chia seeds, promote regular bowel movements and help eliminate toxins from the digestive tract.

Herbal Supplements

Certain herbs and supplements can support detoxification by enhancing liver function and promoting the elimination of toxins. Milk thistle is well-known for its liver-protective properties and can aid in detoxification by boosting liver detox enzymes. Dandelion root acts as a natural diuretic, supporting kidney function and promoting eliminating waste products through urine. Consider incorporating these herbs into your daily routine through teas or as supplements, following recommended dosages.

Sweating

Sweating is a natural way for the body to eliminate toxins through the skin. Engage in regular physical activity, such as aerobic exercise, yoga, or even brisk walking, to promote sweating and enhance detoxification. Additionally, using saunas or steam rooms can further support detoxification by increasing sweat production and promoting the removal of toxins from the body. Remember to stay hydrated before, during, and after sweating to replenish lost fluids and support detoxification pathways.

Deep Breathing and Relaxation Techniques

Stress can impair the body's detoxification processes and contribute to toxin buildup. To promote relaxation and reduce stress levels, incorporate deep breathing exercises, meditation, or yoga into your daily routine. Deep breathing techniques, such as diaphragmatic breathing or alternate nostril breathing, help oxygenate the body and support lymphatic circulation, which aids in toxin removal.

Dry Brushing

Dry brushing is a simple yet effective technique stimulating the lymphatic system and promoting detoxification. Use a natural bristle brush to gently brush your skin in circular motions, starting from your feet and moving upwards towards your heart. Dry brushing helps exfoliate dead skin cells, improve circulation, and stimulate lymphatic drainage, which supports the removal of toxins from the body. Practice dry brushing before showering, and follow it with a soothing bath or shower to rinse off exfoliated skin cells.

Mindful Eating Practices

Mindful eating involves paying attention to your food choices and eating habits, which can support digestion and detoxification. Chew your food thoroughly and eat slowly to aid digestion and nutrient absorption. Avoid eating large meals late at night, as this can burden digestion and impair detoxification processes during sleep. Be mindful of portion sizes and avoid overeating, which can strain the digestive system and hinder detoxification.

Adequate Sleep

Quality sleep is essential for overall health and supports detoxification processes. Aim for 7-9 hours of uninterrupted sleep each night to allow your body time to repair and regenerate. During sleep, the body undergoes cellular repair and detoxification, eliminating waste products accumulated throughout the day. Establish a regular sleep schedule, practice good sleep hygiene, and create a relaxing bedtime routine to promote restful sleep and optimize detoxification.

Incorporating these simple detox practices into your daily routine can promote overall health and well-being by supporting the body's natural detoxification pathways. Start with small changes and gradually build upon them to create a holistic approach to detoxification. By prioritizing hydration, nutrient-dense eating, herbal supplements, sweating, relaxation techniques, dry brushing, mindful eating, and adequate sleep, you can enhance your body's ability to cleanse, rejuvenate, and thrive. These practices support detoxification and contribute to increased energy levels, improved digestion, clearer skin, enhanced immune function, and overall vitality.

Book 3: Common Natural Remedies and Their Uses

A Practical Handbook for Everyday Health and Healing

Chapter 1: Herbal Remedies

Herbal remedies are integral to natural healing practices, offering a holistic approach to promoting health and well-being through plant-based medicines. Throughout history, herbs have been valued for their therapeutic properties, providing remedies for various ailments and supporting overall vitality. Herbal remedies can be used in multiple forms, including teas, tinctures, capsules, and topical applications, each harnessing the medicinal qualities of plants to enhance physical, mental, and emotional health.

Herbal remedies offer numerous benefits that distinguish them from conventional medicine. They are often gentler on the body, with fewer side effects than synthetic pharmaceuticals. Many herbs contain a complex array of active compounds that work synergistically to promote healing, addressing underlying causes rather than just alleviating symptoms. Additionally, herbal remedies can support the body's natural healing processes, enhance immune function, and contribute to overall vitality, all while being safe and natural.

1.1 Common Herbal Remedies

Echinacea: Known for its immune-boosting properties, echinacea is commonly used to prevent and treat the common cold and flu. It stimulates the immune system and has antiviral and antibacterial properties.

Ginger: Ginger is prized for its anti-inflammatory and digestive benefits. It can help alleviate nausea, improve digestion, and reduce muscle soreness and joint pain.

Turmeric: Turmeric contains curcumin, a potent anti-inflammatory compound. It supports joint health, reduces inflammation, and promotes overall well-being.

Chamomile: Chamomile is renowned for its calming and relaxing effects. It is often used to promote sleep, reduce anxiety, and soothe digestive discomfort.

Peppermint: Peppermint benefits digestive health, relieving symptoms such as bloating, indigestion, and gas. It also has antimicrobial properties.

Valerian Root: Valerian root is used as a natural remedy for insomnia and sleep disorders. It promotes relaxation and improves sleep quality.

St. John's Wort: St. John's Wort is traditionally used to alleviate symptoms of mild to moderate depression and anxiety. It may also support nerve health.

Garlic: Garlic has antimicrobial and immune-boosting properties. It supports cardiovascular health, lowers cholesterol levels, and promotes overall immunity.

1.2 Choosing and Using Herbal Remedies

When selecting herbal remedies, factors such as their intended purpose, dosage, and potential interactions with medications or existing health conditions must be considered. Consulting with a qualified herbalist or healthcare provider can help ensure the safe and effective use of herbal remedies.

Teas: Herbal teas are one of the simplest and most traditional forms of herbal remedies. Brewing herbs in hot water extracts their medicinal properties, which can then be consumed for various health benefits.

Tinctures: Tinctures are concentrated extracts of herbs, usually preserved in alcohol or glycerin. They are potent and fast-acting, making them convenient for precise dosing.

Capsules: Herbal supplements in capsule form provide a convenient way to consume standardized doses of herbs. They are often used for conditions requiring long-term support.

Topical Applications: Some herbs are applied topically in creams, ointments, or essential oils. This method is beneficial for treating skin conditions, muscle soreness, and other localized issues.

1.3 Integrating Herbal Remedies into Your Wellness Routine

Incorporating herbal remedies into your daily wellness routine can support overall health and enhance quality of life. Start by identifying your health goals and selecting herbs that align with those objectives. Experimenting with different herbal remedies can be an exciting journey of discovery, helping you find what works best for you. Remember to source high-quality herbs from reputable suppliers to ensure purity and effectiveness.

Herbal remedies offer a natural and holistic approach to promoting health and well-being. With their diverse therapeutic properties and minimal side effects, herbs provide valuable options for supporting immune function, relieving symptoms, and enhancing overall vitality. Whether used as teas, tinctures, capsules, or topical treatments, herbal remedies can significantly complement a balanced lifestyle and foster long-term wellness. By integrating herbal remedies into your wellness routine and seeking guidance from qualified practitioners, you can harness the healing power of plants to optimize your health and cultivate a vibrant life.

Chapter 2: Popular Herbs and Their Benefits

Herbs have been valued for centuries for their medicinal properties, offering natural remedies for various health concerns. From enhancing immune function to supporting digestion and promoting relaxation, popular herbs play a vital role in holistic health practices. Here are some well-known herbs and their associated benefits:

Echinacea

Echinacea is renowned for its immune-boosting properties, making it a popular choice during cold and flu season. This herb stimulates the immune system by increasing the production of white blood cells, which are crucial for fighting infections. Echinacea is often used to shorten the duration and severity of colds and respiratory diseases. It also possesses antiviral and anti-inflammatory properties, further supporting immune health.

Ginger

Ginger is a versatile herb known for its potent anti-inflammatory and digestive benefits. It contains bioactive compounds such as gingerol, which helps reduce inflammation and oxidative stress. Ginger is commonly used to alleviate nausea, whether due to motion sickness, pregnancy, or chemotherapy. It also aids digestion by stimulating the production of digestive enzymes, improving nutrient absorption, and reducing gastrointestinal discomfort like bloating and gas.

Turmeric

Turmeric is prized for its vibrant yellow-orange color and powerful anti-inflammatory properties, primarily due to its active compound, curcumin. This herb has been used traditionally in Ayurvedic and Chinese medicine to treat inflammatory conditions such as arthritis and joint pain. Turmeric also supports liver health by aiding in detoxification processes and promoting bile production, which aids in fat digestion. Its antioxidant properties protect cells from damage caused by free radicals, contributing to overall well-being.

Chamomile

Chamomile is well-known for its calming and soothing effects, making it a popular herb for promoting relaxation and improving sleep quality. It contains compounds like apigenin, which binds to receptors in the brain that may reduce anxiety and initiate sleep. Chamomile tea is often consumed before bedtime to induce relaxation and support a restful night's sleep. Chamomile has anti-inflammatory and antioxidant properties that can benefit skin health when used topically.

Peppermint

Peppermint is a refreshing herb with multiple health benefits, particularly for digestive health. It contains menthol, which helps relax muscles in the digestive tract and alleviates irritable bowel syndrome (IBS) symptoms, such as abdominal pain and bloating. Peppermint tea is commonly consumed after meals to aid digestion and relieve indigestion. Its antimicrobial properties also help combat bacteria that can contribute to bad breath and digestive discomfort.

Valerian Root

Valerian root is a natural remedy for promoting relaxation and improving sleep quality. It contains compounds that interact with gamma-aminobutyric acid (GABA) receptors in the brain, reducing nerve activity and inducing feelings of calmness. Valerian root is often used to alleviate insomnia and other sleep disorders, allowing for deeper and more restorative sleep without the side effects of pharmaceutical sleep aids.

Garlic

Garlic is a culinary staple and a potent medicinal herb with numerous health benefits. It has antimicrobial, antiviral, and immune-boosting properties that support overall immune function and help the body fight infections. Garlic is beneficial for cardiovascular health by lowering blood pressure and cholesterol levels and reducing the risk of heart disease. It also has antioxidant properties that protect cells from oxidative damage and support healthy aging.

These popular herbs represent just a glimpse into the vast world of herbal medicine, each offering unique therapeutic benefits that contribute to holistic health and well-being. Whether used individually or in combination, herbs can complement a balanced lifestyle and provide natural alternatives to support immune function, digestive health, relaxation, and more. When incorporating herbs into your wellness routine, consider consulting with a qualified herbalist or healthcare provider to ensure safe and effective use, especially if you have existing health conditions or are taking medications. Embracing the healing power of herbs allows individuals to cultivate a proactive approach to health, enhancing vitality and fostering a deeper connection with natural remedies for long-term wellness.

2.1 How to Use Herbs Safely

Using herbs safely and effectively is essential to maximize their therapeutic benefits while minimizing potential risks. Herbs are potent natural substances that can interact with medications, exacerbate certain health conditions, or cause adverse reactions if misused. By empowering yourself with the understanding of proper usage guidelines and consulting with qualified practitioners, you can integrate herbs into your wellness routines with confidence and control, ensuring safety and effectiveness.

1) Research and Education

Before using any herb, conduct thorough research to understand its properties, potential benefits, and possible side effects. Reliable sources such as reputable books, scientific journals, and trusted websites can provide valuable information. Look for studies or clinical trials supporting the herb's use for specific health concerns. Additionally, consider consulting with a qualified herbalist or healthcare provider who can offer personalized guidance based on your health status and individual needs.

2) Quality and Sourcing

Ensure the safety and effectiveness of the herbs you use by choosing high-quality products from reputable suppliers. Organic or wildcrafted herbs are preferable, as they are less likely to contain pesticides, heavy metals, or other contaminants. Avoid purchasing herbs from uncertain sources or those with unclear labeling. Look for certifications or third-party testing that verify the quality and authenticity of the herbs.

3) Dosage Guidelines

Follow recommended dosage guidelines from herbalists, healthcare providers, or reputable sources. Dosage recommendations can vary based on age, weight, health status, and the herb used. Start with the lowest effective dose and gradually increase as needed, monitoring your body's response to the herb. Avoid exceeding recommended doses, as this can increase the risk of adverse effects.

4) Methods of Administration

Herbs can be consumed in various forms, including teas, tinctures, capsules, extracts, and topical preparations. Choose a method of administration that best suits your preferences and health needs. For example, teas are ideal for promoting relaxation or supporting digestion, while tinctures provide a concentrated dose for specific therapeutic purposes. Topical applications, such as herbal ointments or essential oils, can be used for skin conditions or localized pain relief.

5) Considerations for Special Populations

Specific populations, such as pregnant or breastfeeding women, children, and individuals with pre-existing health conditions, may require special considerations when using herbs. Some herbs are contraindicated during pregnancy due to potential effects on fetal development or hormonal balance. Children may require lower doses or specific herbs safe for pediatric use. Individuals with chronic health conditions or those taking medications should consult with a healthcare provider before starting any herbal regimen to avoid interactions or complications.

6) Monitoring and Adjustments

Pay attention to how your body responds to herbal remedies and adjust as needed. Monitor for any adverse reactions, such as allergic symptoms, digestive upset, or changes in mood or energy levels. If you experience any negative effects, discontinue use and consult with a healthcare provider. Keep a journal to track your herbal usage, noting dosage, frequency, and observed effects to inform future decisions about herb selection and dosage adjustments.

7) Interactions with Medications

Herbs can interact with prescription medications, over-the-counter drugs, and supplements, potentially altering their effectiveness or causing adverse reactions. Before using herbs alongside medications, consult a healthcare provider to identify potential interactions and ensure safe co-administration. Some herbs may potentiate or inhibit certain medications' effects, requiring dosage or timing adjustments to avoid complications.

2.2 Essential Oils

Essential oils are highly concentrated plant extracts that capture the aromatic and therapeutic properties of various botanicals. They have been used for centuries in aromatherapy, a holistic healing practice that utilizes aromatic compounds to promote physical, emotional, and spiritual well-being. Essential oils are derived through steam distillation, cold pressing, or solvent extraction from flowers, leaves, roots, and other plant parts, resulting in potent extracts that offer a wide range of therapeutic benefits.

2.2.1 Therapeutic Uses

Essential oils are prized for their versatile therapeutic uses. They can be used aromatically, topically, or even internally, depending on the oil and its intended purpose. Aromatic use involves inhaling the oil's fragrance through methods such as diffusers, steam inhalation, or direct inhalation from the bottle. This method can promote relaxation, improve mood, and support respiratory health.

Topical application involves diluting essential oils with a carrier oil and applying them directly to the skin. This allows for absorption of the oil's beneficial compounds, which can help alleviate muscle tension, soothe skin irritations, and support overall skin health. Common carrier oils include coconut oil, jojoba oil, and almond oil, which help to dilute the potent essential oils and prevent skin irritation.

2.2.2 Popular Essential Oils and Their Benefits

Lavender: Lavender essential oil is renowned for its calming and soothing properties. It promotes relaxation, reduces stress and anxiety, and supports sleep quality. Lavender oil is also used topically to soothe minor burns, cuts, and insect bites due to its anti-inflammatory and antiseptic properties.

Peppermint: Peppermint essential oil is invigorating and refreshing. It helps to relieve headaches, improve mental clarity, and alleviate digestive discomfort such as bloating and indigestion. Peppermint oil can also be used topically to cool sore muscles and joints.

Tea Tree: Tea tree essential oil is known for its powerful antimicrobial and antiseptic properties. It is commonly used to treat acne, fungal infections, and minor skin irritations. Tea tree oil can also support immune function and promote clear, healthy skin.

Eucalyptus: Eucalyptus essential oil has a fresh, clean scent and is excellent for respiratory health. It helps to clear congestion, ease sinusitis symptoms, and support overall respiratory function. Eucalyptus oil is often used in steam inhalations during cold and flu season.

Frankincense: Frankincense essential oil is valued for its grounding and calming effects. It promotes emotional balance, reduces stress, and supports meditation practices. Frankincense oil also has anti-inflammatory properties and can be used topically to rejuvenate the skin and reduce signs of aging.

2.2.3 Safety Considerations

While essential oils offer numerous benefits, they are potent substances that require careful use. Always dilute essential oils with a carrier oil before applying to the skin, as direct application can cause irritation or sensitivity reactions. Perform a patch test on a small area of skin before using a new essential oil, especially if you have sensitive skin or allergies.

Avoid ingesting essential oils unless under the guidance of a qualified healthcare provider, as some oils can be toxic if consumed orally. Keep essential oils out of reach of children and pets, as they are highly concentrated and should be used with caution.

Essential oils are valuable tools in promoting holistic health and well-being. Whether used for relaxation, skincare, respiratory support, or emotional balance, their aromatic and therapeutic properties can enhance daily wellness routines. By understanding their uses, benefits, and safety considerations, individuals can incorporate essential oils effectively into their lifestyles, harnessing the natural power of plants for optimal health and vitality.

2.3 Creating Your Own Blends

Creating your own essential oil blends allows for customization to address specific needs and preferences, enhancing the therapeutic benefits of aromatherapy. By combining different essential oils, you can create unique synergies that promote relaxation, boost energy, support immune function, or address specific emotional or physical concerns. Here are some tips to help you create effective and personalized essential oil blends:

Each essential oil has its own aromatic profile and therapeutic properties. Some oils are known for their calming effects (e.g., lavender, chamomile), while others are invigorating (e.g., peppermint, citrus oils). Begin by familiarizing yourself with the properties and uses of individual essential oils to determine which ones will complement each other in your blend.

Decide on the purpose or theme of your blend based on your desired outcome. Are you creating a blend to promote relaxation and reduce stress? Or perhaps you want to create an uplifting blend to boost mood and energy levels. Having a clear intention will guide your selection of essential oils and their proportions in the blend.

Select essential oils that align with your chosen purpose or theme. For relaxation, consider oils like lavender, chamomile, and frankincense. For an energizing blend, peppermint, citrus oils (such as lemon or orange), and rosemary are excellent choices. Experiment with different combinations to find the aroma and effect that resonate with you.

When creating blends, consider the potency and intensity of each essential oil. Start with a base note oil (e.g., cedarwood, patchouli) as the foundation of your blend, followed by middle notes (e.g., lavender, rosemary) and top notes (e.g., citrus oils, peppermint) to create a balanced aroma. A common ratio for blending is 30% base note, 50% middle note, and 20% top note, but adjust according to your preferences and the specific oils used.

Always perform a patch test on a small area of skin to ensure you do not have a sensitivity or allergic reaction to the blend. Once you are satisfied with the blend's aroma and effect, you can adjust the ratios of essential oils to fine-tune the blend to your liking. Keep notes of your blends and adjustments for future reference.

Once your blend is finalized, consider different application methods based on its intended use. Diffusing the blend in a room can provide continuous aromatic benefits. Dilute the blend in a carrier oil for topical application, such as massage or applying to pulse points. You can also add a few drops of the blend to bathwater for a relaxing soak.

Store your essential oil blends in dark glass bottles away from direct sunlight and heat to preserve their potency. Properly stored blends can last several months to a year, depending on the oils used. Label each blend with its ingredients and intended purpose for easy identification.

Creating your own essential oil blends allows for personalization and customization in aromatherapy practices. Whether you are seeking relaxation, energy enhancement, emotional support, or other therapeutic benefits, experimenting with different essential oils and blending techniques empowers you to harness the natural healing properties of plants. By understanding essential oil profiles, selecting oils purposefully, and experimenting with blending ratios, you can create effective and enjoyable blends that enrich your holistic wellness journey.

Chapter 3: Building a Natural Healing Toolkit

3.1 Essential Tools and Supplies

Building a natural healing toolkit requires essential tools and supplies to support your journey toward holistic wellness. Whether you are exploring herbal remedies, essential oils, or other natural healing practices, having the right tools at your disposal enhances efficacy and convenience. Here are crucial tools and supplies to consider for your natural healing toolkit:

1) Herb Storage Containers

Proper storage is crucial to maintaining herbs' potency and freshness. Choose dark glass jars or containers with tight-sealing lids to protect herbs from light and moisture. Label each container with the herb's name and date of purchase or harvest for easy identification and tracking of expiration dates.

2) Infusers and Strainers

Infusers and strainers are essential for preparing herbal teas and infusions. Invest in stainless steel or silicone infusers that fit various cup sizes for brewing loose herbs. Fine-mesh strainers are ideal for filtering herbal extracts and teas to remove plant particles and debris.

3) Essential Oil Diffuser

An essential oil diffuser disperses aromatic essential oils into the air, creating a therapeutic atmosphere and promoting relaxation or other desired effects. Choose diffusers that use ultrasonic technology to maintain the integrity of essential oils without overheating them.

4) Carrier Oils

Carrier oils dilute essential oils for safe topical application and nourish the skin. Common carrier oils include jojoba, coconut, sweet almond, and olive oil. Choose organic, cold-pressed carrier oils free from additives or synthetic ingredients.

5) Glass Dropper Bottles

Glass dropper bottles are essential for safely storing and dispensing essential oils, herbal extracts, and custom blends. Amber or cobalt blue glass bottles help protect oils from light degradation. Choose bottles with graduated droppers for precise measurement and application.

6) Herbal Books and References

Invest in reputable herbal books, guides, or references that provide comprehensive information on medicinal herbs, their uses, dosage guidelines, and safety precautions. Look for books written by experienced herbalists or experts in natural healing to expand your knowledge and skills.

7) Salve Tins and Lip Balm Containers

If you plan to make herbal salves, balms, or lip balms, stock up on small tin or glass containers with secure lids. These containers are ideal for storing and carrying homemade herbal remedies, providing convenient access to natural healing solutions.

8) Digital Scale

A digital scale accurately measures dried herbs, botanical powders, and other ingredients when preparing herbal formulations or recipes. Choose a scale with precision measurements in grams or ounces to ensure consistency in herbal preparations.

9) Labeling Supplies

Keep your herbal creations organized and easily identifiable with labeling supplies. Use waterproof labels or marker pens to label herb jars, essential oil bottles, and homemade products with ingredient lists, expiration dates, and usage instructions.

10) Storage and Organization

Designate a dedicated space for storing herbs, essential oils, and natural healing supplies. Organize your toolkit in a cool, dry area away from direct sunlight to preserve the quality and potency of herbs and oils. Use shelves, bins, or drawers to keep supplies neatly arranged and accessible.

3.2 Creating a Healing Environment at Home

Establishing a healing environment at home enhances the effectiveness of natural healing practices and promotes overall well-being. A nurturing space encourages relaxation, reduces stress, and supports the body's natural healing processes. Here are essential elements to consider when creating a healing environment at home:

Natural Light and Fresh Air

Maximize natural light and fresh air in your home to create a bright and refreshing atmosphere. Open windows regularly to ventilate indoor spaces and promote air circulation. Natural light uplifts mood and supports the body's circadian rhythm, promoting better sleep and overall health.

Clean and Clutter-Free Spaces

Maintain clean and clutter-free spaces to foster a sense of calm and serenity. Regular cleaning and decluttering minimize distractions and promote a peaceful environment conducive to relaxation and healing. Use natural cleaning products or homemade solutions with essential oils for a non-toxic and pleasant cleaning experience.

Nature-Inspired Decor

Incorporate elements of nature into your home decor to evoke a sense of connection with the natural world. Display indoor plants, botanical artwork, or natural materials such as wood and stone to create a soothing and grounding ambiance. Nature-inspired decor enhances relaxation and reduces stress, contributing to a healing environment.

Aromatherapy and Essential Oils

Use aromatherapy to infuse your home with therapeutic scents, promoting relaxation and emotional well-being. Place essential oil diffusers in critical areas such as bedrooms, living rooms, or home offices to disperse aromatic essential oils like lavender, chamomile, or citrus blends. Adjust the diffuser settings to create a personalized sensory experience that supports relaxation and stress relief.

Comfortable and Cozy Spaces

Create comfortable and cozy spaces where you can unwind and relax. Invest in supportive furniture, plush cushions, and soft textiles to enhance comfort and encourage relaxation. Designate a quiet corner or reading nook with comfortable seating and soft lighting for moments of introspection and rejuvenation.

Healing Sounds and Music

Integrate healing sounds or soothing music into your home environment to enhance relaxation and promote mental clarity. Play calming music, nature sounds, or meditation tracks to create a tranquil atmosphere conducive to stress reduction and emotional balance. Use soundscapes to mask noise disturbances and create a peaceful sanctuary for relaxation and healing.

Mindfulness and Meditation Spaces

Designate a dedicated space for mindfulness practices such as meditation, yoga, or deep breathing exercises. Set up a meditation cushion, yoga mat, or comfortable seating in a quiet area free from distractions. Decorate the space with calming colors, candles, or inspirational artwork to inspire mindfulness and inner peace.

Personalized Healing Rituals

Establish personalized healing rituals that align with your wellness goals and preferences. Incorporate daily practices such as herbal tea rituals, aromatherapy sessions, or journaling exercises to promote self-care and emotional well-being. Consistent rituals create a sense of structure and mindfulness, supporting your journey toward holistic health and healing.

Positive Affirmations and Inspirational Quotes

Display positive affirmations, inspirational quotes, or affirming artwork throughout your home to cultivate a positive mindset and uplift your spirits. Choose messages that resonate with your intentions for health, healing, and personal growth. Surrounding yourself with affirming words and imagery reinforces a nurturing and supportive environment for holistic wellness.

Sacred Space for Reflection and Renewal

Create a sacred space within your home to retreat for quiet reflection and spiritual renewal. This space may include a personal altar, sacred objects, or meaningful symbols that hold significance for your spiritual practice or healing journey. Use this space for meditation, prayer, or simply moments of introspection and gratitude.

Creating a healing environment at home involves integrating elements that nurture physical, emotional, and spiritual well-being. By incorporating natural light, clean spaces, nature-inspired decor, aromatherapy, comfortable surroundings, and personalized healing rituals, you cultivate a sanctuary that supports relaxation, reduces stress, and enhances the effectiveness of natural healing practices. Embrace the opportunity to design your home as a haven for holistic wellness, where you can rejuvenate your mind, body, and spirit in alignment with your wellness goals and aspirations.

3.3 Daily Practices for Maintaining Health

Incorporating daily practices into your routine supports overall health, vitality, and well-being. These practices focus on nurturing your life's physical, emotional, and mental aspects, promoting a holistic approach to health maintenance. Integrating these practices into your daily life can cultivate resilience, balance, and vitality. Here are essential daily practices for maintaining health:

1) Hydration

Start your day with a glass of water to hydrate your body and kickstart your metabolism. Aim to drink plenty of water throughout the day to support digestion, circulation, and overall hydration. Carry a reusable water bottle with you as a reminder to stay hydrated, especially during busy periods or physical activities.

2) Nutritious Diet

Eat a balanced diet rich in whole foods, including fruits, vegetables, lean proteins, whole grains, and healthy fats. Prioritize nutrient-dense foods that provide essential vitamins, minerals, and antioxidants to support immune function, energy levels, and overall health. Choose organic and locally sourced foods whenever possible for optimal nutrition and sustainability.

3) Physical Activity

Incorporate regular physical activity into your daily routine to support cardiovascular health, muscular strength, and flexibility. Engage in activities you enjoy, such as walking, jogging, yoga, or dancing, for at least 30 minutes most days of the week. Physical exercise promotes circulation, releases endorphins, and reduces stress, contributing to a balanced and healthy lifestyle.

4) Mindful Eating

Practice mindful eating by savoring each bite, chewing slowly, and paying attention to hunger and fullness cues. Avoid distractions such as screens or multitasking during meals to foster awareness of food choices and eating habits. Mindful eating promotes digestion, prevents overeating, and enhances the enjoyment of meals.

5) Stress Management

Incorporate stress management techniques such as deep breathing, meditation, yoga, or progressive muscle relaxation into your daily routine. These practices help reduce cortisol levels, alleviate tension, and promote relaxation response in the body. Find moments throughout the day to pause, breathe deeply, and center yourself amidst daily challenges.

6) Quality Sleep

Establish a consistent sleep schedule and create a relaxing bedtime routine to prioritize adequate sleep. Aim for 7-9 hours of quality sleep each night to support cognitive function, immune health, and overall well-being. Create a sleep-friendly environment by dimming lights, minimizing noise, and keeping electronic devices away from the bedroom.

7) Personal Care and Hygiene

Maintain personal hygiene by practicing regular handwashing, dental care, and skincare routines to prevent infections and promote skin health. Use natural and non-toxic personal care products that align with your skin type and preferences. Incorporate self-care practices such as dry brushing, aromatherapy baths, or herbal skincare rituals to nurture your body and enhance relaxation.

8) Connection and Social Support

Cultivate meaningful connections with friends, family, and community members to foster a sense of belonging and emotional well-being. Schedule time for social activities, hobbies, or volunteering to nurture relationships and reduce feelings of loneliness or isolation. Share experiences, laughter, and support with loved ones to enhance happiness and resilience.

9) Gratitude and Positive Mindset

Practice gratitude by reflecting on positive aspects of your life and expressing appreciation for small moments of joy and abundance. Keep a gratitude journal or practice daily affirmations to cultivate a positive mindset and resilience in facing challenges. Embrace an optimistic outlook that promotes emotional well-being and enhances overall life satisfaction.

10) Continual Learning and Growth

Engage in lifelong learning by exploring new interests, hobbies, or skills stimulating your mind and creativity. Stay curious and open to new experiences, whether reading books, taking classes, or participating in workshops. Continuous learning fosters personal growth, expands perspective, and promotes mental agility and resilience.

Chapter 4: Integrating Natural Healing into Daily Life

4.1 Developing a Personal Health Plan

Creating a personalized health plan empowers you to take proactive steps toward achieving and maintaining optimal health and well-being. A well-rounded health plan considers your unique needs, goals, and lifestyle preferences, integrating holistic approaches to support physical, mental, and emotional wellness. Follow these steps to develop a personalized health plan tailored to your individual needs:

4.1.1 Assess Your Current Health Status

Begin by assessing your current health status through reflection, self-assessment tools, or consultations with healthcare professionals. Identify areas of strength and areas for improvement in physical health, mental well-being, emotional resilience, and lifestyle habits. Consider factors such as nutrition, exercise habits, stress levels, sleep quality, and overall life satisfaction.

4.1.2 Set SMART Goals

Setting specific, measurable, achievable, relevant, and time-bound (SMART) goals is a crucial step in your health journey. These goals serve as a roadmap, guiding you towards your health aspirations. Whether it's improving fitness levels, managing stress effectively, achieving a healthy weight, or enhancing emotional resilience, these objectives keep you focused and determined. Breaking down larger goals into smaller, actionable steps helps you maintain motivation and track progress over time.

4.1.3 Identify Health Priorities

Based on your assessment and goals, prioritize areas of health that require attention or enhancement. Focus on key aspects such as nutrition, physical activity, stress management, sleep hygiene, mental health, and preventive care. Tailor your health plan to address specific concerns or challenges while promoting overall well-being and longevity.

4.1.4 Create a Holistic Approach

Integrate holistic approaches to health that encompass physical, mental, emotional, and spiritual dimensions. For instance, incorporate mindfulness practices like meditation or yoga to manage stress and promote mental clarity. Explore natural healing modalities such as herbal remedies or aromatherapy to support physical health and vitality. Cultivate supportive relationships and engage in social activities to foster emotional well-being and connection.

4.1.5 Establish Healthy Habits

Develop daily routines and habits that align with your health goals and promote sustainable lifestyle changes. Adopt nutritious eating habits by incorporating whole foods, balanced meals, and mindful eating practices. Commit to regular physical activity, including cardiovascular exercise, strength training, flexibility exercises, or outdoor activities for overall fitness and vitality. Prioritize adequate sleep and establish a bedtime routine that supports restorative rest and optimal cognitive function.

4.1.6 Monitor Progress and Adjust Accordingly

Regularly monitor your progress toward achieving your health goals by tracking weight, fitness levels, emotional well-being, and lifestyle habits. Keep a health journal or use digital apps to record daily activities, mood changes, dietary choices, and exercise routines. Evaluate your achievements, identify areas for improvement, and adjust your health plan accordingly to maintain motivation and momentum.

4.1.7 Seek Professional Guidance

Consult healthcare professionals, nutritionists, fitness trainers, or holistic practitioners for personalized guidance and support. Discuss any health concerns, receive recommendations for preventive care, and explore complementary therapies or treatments that align with your health goals. Collaborate with experts to develop strategies for overcoming challenges, managing chronic conditions, or optimizing overall well-being.

4.1.8 Celebrate Milestones and Successes

Celebrate your achievements, milestones, and successes along your health journey to reinforce positive behaviors and maintain motivation. Acknowledge progress, no matter how small, and reward yourself for reaching milestones or achieving significant goals. Celebrating successes boosts self-confidence, reinforces commitment, and encourages continued effort toward long-term goals. It's important to recognize and appreciate the effort you put into your health journey, as this can help you stay motivated and committed to your plan.

Developing a personalized health plan empowers you to take proactive control of your well-being, promoting physical vitality, mental clarity, and emotional resilience. By assessing your current health status, setting SMART goals, prioritizing health needs, integrating holistic approaches, establishing healthy habits, monitoring progress, seeking professional guidance, and celebrating successes, you create a comprehensive framework for achieving optimal health and longevity. Embrace your health plan as a roadmap to cultivate a balanced and fulfilling lifestyle that supports your wellness goals with intention, mindfulness, and commitment to lifelong well-being.

4.2 Overcoming Challenges and Staying Motivated

Embarking on a journey toward improved health and well-being is rewarding but can also present challenges along the way. Overcoming obstacles and maintaining motivation is essential for staying committed to your health plan and achieving long-term success. Here are strategies to overcome challenges and stay motivated on your wellness journey:

Anticipate potential challenges on your health journey, such as time constraints, stress triggers, temptation for unhealthy habits, or unexpected setbacks. Recognize common barriers to achieving your health goals and prepare proactive strategies to address them effectively.

Cultivate a resilient mindset that embraces setbacks as learning opportunities rather than failures. Practice self-compassion and patience with yourself during times of difficulty or slow progress. Focus on positive affirmations, visualization techniques, or gratitude practices to maintain optimism and motivation.

Set realistic expectations for your health journey by acknowledging that progress takes time and consistency. Avoid comparing yourself to others and recognize that each person's path to wellness is unique. Break larger goals into smaller, achievable milestones to celebrate incremental progress and maintain momentum.

Remain adaptable and flexible in adjusting your health plan as needed to accommodate changes in circumstances or priorities. Be open to modifying goals, routines, or strategies based on feedback from your body, new information, or shifting life circumstances. Embrace a growth mindset that embraces continuous improvement and adaptation.

Establish accountability measures to stay committed to your health goals. Share your goals with supportive friends, family members, or a health coach who can provide encouragement, feedback, and accountability. Join online communities, support groups, or fitness classes to connect with like-minded individuals and share experiences.

Celebrate small victories and milestones along your health journey to reinforce positive behaviors and maintain motivation. Recognize and reward yourself for achieving goals, making progress, or adopting healthy habits. Celebrating successes boosts self-confidence, reinforces commitment, and encourages continued effort toward long-term goals.

Prioritize self-care practices that nurture your physical, emotional, and mental well-being. Incorporate activities such as relaxation techniques, massage, aromatherapy, or hobbies that bring joy and relaxation. Take regular breaks, practice mindfulness, and listen to your body's signals for rest and rejuvenation.

Regularly reflect on your experiences, challenges, and achievements to gain insights into your health journey. Keep a journal or diary to track progress, record thoughts and emotions, and identify patterns in behavior or outcomes. Learn from setbacks or obstacles by exploring alternative strategies and adjusting your approach as needed.

Seek guidance from healthcare professionals, nutritionists, or counselors to address specific challenges or obstacles. Discuss concerns, receive personalized recommendations, and explore additional resources or therapies that align with your health goals. Professional support provides expertise, encouragement, and practical solutions to overcome barriers effectively.

Stay inspired by revisiting your reasons for pursuing a healthier lifestyle, whether improving overall well-being, increasing energy levels, or enhancing quality of life. Surround yourself with motivational quotes, success stories, or role models who inspire you to stay committed to your goals. Visualize your desired outcomes and stay focused on the positive impact of your efforts on your health and happiness.

Chapter 5: Case Studies and Testimonials

5.1 Success Stories of Natural Healing

Success stories of natural healing inspire and demonstrate the transformative power of holistic approaches to health and wellness. These stories illustrate real-life experiences where individuals have significantly improved their health through natural healing practices. By sharing these stories, we celebrate the healing potential and encourage others to explore alternative methods that support the body's innate ability to heal. Here are a few compelling success stories of natural healing:

Jane's Journey to Overcoming Chronic Fatigue Syndrome

Jane, a 42-year-old marketing executive, struggled with chronic fatigue syndrome (CFS) for several years. Conventional treatments offered limited relief, leaving her feeling discouraged and fatigued. Jane sought a holistic approach, consulted with a naturopathic doctor who recommended a personalized health plan focused on nutrition, stress management, and herbal supplements. Over several months, Jane adopted a whole foods diet rich in antioxidants and essential nutrients, practiced mindfulness meditation daily, and took herbal remedies known for their adaptogenic and immune-supportive properties. Gradually, Jane noticed improvements in her energy levels, sleep quality, and overall well-being. Today, Jane leads an active lifestyle, free from the debilitating effects of CFS, thanks to her commitment to natural healing practices.

Mark's Recovery from Digestive Issues with Herbal Remedies

Mark, a 35-year-old entrepreneur, struggled with chronic digestive issues characterized by bloating, indigestion, and irregular bowel movements. After consulting with multiple specialists and undergoing various tests with inconclusive results, Mark turned to herbal remedies and dietary adjustments for relief. With guidance from an herbalist, Mark incorporated digestive herbs such as peppermint, ginger, and chamomile into his daily routine. He also eliminated trigger foods such as processed sugars and refined grains, focusing on a whole foods diet rich in fiber and probiotics. Within weeks, Mark experienced significant improvements in his digestive symptoms, including reduced bloating and improved bowel regularity. Today, Mark maintains his digestive health with herbal remedies and mindful eating habits, enjoying a renewed sense of vitality and well-being.

Sarah's Journey to Managing Anxiety with Aromatherapy

Sarah, a 28-year-old teacher, struggled with anxiety and stress-related symptoms that affected her daily life and teaching performance. Seeking a natural approach to managing her anxiety, Sarah explored aromatherapy under the guidance of a certified aromatherapist. She incorporated essential oils such as lavender, bergamot, and frankincense into her self-care routine, using a diffuser at home and creating personalized blends for relaxation and stress relief. Sarah also practiced deep breathing exercises and mindfulness meditation and established a calming bedtime routine. Over time, Sarah noticed reduced anxiety symptoms, improved sleep quality, and greater emotional resilience. Today, Sarah continues to incorporate aromatherapy and mindfulness practices into her daily life, empowering herself to manage anxiety effectively and enjoy a balanced, fulfilling lifestyle.

Tom's Recovery from Sports Injury with Herbal Remedies and Physical Therapy

Tom, a 30-year-old athlete, sustained a severe sports injury that left him with chronic pain and limited mobility. Frustrated with conventional treatments that offered temporary relief, Tom sought a holistic approach to support his recovery. With guidance from a holistic health practitioner, Tom integrated herbal remedies known for their anti-inflammatory and pain-relieving properties, such as turmeric, devil's claw, and arnica. He also incorporated physical therapy exercises to improve flexibility, strength, and range of motion in the affected area. Over several months of consistent herbal treatment and rehabilitation, Tom experienced a significant reduction in pain, improved mobility, and accelerated healing of the injured tissues. Today, Tom continues to maintain his active lifestyle, supported by herbal remedies and ongoing physical therapy, with a renewed sense of resilience and vitality.

5.2 Real-Life Applications of Barbara O'Neill's Methods

Barbara O'Neill's holistic methods have empowered individuals worldwide to embrace natural healing practices and achieve significant improvements in their health and well-being. Through her teachings on nutrition, herbal remedies, detoxification, and lifestyle adjustments, Barbara O'Neill has inspired countless individuals to adopt sustainable health practices rooted in holistic principles. Here are real-life applications of Barbara O'Neill's methods that illustrate their transformative impact:

5.2.1 Nutrition and Whole Foods Diet

Barbara O'Neill emphasizes the importance of nutrition as a cornerstone of health and vitality. Her advocacy for a whole-foods diet encourages individuals to prioritize nutrient-dense foods that support optimal health. Many individuals have applied Barbara O'Neill's principles by adopting diets rich in fruits, vegetables, whole grains, lean proteins, and healthy fats. By eliminating processed foods and refined sugars, individuals experience improved digestion, increased energy levels, and enhanced overall well-being. Real-life examples include individuals who have successfully managed chronic conditions such as diabetes, obesity, and cardiovascular disease through dietary changes inspired by Barbara O'Neill's teachings.

5.2.2 Herbal Remedies and Natural Therapies

Barbara O'Neill's expertise in herbal remedies and natural therapies offers practical solutions for managing various health concerns. Many individuals have integrated herbal remedies such as turmeric for its anti-inflammatory properties, ginger for digestive support, and echinacea for immune enhancement into their health routines. By consulting with herbalists or following Barbara O'Neill's guidance, individuals have experienced relief from symptoms associated with arthritis, allergies, digestive disorders, and respiratory ailments. Real-life applications demonstrate how herbal remedies complement conventional treatments or serve as alternatives for individuals seeking natural health maintenance and symptom management approaches.

5.2.3 Detoxification and Cleansing Practices

Detoxification and cleansing practices recommended by Barbara O'Neill promote the elimination of toxins from the body and support organ function. Real-life applications include individuals who have benefited from periodic fasting, juice cleanses, or liver detox protocols advocated by Barbara O'Neill. By reducing exposure to environmental toxins, optimizing nutrition, and supporting the body's natural detoxification pathways, individuals report increased energy, clearer skin, improved digestion, and enhanced mental clarity. Barbara O'Neill's methods encourage individuals to adopt sustainable detoxification practices that promote long-term health benefits and support overall wellness.

5.2.4 Stress Management and Mind-Body Techniques

Barbara O'Neill emphasizes the importance of stress management and mind-body techniques in promoting holistic health. Real-life applications include individuals who have incorporated mindfulness meditation, deep breathing exercises, yoga, or tai chi into their daily routines. By practicing these techniques regularly, individuals report reduced stress levels, improved sleep quality, and greater emotional resilience. Barbara O'Neill's teachings encourage a holistic approach to managing stress that addresses the interconnectedness of mind, body, and spirit, promoting overall well-being and a balanced lifestyle.

5.2.5 Lifestyle Adjustments for Longevity

Barbara O'Neill advocates for lifestyle adjustments that promote longevity and vitality. Real-life applications include individuals who have embraced habits such as regular physical activity, adequate sleep, hydration, and positive social connections. By prioritizing self-care practices and adopting a balanced approach to work-life balance, individuals experience enhanced quality of life, reduced risk of chronic diseases, and increased longevity. Barbara O'Neill's methods inspire individuals to cultivate sustainable lifestyle habits supporting overall health and well-being.

Book 4: Understanding Herbal Medicine

Discovering the Power of Nature's Remedies

Chapter 1: History and evolution of herbal medicine

<u>History and Evolution of Herbal Medicine</u>

Herbal medicine, one of the oldest forms of healthcare known to humanity, has a rich and diverse history that spans thousands of years. This ancient practice involves using plants and their extracts to treat various ailments and maintain health. The evolution of herbal medicine is a testament to the enduring relationship between humans and nature and the continuous quest for healing and well-being.

<u>Ancient Origins</u>

The roots of herbal medicine trace back to prehistoric times when early humans discovered that certain plants had medicinal properties. Archaeological evidence shows that even Neanderthals used plants like yarrow and chamomile, indicating that the knowledge of healing herbs predates written history. As societies evolved, so did their understanding and documentation of herbal remedies.

In ancient Mesopotamia, clay tablets dating back to 2600 BCE record the use of medicinal plants. Similarly, ancient Egyptian texts, such as the Ebers Papyrus (circa 1550 BCE), list hundreds of herbal remedies. These early civilizations laid the foundation for systematically studying plants and their medicinal uses.

<u>Classical Antiquity</u>

The Greeks and Romans made significant contributions to herbal medicine. Hippocrates, often called the "Father of Medicine," emphasized using diet, lifestyle, and herbal remedies to treat diseases. His holistic approach influenced subsequent medical traditions. Dioscorides, a Greek physician in the 1st century CE, compiled "De Materia Medica," an extensive pharmacopeia that described the properties and uses of over 600 plants. This work remained a cornerstone of herbal knowledge for over a millennium.

In ancient China, herbal medicine developed independently and became a key component of Traditional Chinese Medicine (TCM). The "Shennong Ben Cao Jing," attributed to the mythical emperor Shennong, is one of the earliest Chinese texts on medicinal plants. Later, during the Han dynasty, Zhang Zhongjing's "Shang Han Lun" further advanced the understanding of herbal treatments.

<u>Medieval Period</u>

During the Middle Ages, herbal medicine flourished, particularly in the Islamic world. Scholars like Avicenna (Ibn Sina) and Al-Razi (Rhazes) preserved and expanded upon Greek and Roman knowledge. Avicenna's "The Canon of Medicine" included detailed descriptions of numerous herbs and their therapeutic uses.

In medieval Europe, monasteries became centers of herbal knowledge. Monastic gardens cultivated medicinal plants, and monks compiled herbals—manuscripts detailing the medicinal properties of plants. The "Hildegard of Bingen" texts, written by a German Benedictine abbess, combined spiritual and herbal healing, reflecting the intertwined nature of faith and medicine during this period.

<u>Renaissance and Enlightenment</u>

The Renaissance brought renewed interest in classical texts and the natural world. Herbalists like Nicholas Culpeper in England democratized herbal knowledge by writing in vernacular languages and making it accessible to the public. Culpeper's "Complete Herbal" remains a popular reference for herbalists today.

The Age of Exploration expanded the repertoire of medicinal plants as explorers encountered new flora in the Americas, Africa, and Asia. Indigenous knowledge of these plants was integrated into European herbal medicine, enriching the pharmacopeia with new remedies.

Modern Era

The 19th and 20th centuries saw the rise of modern pharmacology and synthetic drugs, which led to a decline in the use of herbal medicine in mainstream healthcare. However, herbal medicine never disappeared; it continued to be practiced in many cultures and regions worldwide.

The late 20th century witnessed a resurgence of interest in natural and holistic health practices, including herbal medicine. Growing concerns about the side effects of pharmaceutical drugs and a desire for more natural approaches to health drove this revival. Scientific research began to validate the efficacy of many traditional herbal remedies, bridging the gap between ancient wisdom and modern science.

Contemporary Herbal Medicine

Today, herbal medicine is recognized as a complementary and alternative medicine (CAM) practice. It is integrated into holistic health approaches that emphasize the whole person—body, mind, and spirit. Modern herbalists combine traditional knowledge with scientific research to provide safe and effective treatments. Regulatory bodies in many countries oversee the use of herbal medicines to ensure quality and safety.

The history and evolution of herbal medicine illustrate a dynamic and enduring tradition. From ancient roots to modern applications, herbal medicine reflects humanity's continuous quest for healing through nature. It remains a vital part of healthcare for millions worldwide, offering a natural and holistic approach to well-being.

Chapter 2: Basics of plant properties and their medicinal uses

Understanding the basics of plant properties and their medicinal uses is fundamental to the practice of herbal medicine. Plants have been used for centuries to treat a variety of ailments, and modern research continues to uncover the complex chemistry behind their healing properties. The medicinal uses of plants are based on the active compounds they contain, which can have diverse and potent effects on the human body.

2.1 Active Compounds in Plants

Plants produce a wide array of chemical compounds that can be harnessed for medicinal purposes. These active compounds include:

- Alkaloids: These are nitrogen-containing compounds that often have potent effects on the body. Examples include morphine from the opium poppy, which is used for pain relief, and quinine from cinchona bark, which is used to treat malaria.

- Flavonoids: These are a group of antioxidants found in many fruits and vegetables. They have anti-inflammatory, antiviral, and anticancer properties. Examples include quercetin, found in onions and apples, and catechins, found in green tea.

- Tannins: These compounds have astringent properties and can help to reduce inflammation and combat infection. They are found in plants like witch hazel and oak bark.

- Terpenoids: These are a diverse class of organic chemicals that can have antibacterial, antiviral, and anti-inflammatory effects. Examples include menthol from peppermint and artemisinin from sweet wormwood.

- Glycosides: These compounds can have a variety of effects, including heart stimulation and laxative action. Digitalis glycosides from foxglove are used to treat heart failure, and anthraquinone glycosides from senna are used as laxatives.

- Saponins: These compounds can enhance immune function and reduce inflammation. They are found in plants like ginseng and licorice root.

2.2 Medicinal Uses of Plants

The medicinal uses of plants are as varied as the plants themselves. Here are some common applications of herbal medicine based on the properties of different plants:

- Anti-inflammatory: Many plants have anti-inflammatory properties that can help reduce swelling and pain. For example, turmeric contains curcumin, which has strong anti-inflammatory effects and is used to treat conditions like arthritis.

- Antimicrobial: Some plants can fight bacterial, viral, and fungal infections. Garlic, for instance, contains allicin, which has been shown to have antibacterial and antiviral properties.

- Digestive Health: Certain herbs can aid digestion and alleviate gastrointestinal issues. Peppermint, with its menthol content, is commonly used to relieve irritable bowel syndrome (IBS) symptoms, and ginger is widely known for its ability to reduce nausea and improve digestion.

- Cardiovascular Health: Some plants support heart health and improve circulation. Hawthorn, which contains flavonoids and proanthocyanidins, is used to treat heart conditions such as congestive heart failure and hypertension.

- Respiratory Health: Herbal remedies can also address respiratory issues. Eucalyptus, containing eucalyptol, is often used in cough syrups and lozenges to help clear mucus and ease breathing.

- Immune Support: Certain herbs can boost the immune system. Echinacea is well-known for its immune-enhancing properties, making it a popular remedy for colds and flu.

- Skin Health: Many plants are beneficial for skin health, providing relief from conditions like eczema, psoriasis, and acne. Aloe vera, with its soothing and anti-inflammatory properties, is commonly used to treat burns and skin irritations.

- Mental Health: Some plants have calming and mood-enhancing effects. St. John's Wort, for example, is used to treat mild to moderate depression, and valerian root is often used to promote relaxation and improve sleep.

2.3 Preparation and Dosage

The effectiveness of herbal medicine depends not only on the choice of plant but also on its preparation and dosage. Common methods of preparation include:

- Teas and Infusions: These are made by steeping herbs in hot water. This method is suitable for extracting water-soluble compounds, such as those found in chamomile or peppermint.

- Tinctures: These are concentrated liquid extracts made by soaking herbs in alcohol or glycerin. Tinctures are potent and have a longer shelf life than teas.

- Capsules and Tablets: These provide a convenient way to consume herbs in measured doses. They are often used for powdered herbs or standardized extracts.

- Topical Applications: Creams, ointments, and poultices are applied directly to the skin. They are used for conditions like rashes, wounds, and muscle pain.

- Essential Oils: These are concentrated extracts obtained through distillation. Essential oils are used in aromatherapy and can be applied topically with a carrier oil or diffused for inhalation.

While herbal medicine can offer significant health benefits, it is important to use herbs safely and effectively. This involves understanding potential side effects, interactions with other medications, and appropriate dosages.

Consulting with a knowledgeable healthcare provider, such as a certified herbalist or a naturopathic doctor, can help ensure the safe use of herbal remedies.

The basics of plant properties and their medicinal uses encompass a wide range of compounds and applications. From anti-inflammatory and antimicrobial properties to supporting cardiovascular and mental health, plants offer a natural and holistic approach to healthcare. By understanding the active compounds in plants and how to prepare and use them safely, individuals can harness the healing power of nature to support their well-being.

Chapter 3: The importance of holistic health

Holistic health is an approach to wellness that considers the whole person—body, mind, and spirit—rather than focusing solely on individual symptoms or illnesses. This perspective is essential for achieving optimal health and well-being because it recognizes the interconnectedness of various aspects of a person's life. The importance of holistic health lies in its comprehensive approach, which aims to promote balance and harmony in all areas of life.

Comprehensive Care

Holistic health emphasizes comprehensive care, which means addressing the root causes of health issues rather than just treating symptoms. By examining a person's physical, emotional, mental, and spiritual aspects, holistic health practitioners can develop personalized treatment plans that promote overall well-being. This approach often involves a combination of conventional medical treatments and alternative therapies such as nutrition, exercise, stress management, and herbal medicine.

Physical Health: This includes regular exercise, a balanced diet, adequate sleep, and routine medical check-ups. Physical health is the foundation of holistic health, and maintaining it requires a proactive approach to wellness.

Emotional Health: Emotional well-being is crucial for overall health. It involves understanding and managing emotions, developing resilience, and fostering healthy relationships. Techniques like mindfulness, meditation, and counseling can help improve emotional health.

Mental Health: Mental health encompasses cognitive functions, mental clarity, and psychological well-being. Lifelong learning, problem-solving, and creative pursuits can support mental health.

Spiritual Health: Spiritual health involves finding purpose and meaning in life, which can provide a sense of fulfillment and peace. This aspect of health can be nurtured through practices such as meditation, prayer, or spending time in nature.

Preventative Approach

Holistic health strongly emphasizes prevention, aiming to maintain health and prevent disease before it occurs. This preventative approach involves lifestyle changes and practices that support the body's natural ability to heal and maintain balance. By focusing on healthy habits and early intervention, holistic health can reduce the risk of chronic diseases and improve quality of life.

Nutrition: A balanced diet rich in fruits, vegetables, whole grains, and lean proteins provides the essential nutrients for optimal health. Avoiding processed foods and excessive sugars can prevent many health issues.

Exercise: Regular physical activity is vital for maintaining physical health, reducing stress, and improving mood. It helps to strengthen the cardiovascular system, build muscle, and enhance flexibility.

Stress Management: Chronic stress can lead to a variety of health problems, including heart disease, depression, and weakened immune function. Techniques such as yoga, meditation, deep breathing exercises, and time in nature can help manage stress.

Adequate Sleep: Quality sleep is crucial for physical and mental health. It allows the body to repair itself and the mind to consolidate memories and process information.

Empowerment and Education

Holistic health empowers individuals to take an active role in their health. Education is a critical component of this empowerment, providing people with the knowledge and tools they need to make informed decisions about their health and lifestyle. By understanding the principles of holistic health, individuals can implement changes that lead to lasting improvements in their well-being.

Self-Care: Holistic health encourages self-care practices that promote well-being. This can include regular exercise, healthy eating, adequate rest, and activities that bring joy and relaxation.

Informed Choices: Being informed about different health options, from conventional treatments to alternative therapies, allows individuals to make choices that best suit their needs and preferences.

Personal Responsibility: Taking responsibility for one's health involves making proactive choices and seeking resources and support when needed. This proactive approach can lead to better health outcomes and greater control over one's life.

Community and Connection

Holistic health recognizes the importance of community and social connections in maintaining health. Positive relationships and a strong support network can provide emotional support, reduce stress, and improve overall well-being. Engaging with a community can also provide opportunities for shared learning and mutual support in pursuing health goals.

A network of friends, family, and healthcare providers can provide emotional and practical support, essential for coping with life's challenges. Participating in community activities and organizations can foster a sense of belonging and purpose, enhancing overall well-being.

Holistic health is essential because of its comprehensive and integrative approach to well-being. Holistic health promotes balance, prevention, and empowerment by considering all aspects of a person's life and addressing the root causes of health issues. This approach helps prevent disease and enhances the overall quality of life, making it a vital aspect of modern healthcare.

Chapter 4: Benefits of herbal remedies

Herbal remedies have been used for centuries across various cultures to treat illnesses and promote health. Today, they continue to be popular due to their numerous benefits, which are increasingly validated by scientific research. Understanding these benefits can help individuals make informed decisions about integrating herbal remedies into their healthcare routines.

4.1 Natural and Holistic Approach

One of the primary benefits of herbal remedies is that they offer a natural and holistic approach to health. Unlike synthetic drugs, herbal remedies are derived from natural sources, which can be more compatible with the body's systems. They often work harmoniously with the body's natural processes, supporting overall health rather than just targeting specific symptoms.

Whole-Plant Benefits. Herbal remedies often utilize the whole plant or a combination of plant parts, such as leaves, roots, flowers, and seeds. This holistic use can provide a broader range of therapeutic benefits because the various compounds in the plant can work synergistically.

Fewer Side Effects. Because herbal remedies are natural, they typically have fewer and less severe side effects than synthetic pharmaceuticals. When used appropriately, they are generally well-tolerated by the body.

4.2 Prevention and Maintenance

Herbal remedies are not just for treating illnesses; they are also effective for preventing and maintaining good health. Many herbs contain compounds that support the immune system, reduce inflammation, and promote overall wellness.

Immune Support. Herbs like echinacea and elderberry are known for their immune-boosting properties, helping to ward off infections and illnesses.

Anti-Inflammatory. Turmeric and ginger are powerful anti-inflammatory agents that can help prevent inflammation-related chronic diseases, such as arthritis and heart disease.

Antioxidant Properties. Many herbs are rich in antioxidants, which protect the body from oxidative stress and free radical damage. Examples include green tea and rosemary.

4.3 Accessibility and Cost-Effectiveness

Herbal remedies are often more accessible and cost-effective than conventional medications. Many herbs can be grown at home or purchased inexpensively, making them a viable option for those with limited access to healthcare.

Ease of Access. Herbal remedies are available in various forms, including teas, capsules, tinctures, and essential oils. This variety makes it easy for individuals to find and use herbal treatments that suit their preferences and needs.

Affordability. Growing herbs at home or purchasing them in bulk can significantly reduce healthcare costs. This is especially beneficial for managing chronic conditions that require ongoing treatment.

4.4 Customizable and Personalized Treatment

Another significant benefit of herbal remedies is their ability to be customized and personalized. Herbalists can tailor treatments to address specific health issues, considering an individual's unique needs and health history.

Individualized Formulations. Herbal practitioners can create personalized blends that target multiple aspects of a health condition. For example, a blend for digestive health might include peppermint for soothing the stomach, ginger for reducing nausea, and fennel for relieving gas.

Adjustable Dosages. Herbal remedies allow for flexible dosing. Dosages can be adjusted based on an individual's response to treatment, providing a more nuanced approach to healthcare.

4.5 Supporting Conventional Treatments

Herbal remedies can complement and enhance conventional medical treatments. They can be used alongside prescription medications to support overall health and well-being, often reducing the need for higher doses of pharmaceuticals.

Complementary Use. Herbs like milk thistle can support liver function during pharmaceutical treatments, while others like valerian root can help manage anxiety and improve sleep without additional medication.

Synergistic Effects. Some herbs can enhance the efficacy of conventional drugs. For instance, combining certain antibiotics with antimicrobial herbs like oregano oil can improve infection control.

4.6 Promoting Long-Term Health

Herbal remedies focus on promoting long-term health rather than providing quick fixes. This approach encourages sustainable health practices and lifestyle changes that contribute to well-being.

Lifestyle Integration. Using herbal remedies often involves adopting healthier lifestyle habits, such as improved diet, regular exercise, and stress management techniques.

Chronic Condition Management. Herbs like ginseng and ashwagandha help manage stress and improve energy levels, supporting individuals with chronic conditions to maintain better health over time.

Herbal remedies offer multifaceted benefits, offering a natural, accessible, and holistic approach to health and wellness. They support prevention and maintenance, provide customizable treatments, and can be used alongside conventional medicine. As more people seek out natural alternatives, the enduring benefits of herbal remedies continue to play a significant role in promoting long-term health and well-being.

Book 5: Herbal Remedies and Therapies by Barbara O'Neill

Comprehensive Guide to Natural Healing, Immune Support, and Everyday Wellness Through the Power of Plants

Chapter 1: The Basics of Herbal Medicine

1.1 Introduction to Herbal Medicine

Herbal medicine, also known as botanical medicine or phytotherapy, is a time-honored practice that harnesses the therapeutic properties of plants to promote health and treat various ailments. Throughout history, cultures around the world have relied on plants for their healing properties, recognizing their ability to address both acute and chronic health conditions. Barbara O'Neill's exploration of herbal remedies integrates traditional wisdom with modern scientific understanding, offering a comprehensive approach to natural healing.

<u>Historical Significance and Cultural Roots</u>

The use of herbs for medicinal purposes dates back to ancient civilizations, where healers and shamans relied on the knowledge passed down through generations. In ancient Egypt, herbal preparations were documented for their efficacy in treating ailments ranging from digestive disorders to skin conditions. Traditional Chinese Medicine (TCM) similarly emphasizes the balance of energies or "qi" within the body, using herbs like ginseng and astragalus to strengthen vitality and resilience against disease.

Similarly, Ayurveda, the traditional medicine of India, categorizes herbs based on their effects on the body's three doshas: Vata, Pitta, and Kapha. This system utilizes herbs like ashwagandha and turmeric to restore balance and promote overall health. Indigenous cultures across the globe, from the Amazon rainforest to the Australian Outback, have also developed extensive knowledge of local plants and their medicinal properties, illustrating the universality of herbal medicine's enduring appeal.

<u>Principles of Herbal Medicine</u>

Herbal medicine operates on the principle that plants contain compounds that interact with the body's physiological systems to promote healing and restore balance. These bioactive compounds, such as alkaloids, flavonoids, and essential oils, contribute to the therapeutic effects of herbs. Barbara O'Neill advocates for a holistic approach to herbal medicine, emphasizing the importance of considering the whole person—body, mind, and spirit—in the treatment and prevention of disease.

<u>Modern Scientific Validation</u>

Advancements in scientific research have validated many traditional uses of herbs and provided insights into their mechanisms of action. For example, studies have demonstrated the anti-inflammatory properties of herbs like ginger and turmeric, which are used to alleviate pain and support joint health. Similarly, the adaptogenic effects of herbs such as ashwagandha and rhodiola have been studied for their ability to enhance resilience to stress and improve overall well-being.

Barbara O'Neill integrates this scientific understanding with her practical experience and traditional knowledge, offering evidence-based recommendations for the safe and effective use of herbal remedies. Her approach emphasizes the importance of quality sourcing, proper preparation, and individualized dosing to maximize therapeutic benefits while minimizing potential risks.

Herbal medicine encompasses a wide range of applications, from everyday wellness support to the management of chronic conditions. Herbs can be used in various forms, including teas, tinctures, capsules, and topical preparations, allowing for flexibility in administration based on individual preferences and therapeutic goals.

1.2 History and Traditions of Herbal Remedies

The history of herbal remedies spans millennia, rooted in the rich traditions and wisdom of ancient civilizations across the globe. From the fertile valleys of Mesopotamia to the lush rainforests of the Amazon, cultures have cultivated a profound understanding of plants and their therapeutic properties for promoting health and treating ailments.

1.2.1 Ancient Civilizations and Herbal Knowledge

Ancient civilizations such as Egypt, Mesopotamia, China, and India played pivotal roles in developing herbal medicine practices. In ancient Egypt, medicinal plants like aloe vera and garlic were used for their healing properties, documented in papyrus scrolls that serve as early medical texts. The Ebers Papyrus, dated around 1550 BCE, contains references to over 700 herbal remedies for various conditions, illustrating the advanced medical knowledge of ancient Egyptian healers.

In Mesopotamia, the Sumerians and Babylonians utilized herbs such as licorice and myrrh in medicinal preparations, addressing ailments ranging from digestive disorders to skin infections. Clay tablets from this era provide insights into herbal remedies prescribed by early healers, emphasizing the integration of botanical knowledge with spiritual beliefs.

1.2.2 Traditional Chinese Medicine (TCM) and Ayurveda

Traditional Chinese Medicine (TCM) dates back over 5,000 years and is grounded in the concept of balancing qi, or life force, within the body. Herbal medicine plays a central role in TCM, where practitioners use plants like ginseng, astragalus, and goji berries to strengthen the body's vitality and resilience against disease. TCM categorizes herbs according to their energetic properties and uses complex formulas to treat imbalances and restore health.

Similarly, Ayurveda, the traditional medicine of India, emphasizes the interconnectedness of body, mind, and spirit. Ayurvedic texts such as the Charaka Samhita and Sushruta Samhita detail herbal remedies like turmeric, ashwagandha, and holy basil for promoting longevity and treating specific health conditions based on individual constitution or dosha.

1.2.3 Indigenous Healing Traditions

Indigenous cultures around the world possess profound knowledge of local plants and their medicinal properties, passed down through oral traditions and practical experience. In the Amazon rainforest, indigenous tribes like the Shipibo-Conibo have developed extensive botanical knowledge, using plants like cat's claw and ayahuasca for healing ceremonies and medicinal purposes. Similarly, Aboriginal Australians have a deep understanding of bush medicine, utilizing plants such as eucalyptus and tea tree for their antiseptic and healing properties.

1.2.4 Continuity and Evolution

The traditions of herbal remedies have continued to evolve over time, integrating insights from scientific research with traditional knowledge. Modern herbalists and practitioners like Barbara O'Neill draw upon this rich tapestry of history and tradition, advocating for the safe and effective use of herbs in promoting holistic health. By honoring ancient wisdom while embracing contemporary advancements, Barbara O'Neill invites individuals to explore the transformative potential of herbal remedies in supporting well-being and vitality.

1.3 How Herbs Work in the Body

Understanding the mechanisms by which herbs exert their effects in the body is fundamental to appreciating their therapeutic potential in herbal medicine. Herbs contain a diverse array of bioactive compounds, each with specific properties that interact with physiological systems to promote health and well-being. Barbara O'Neill's holistic approach integrates traditional wisdom with modern scientific insights, providing a comprehensive understanding of how herbs work within the body.

1.3.1 Bioactive Compounds and Their Actions

Herbs contain bioactive compounds such as alkaloids, flavonoids, terpenes, and phenolic acids, among others, which contribute to their medicinal properties. These compounds are synthesized by plants to defend against pathogens, attract pollinators, or regulate growth, and humans have learned to harness their benefits for therapeutic purposes.

Alkaloids are nitrogen-containing compounds found in plants like caffeine (stimulant), morphine (analgesic), and quinine (antimalarial). These compounds can affect neurotransmitter activity in the nervous system, alter cellular metabolism, or even act as toxins to deter herbivores.

Flavonoids are polyphenolic compounds found in fruits, vegetables, and herbs like chamomile and ginkgo. They possess antioxidant, anti-inflammatory, and immune-modulating properties. Flavonoids interact with enzymes and cell signaling pathways, helping to regulate gene expression and modulate cellular functions.

Terpenes are aromatic compounds found in essential oils of plants like lavender, peppermint, and eucalyptus. They contribute to the characteristic fragrance of plants and have diverse biological activities, including antimicrobial, anti-inflammatory, and analgesic effects. Terpenes can also enhance the absorption of other compounds and influence neurotransmitter activity in the brain.

Phenolic acids are another group of compounds found in herbs such as sage, rosemary, and thyme. They possess antioxidant properties and contribute to the bitter or astringent taste of some plants. Phenolic acids have been studied for their potential role in reducing oxidative stress and inflammation in the body.

1.3.2 Mechanisms of Action

The bioactive compounds in herbs exert their effects through various mechanisms within the body:

Interaction with Cell Receptors: Many herbal compounds interact with specific receptors on cell membranes, influencing cellular responses. For example, cannabinoids from cannabis plants interact with cannabinoid receptors in the endocannabinoid system, which regulates mood, appetite, and pain sensation.

Enzyme Inhibition or Activation: Some herbs contain compounds that inhibit or activate enzymes involved in metabolic pathways. For instance, garlic contains allicin, which inhibits enzymes involved in bacterial cell wall synthesis, contributing to its antimicrobial properties.

Modulation of Gene Expression: Certain herbal compounds can modulate gene expression, altering the production of proteins involved in various physiological processes. This molecular-level regulation can affect inflammation, immune response, and cellular repair mechanisms.

Antioxidant and Anti-inflammatory Effects: Many herbs are rich in antioxidants, which neutralize free radicals and reduce oxidative stress in cells. This antioxidant activity helps protect cells from damage and supports overall cellular health. Additionally, herbs with anti-inflammatory properties can help mitigate chronic inflammation, a contributing factor to many chronic diseases.

1.3.3 Holistic Approach to Herbal Medicine

Barbara O'Neill advocates for a holistic approach to herbal medicine, considering the interconnectedness of body, mind, and spirit in achieving optimal health. By understanding the biochemical actions of herbs and their broader effects on health systems, individuals can make informed choices about incorporating herbal remedies into their wellness routines. This approach encourages personalized treatment plans that address individual health needs while respecting the traditional wisdom and scientific evidence supporting herbal medicine.

Herbs represent a treasure trove of bioactive compounds that interact synergistically with the body's physiological systems to promote health and well-being. Barbara O'Neill's integration of traditional herbal knowledge with contemporary scientific insights underscores the potency and versatility of herbal medicine in supporting holistic health. By exploring the mechanisms of action of herbs, individuals can harness their therapeutic potential to enhance vitality, manage health conditions, and foster overall wellness naturally.

Chapter 2: Getting Started with Herbal Remedies

2.1 Choosing the Right Herbs

Selecting the appropriate herbs for health and wellness requires careful consideration of individual needs, health goals, and the specific properties of each herb. Barbara O'Neill advocates for a thoughtful and informed approach to choosing herbs, emphasizing the importance of quality, safety, and effectiveness in herbal medicine.

Herbs vary widely in their medicinal properties, which include but are not limited to:

<u>Primary Actions</u>: Each herb typically has one or more primary actions or effects on the body. For example, chamomile is known for its calming and anti-inflammatory properties, making it suitable for promoting relaxation and soothing digestive discomfort. Conversely, herbs like ginger are renowned for their warming and digestive stimulant actions, aiding in digestion and alleviating nausea.

<u>Secondary Actions</u>: Many herbs possess secondary actions that complement their primary effects. For instance, while St. John's Wort is primarily recognized for its antidepressant properties, it also exhibits antiviral and anti-inflammatory effects, broadening its therapeutic applications.

<u>Energetics</u>: In traditions such as Traditional Chinese Medicine (TCM) and Ayurveda, herbs are classified based on their energetic qualities, which influence their effects on the body. Herbs may be categorized as warming or cooling, moistening or drying, and can be selected to balance specific constitutional imbalances.

2.1.1 Individual Health Needs

When selecting herbs, it is crucial to consider individual health needs and goals. Some key factors to consider include:

Health Conditions: Choose herbs that target specific health concerns or conditions. For instance, individuals with insomnia may benefit from herbs like valerian or passionflower, known for their sedative properties, while those seeking immune support may opt for herbs like echinacea or elderberry.

Contraindications and Interactions: Take into account any contraindications or potential herb-drug interactions. Certain herbs may not be suitable for individuals with specific medical conditions or those taking medications. Consulting with a qualified herbalist or healthcare provider can help navigate these considerations.

Quality and Sourcing: Ensure the herbs are sourced from reputable suppliers who adhere to quality standards. Organic certification, sustainable harvesting practices, and third-party testing for purity and potency are essential factors to consider when choosing herbal products.

2.1.2 Forms of Herbal Preparations

Herbs can be prepared and administered in various forms to suit individual preferences and therapeutic needs:

Teas and Infusions: Herbal teas are popular for their simplicity and ease of preparation. They involve steeping dried herbs in hot water to extract their medicinal properties. Teas can be consumed daily to support overall health or used as needed for acute conditions.

Tinctures: Tinctures are concentrated liquid extracts of herbs, typically made by soaking herbs in alcohol or glycerin to extract their active constituents. Tinctures offer a convenient and potent way to administer herbs, allowing for precise dosing and longer shelf life.

Capsules and Tablets: Herbal supplements in capsule or tablet form provide standardized doses of herbs, ensuring consistency in potency and effectiveness. This format is convenient for individuals who prefer a measured and easily portable option.

Barbara O'Neill promotes a holistic approach to herbal selection, emphasizing the importance of integrating herbs into a comprehensive wellness plan that includes nutrition, lifestyle modifications, and mindfulness practices. By addressing the root causes of health imbalances and supporting the body's innate healing mechanisms, herbal medicine can play a pivotal role in achieving and maintaining optimal health.

2.2 Sourcing and Storing Herbs

Sourcing and storing herbs correctly are crucial steps in maintaining their potency, effectiveness, and safety for therapeutic use. Barbara O'Neill emphasizes the importance of selecting high-quality herbs and ensuring proper storage practices to preserve their medicinal properties.

Choosing high-quality herbs begins with selecting reputable suppliers who prioritize quality, sustainability, and ethical sourcing practices. Consider the following factors when sourcing herbs.

1) Organic Certification

Opt for herbs that are certified organic whenever possible. Organic certification ensures that herbs are grown without synthetic pesticides, herbicides, or genetically modified organisms (GMOs), minimizing exposure to potentially harmful chemicals.

2) Sustainable Harvesting

Choose herbs that are sustainably harvested to support biodiversity and environmental conservation. Sustainable harvesting practices ensure that wildcrafted herbs are harvested in a manner that allows populations to regenerate naturally, preserving their availability for future generations.

3) Quality Standards

Look for herbs that undergo rigorous quality testing for purity, potency, and contaminants. Third-party testing by reputable laboratories can verify the authenticity of herbal products and ensure they meet safety and efficacy standards.

Barbara O'Neill advocates for ethical sourcing practices that prioritize fair trade principles and support local communities. When purchasing herbs, consider suppliers who engage in fair trade partnerships with growers and communities, ensuring equitable compensation and sustainable livelihoods for those involved in herb cultivation and harvesting.

Proper storage is essential to maintain the potency and freshness of herbs over time. Follow these guidelines for storing herbs:

Keep Herbs Dry. Store dried herbs in airtight containers away from moisture and humidity. Exposure to moisture can cause herbs to degrade and lose their medicinal properties. Use glass jars or containers with tight-fitting lids to protect herbs from environmental exposure.

Store in a Cool, Dark Place. Store herbs in a cool, dark location away from direct sunlight and heat sources. Light and heat can accelerate the degradation of herbal compounds, reducing their efficacy. A pantry or cupboard is ideal for storing dried herbs, maintaining optimal conditions for long-term storage.

Label and Date Containers. Label herb containers with the herb's name and date of purchase or harvest. Proper labeling ensures you can easily identify herbs and track their freshness. Rotate herbs regularly to use older stock first and maintain a fresh supply.

Avoid Contamination. Prevent cross-contamination by storing different herbs separately. Strongly aromatic herbs like peppermint or garlic should be stored in separate containers to prevent flavors from mingling.

2.3 Basic Equipment and Supplies for Herbal Preparations

Effective herbal preparations require the right tools and supplies to ensure safety, potency, and ease of use. Barbara O'Neill emphasizes the importance of having basic equipment on hand for preparing and administering herbs, whether for teas, tinctures, or topical applications.

Essential Equipment

1. Mortar and Pestle: A mortar and pestle are fundamental tools for grinding and crushing dried herbs into powder or coarse consistency. This traditional method allows for controlled preparation of herbs and helps release their active constituents for extraction.

2. Herb Grinder: An herb grinder is an alternative to a mortar and pestle, particularly useful for grinding larger quantities of herbs quickly and efficiently. Herb grinders come in various sizes and designs, including manual and electric options, catering to different preparation needs.

3. Strainer or Cheesecloth: Strainers and cheesecloth are essential for filtering herbal infusions, decoctions, and tinctures. Fine-mesh strainers or cheesecloth remove plant material from liquid extracts, ensuring clarity and purity of herbal preparations.

4. Glass Jars and Containers: Glass jars with tight-sealing lids are ideal for storing dried herbs, herbal teas, tinctures, and infused oils. Glass containers protect herbs from moisture, light, and contaminants, preserving their freshness and potency over time.

5. Double Boiler or Bain-Marie: A double boiler or bain-marie is used for gently heating herbs in oil or water-based preparations without direct exposure to high heat. This method helps preserve delicate herbal compounds and prevents overheating during extraction processes.

6. Weighing Scale: A precise weighing scale is essential for accurately measuring herbal ingredients when preparing formulations and ensuring consistency in dosing. Digital scales are recommended for their accuracy and ease of use in herbal preparations.

7. Funnel: A funnel facilitates transferring herbal preparations, such as tinctures or oils, into storage containers without spills or waste. Choose funnels made of stainless steel or food-grade plastic for durability and ease of cleaning.

Additional Supplies

1. Labels and Markers: Labeling herbal containers with the herb's name, date of preparation, and dosage instructions ensures clarity and safety. Use waterproof labels and permanent markers to prevent smudging and ensure information remains legible.

2. Storage Racks or Shelves: Organize herbs, equipment, and supplies on storage racks or shelves in a cool, dry location. Proper storage helps maintain order and accessibility while protecting herbs from environmental factors that could degrade their quality.

3. Herb Drying Rack: For those who harvest fresh herbs, a drying rack allows herbs to dry naturally while maintaining their medicinal properties. Drying racks promote airflow around herbs, preventing mold and ensuring even drying for optimal preservation.

4. Herb Scissors or Shears: Herb scissors or shears are handy for harvesting fresh herbs and cutting them into smaller pieces for drying or immediate use. Stainless steel blades are preferred for their durability and ease of cleaning after use.

Proper maintenance and cleaning of equipment are essential to prevent cross-contamination and ensure longevity. Regularly inspect and replace supplies as needed to maintain optimal conditions for herbal medicine practices.

Chapter 3: Herbal Preparation Techniques

3.1 Infusions and Teas

Infusions and teas are foundational methods for extracting medicinal properties from herbs. They offer convenient and versatile ways to incorporate herbal remedies into daily wellness routines. Barbara O'Neill advocates using infusions and teas due to their simplicity, efficacy, and accessibility in supporting holistic health.

Infusions

An infusion involves steeping dried herbs in hot water to extract their medicinal constituents. This gentle extraction method is suitable for delicate plant parts such as leaves, flowers, and aerial parts. To prepare an infusion, pour boiling water over the herbs in a covered vessel and allow them to steep for 5-15 minutes. Strain the liquid and drink the infusion, either hot or cold. Examples of herbs commonly used in infusions include chamomile for relaxation, peppermint for digestion, and nettle for nutrition.

Teas

Herbal teas are similar to infusions but often involve a longer steeping to extract more potent flavors and medicinal compounds. Teas can be made from various parts of plants, including leaves, flowers, roots, and berries. To prepare a tea, boil water and pour it over the herbs in a teapot or mug. Cover and steep for 10-20 minutes, depending on the desired strength. Strain and enjoy the hot tea or allow it to cool for a refreshing beverage. Popular herbal teas include ginger tea for digestion, echinacea tea for immune support, and hibiscus tea for cardiovascular health.

3.1.1 Benefits of Infusions and Teas

Nutrient Extraction. Infusions and teas effectively extract water-soluble vitamins, minerals, antioxidants, and other beneficial compounds from herbs. This gentle extraction method preserves herbs' delicate flavors and therapeutic properties, providing a nourishing beverage that supports overall health.

Hydration. Drinking infusions and teas contributes to daily hydration goals while offering additional health benefits from herbal constituents. Herbal teas are caffeine-free options that can be enjoyed throughout the day to stay hydrated and promote well-being.

Digestive Support. Many herbs used in infusions and teas have carminative and digestive-stimulating properties. They can help soothe digestive discomfort, reduce bloating, and support healthy digestion after meals. Examples include peppermint, fennel, and chamomile.

Relaxation and Stress Relief. Certain herbs in infusions and teas possess calming and nervine properties, promoting relaxation and stress relief. Herbal teas like chamomile, lemon balm, and passionflower are popular choices for their ability to calm the mind and support restful sleep.

3.1.2 Practical Tips for Preparation

Use high-quality, organic herbs to ensure purity and potency in infusions and teas. Freshly dried herbs or commercially sourced herbal blends are suitable for preparing flavorful and effective beverages.

Adjust steeping times based on the herb's strength and desired potency. Longer steeping times extract more potent flavors and medicinal compounds, while shorter steeping times provide milder infusions.

Store dried herbs in airtight containers in a cool, dry place to maintain freshness and potency. Properly stored herbs retain their quality for extended periods, ensuring consistent results in herbal infusions and teas.

Infusions and teas offer accessible and effective ways to incorporate herbal medicine into daily life, naturally supporting overall health and well-being. Barbara O'Neill's advocacy for infusions and teas highlights their simplicity, versatility, and therapeutic benefits in promoting holistic health. By exploring different herbs and experimenting with infusions and teas, individuals can discover personalized wellness routines that harness the healing power of plants for vitality and resilience.

3.2 Making Herbal Teas

Herbal teas are beloved for their soothing flavors and therapeutic benefits, making them popular for integrating herbal medicine into daily wellness practices. Barbara O'Neill advocates for preparing herbal teas due to their simplicity, versatility, and ability to deliver medicinal properties effectively.

3.2.1 Steps to Prepare Herbal Teas

1. Selection of Herbs: Select high-quality herbs that align with your health goals and preferences. Choose herbs known for their specific therapeutic properties, such as calming herbs like chamomile or energizing herbs like ginseng. Use dried herbs for consistency and ease of preparation, ensuring they are stored in a cool, dry place to maintain freshness.

2. Boiling Water: Boil fresh, filtered water in a kettle or pot. The quality of water used can influence the overall flavor and extraction of herbal teas, so opt for clean, chlorine-free water whenever possible. Avoid using water that has already been boiled multiple times to ensure optimal extraction of herbal compounds.

3. Preparation: Place the desired amount of dried herbs into a teapot, infuser, or a mug. As a general guideline, use approximately 1 teaspoon of dried herbs per cup of water. Adjust the amount based on personal taste preferences and the desired strength of the tea.

4. Steeping Time: Pour the boiling water over the herbs, ensuring they are fully submerged. Cover the teapot or mug with a lid or saucer to trap the steam and prevent the escape of volatile aromatic compounds. Allow the herbs to steep for 5 to 15 minutes, depending on the herb's strength and the desired potency of the tea. Longer steeping times typically result in stronger-flavored teas with more pronounced medicinal effects.

5. Straining and Serving: Strain the herbal tea to remove the spent herbs and debris once steeping is complete. Use a fine-mesh strainer, cheesecloth, or tea infuser to ensure a clear and smooth beverage. Pour the strained herbal tea into cups or mugs and serve hot. Optionally, add natural sweeteners like honey or a squeeze of lemon to enhance flavor.

3.2.2 Tips for Enhancing Herbal Teas

1. Flavor Combinations: Experiment with different herb combinations to create unique flavor profiles and enhance the therapeutic benefits of herbal teas. For example, combine lavender with lemon balm for a relaxing tea or mix peppermint with ginger for a soothing digestive aid.

2. Cold Infusions: Herbal teas can also be enjoyed cold by steeping herbs in room temperature or cold water for several hours in the refrigerator. Cold-infused herbal teas are refreshing and retain their medicinal properties, making them ideal for hot summer days.

3. Herbal Syrups: Transform herbal teas into herbal syrups by reducing brewed herbal tea with natural sweeteners like honey or maple syrup. Herbal syrups can be drizzled over desserts, added to beverages, or used as a base for homemade herbal sodas.

Making herbal teas is a simple yet effective way to incorporate herbal medicine into daily life, promoting overall health and well-being. Barbara O'Neill's advocacy for herbal teas underscores their versatility, accessibility, and therapeutic benefits in supporting holistic health. By mastering the art of preparing herbal teas and exploring different herbs, individuals can cultivate personalized wellness routines that harness the healing power of plants for vitality and resilience.

3.3 Benefits and Uses of Herbal Infusions

Herbal infusions, known for their simplicity and effectiveness, offer numerous health benefits and therapeutic uses that support holistic well-being. Barbara O'Neill advocates for incorporating herbal infusions into daily wellness practices due to their ability to deliver medicinal properties in a gentle and accessible manner.

Nutrient Extraction

Herbal infusions effectively extract water-soluble vitamins, minerals, antioxidants, and phytochemicals from herbs, making them a nutrient-rich beverage that supports overall health. For example, nettle leaf infusions provide a natural source of vitamins A, C, and K and minerals like iron and calcium, which contribute to optimal nutrition and vitality.

Digestive Support

Many infused herbs possess carminative and digestive-stimulating properties, promoting healthy digestion and alleviating digestive discomfort. Chamomile and peppermint infusions are popular choices for soothing upset stomachs, reducing bloating, and supporting gastrointestinal health.

Relaxation and Stress Relief

Herbal infusions can have calming and nervine properties that help reduce stress and promote relaxation. Infusions of herbs like lavender, lemon balm, and passionflower are known for calming the mind, easing tension, and supporting restful sleep, making them valuable allies in managing stress and anxiety.

Immune Support

Certain herbs used in infusions, such as echinacea and elderberry, possess immune-modulating properties that help strengthen the body's natural defenses against infections and seasonal illnesses. Regular consumption of immune-supportive herbal infusions can bolster overall immune function and promote resilience during stress or exposure to pathogens.

<u>Hydration and Detoxification</u>

Drinking herbal infusions contributes to daily hydration goals while supporting the body's natural detoxification processes. Herbs like dandelion leaf and burdock root promote kidney and liver health, aiding in the elimination of toxins and metabolic waste from the body.

3.3.1 Therapeutic Uses of Herbal Infusions

Respiratory Health. Herbal infusions can benefit respiratory conditions by soothing inflamed airways and promoting respiratory function. Infusions of thyme, licorice root, and mullein leaf are traditionally used to support respiratory health, ease coughs, and clear congestion.

Women's Health. Infusions of herbs such as raspberry leaf and red clover are valued for supporting women's health throughout various life stages. These herbs are known for their toning and nourishing effects on the reproductive system, aiding menstrual health, pregnancy, and menopausal transitions.

Skin Care. Topical application of herbal infusions, such as chamomile or calendula, can benefit skin health by soothing irritation, promoting healing of minor wounds, and supporting overall skin resilience. Additionally, consuming herbal infusions rich in antioxidants can contribute to radiant and healthy-looking skin from within.

3.3.2 Practical Considerations

1. Preparation: To prepare herbal infusions, steep 1-2 teaspoons of dried herbs per cup of hot water in a covered vessel for 5-15 minutes, depending on the desired strength. Strain and drink the infusion while hot or cool for a refreshing beverage throughout the day.

2. Quality and Sourcing: Use high-quality, organic herbs sourced from reputable suppliers to ensure purity and potency in herbal infusions. Proper storage of dried herbs in a cool, dry place maintains their freshness and medicinal properties over time.

3. Personalization: Customize herbal infusions based on individual health needs and taste preferences by blending herbs to create unique flavor profiles and therapeutic benefits. Experimentation with herbal combinations allows for tailored wellness support.

3.4 Decoctions

Decoctions are concentrated herbal preparations made by boiling plant materials, such as roots, bark, and harder seeds, to extract their medicinal properties. Barbara O'Neill emphasizes decoctions as potent remedies that offer specific therapeutic benefits and are particularly useful for extracting active compounds from tougher plant parts.

3.4.1 Preparation Method

1. Selection of Herbs: Choose herbs with woody or tough parts, such as roots, bark, seeds, and thicker leaves, that benefit from prolonged boiling to release their medicinal constituents effectively. Examples of herbs suitable for decoctions include licorice root for respiratory health, ginger root for digestion, and astragalus root for immune support.

2. Boiling Process: To prepare a decoction, place 1-2 tablespoons of chopped or crushed dried herbs (or 2-3 tablespoons of fresh herbs) into a pot with 2-3 cups of cold water. Bring the mixture to a boil over medium heat, then reduce the heat and simmer, covered, for 20-30 minutes. Longer simmering times are necessary to ensure thorough extraction of the herb's active compounds.

3. Straining and Storage: After simmering, remove the pot from heat and allow the decoction to cool slightly. Strain the liquid through a fine-mesh strainer or cheesecloth into a clean container, pressing the herbs to extract as much liquid as possible. Discard the spent herbs and store the decoction in a glass jar or container with a tight-fitting lid. Refrigerate any unused portion and use it within a few days for optimal potency.

3.4.2 Uses and Benefits

Therapeutic Effects: Decoctions are valued for their concentrated nature and ability to deliver potent medicinal benefits. They are often used to address specific health concerns such as chronic conditions, immune support, and acute illnesses where stronger herbal actions are desired.

Digestive and Respiratory Support: Herbs like licorice root and marshmallow root are commonly used in decoctions to soothe and support the digestive tract, relieve inflammation, and promote mucous membrane health. Decoctions of mullein leaf or elecampane root are beneficial for respiratory health, helping to alleviate coughs, congestion, and respiratory discomfort.

Chronic Health Conditions: Decoctions are suitable for chronic health conditions that require ongoing support, such as arthritis, digestive disorders, and hormonal imbalances. Regular consumption of decoctions can provide sustained therapeutic benefits by supporting the body's natural healing processes.

Determine appropriate dosage based on individual health needs and herbal strength. Start with small amounts and gradually increase as needed, following guidance from herbalists or healthcare providers for optimal results.

Customize decoctions by combining herbs to create synergistic blends that address specific health concerns and individual preferences. Experimentation with different herbs allows for tailored herbal support and enhanced therapeutic outcomes.

3.5 How to Prepare Decoctions

Decoctions are concentrated herbal preparations that extract medicinal compounds from tough plant materials like roots, bark, seeds, and woody stems through prolonged boiling. Barbara O'Neill advocates for decoctions due to their potency and efficacy in addressing specific health concerns effectively.

Steps to Prepare Decoctions

1. Selection of Herbs: Choose herbs known for their therapeutic properties and tough plant parts that benefit from boiling to release their medicinal constituents. Examples include:

- Licorice Root: Supports respiratory health and soothes digestive discomfort.

- Ginger Root: Aids digestion, reduces nausea, and supports immune function.

- Dandelion Root: Supports liver health and aids in detoxification.

- Echinacea Root: Boosts immune function and supports overall immune health.

Ensure herbs are dried and chopped or crushed to enhance surface area and facilitate extraction during boiling.

2. Boiling Process:

- Place 1-2 tablespoons of dried herbs (or 2-3 tablespoons of fresh herbs) into a pot with 2-3 cups of cold water.

- Bring the mixture to a boil over medium-high heat, ensuring it covers the herbs completely.

- Once boiling, reduce heat to low and simmer the mixture, covered, for 20-30 minutes. This extended simmering time allows for thorough extraction of medicinal compounds from the herbs.

3. Monitoring and Adjusting:

- Monitor the decoction closely to prevent boiling over, adjusting heat as needed to maintain a gentle simmer.

- Stir occasionally to ensure herbs are evenly distributed and submerged in the water for consistent extraction.

4. Straining and Storage:

- After simmering, remove the pot from heat and allow the decoction to cool slightly.

- Strain the liquid through a fine-mesh strainer or cheesecloth into a clean container, pressing the herbs to extract as much liquid as possible.

- Discard the spent herbs and store the decoction in a glass jar or container with a tight-fitting lid.

- Refrigerate any unused portion and use within a few days to preserve potency and freshness.

5. Dosage and Usage:

- Determine the appropriate dosage based on individual health needs and the herb's strength. Start with smaller amounts and gradually increase as needed.

- Decoctions can be consumed warm or cooled to room temperature, depending on preference and therapeutic use.

- Consider consulting with an herbalist or healthcare provider for personalized guidance on dosage and usage for specific health conditions.

Decoctions offer a potent method for extracting medicinal properties from tough plant materials, supporting digestive health, immune function, and overall well-being. By mastering the art of preparing decoctions and understanding their therapeutic benefits, individuals can incorporate these potent herbal remedies into their holistic health practices with confidence and effectiveness. Barbara O'Neill's advocacy for decoctions underscores their role in promoting natural healing and resilience through the power of medicinal herbs.

3.6 Common Herbs for Decoctions

Decoctions are robust herbal preparations that extract potent medicinal compounds from tough plant materials through extended boiling. Barbara O'Neill recommends several herbs renowned for their therapeutic properties when prepared as decoctions, addressing a variety of health concerns effectively.

Licorice Root (*Glycyrrhiza glabra*)

Licorice root is celebrated for its soothing properties, making it a staple in decoctions aimed at respiratory health and digestive support. It contains glycyrrhizin, a compound known for its anti-inflammatory and expectorant effects, making it beneficial for alleviating coughs, soothing sore throats, and supporting respiratory function. Licorice root decoctions are also used to calm gastrointestinal distress, reduce stomach acid, and support overall digestive health.

Ginger Root (*Zingiber officinale*)

Ginger root is prized for its warming properties and diverse health benefits, making it a popular choice for decoctions aimed at digestive support and immune enhancement. Rich in gingerol and other bioactive compounds, ginger root decoctions stimulate digestion, alleviate nausea, and reduce inflammation in the digestive tract. Additionally, ginger root supports immune function by promoting circulation and providing antioxidant protection against oxidative stress.

Dandelion Root (*Taraxacum officinale*)

Dandelion root is renowned for its detoxifying and liver-supportive properties, making it an essential herb in decoctions aimed at cleansing and supporting overall health. Decoctions of dandelion root stimulate bile production, aiding in the digestion of fats and promoting liver detoxification processes. They also act as a mild diuretic, supporting kidney function and helping to eliminate toxins from the body.

Burdock Root (*Arctium lappa*)

Burdock root is valued for its blood-cleansing and skin-supportive properties, making it a key ingredient in decoctions for promoting detoxification and skin health. Rich in antioxidants and anti-inflammatory compounds, burdock root decoctions support liver function, purify the blood, and promote clear, healthy skin. They are also used to alleviate inflammatory conditions such as arthritis and support overall immune health.

Echinacea Root (*Echinacea purpurea*)

Echinacea root is prized for its immune-strengthening properties, making it a valuable herb in decoctions aimed at supporting immune function and combating infections. Decoctions of echinacea root stimulate the immune system's response to pathogens, helping to shorten the duration and severity of colds, flu, and other respiratory infections. They also possess anti-inflammatory properties that support overall immune health and reduce inflammation in the body.

3.6.1 Preparation Tips

- Dosage: Follow dosage guidelines recommended by herbalists or healthcare providers based on individual health needs and the herb's strength.

- Quality: Use high-quality, organic herbs sourced from reputable suppliers to ensure potency and purity in decoctions.

- Storage: Store decoctions in glass jars or containers with tight-fitting lids in a cool, dark place to preserve potency and freshness.

Decoctions are potent herbal preparations that harness the therapeutic benefits of tough plant materials, providing effective support for digestive health, immune function, detoxification, and overall well-being. Barbara O'Neill's advocacy for common herbs used in decoctions underscores their role in promoting natural healing and resilience through the power of medicinal plants. By incorporating these herbs into decoctions and understanding their specific benefits, individuals can enhance their holistic health practices and support long-term wellness naturally.

3.7 Tinctures and Extracts

Tinctures and extracts are concentrated herbal preparations that extract medicinal compounds using alcohol or another solvent. Barbara O'Neill advocates for tinctures and extracts due to their potency, long shelf life, and convenience in delivering therapeutic benefits.

Alcohol-Based Tinctures

- Selection of Herbs: Choose dried herbs known for their medicinal properties and compatibility with alcohol extraction. Examples include echinacea for immune support, valerian for relaxation, and hawthorn for cardiovascular health.

- Alcohol Selection: Use high-proof alcohol such as vodka or brandy, which effectively extracts and preserves the active constituents of herbs. The alcohol concentration should be 40-60% for optimal extraction.

- Preparation: Place finely chopped or powdered herbs into a glass jar and cover completely with alcohol. Seal the jar tightly and store it in a cool, dark place for 4-6 weeks, shaking daily to facilitate extraction. After steeping, strain the liquid through cheesecloth or a fine-mesh strainer, pressing the herbs to extract as much liquid as possible. Store the tincture in dark glass bottles with dropper tops for easy dosing.

Glycerin-Based Extracts

- Selection of Herbs: Glycerin-based extracts are suitable for herbs with water-soluble constituents or for individuals avoiding alcohol. Herbs like marshmallow root for soothing mucous membranes or lemon balm for calming effects are ideal for glycerin extraction.

- Preparation: Combine finely chopped or powdered herbs with vegetable glycerin in a glass jar, ensuring herbs are fully submerged. Seal the jar and place it in a cool, dark location for 4-6 weeks, shaking daily. After steeping, strain the liquid and store the extract in amber glass bottles with dropper tops. Glycerin extracts have a shorter shelf life compared to alcohol-based tinctures but offer a sweet taste and are suitable for children and those sensitive to alcohol.

3.7.1 Uses and Benefits

1. Ease of Administration: Tinctures and extracts are convenient for administration, allowing for precise dosing and easy incorporation into daily routines. They can be taken directly under the tongue, diluted in water or juice, or added to teas or other beverages.

2. Long Shelf Life: Properly stored tinctures and extracts maintain their potency and efficacy for several years, making them a reliable option for long-term herbal support.

3. Concentrated Effects: Tinctures and extracts deliver concentrated doses of medicinal compounds, providing potent therapeutic effects that may be more pronounced compared to teas or infusions.

4. Versatility: Tinctures and extracts offer versatility in herbal use, allowing for customization of blends and formulations to address specific health concerns or support individual wellness goals.

Practical Considerations

Dosage: Follow dosage recommendations provided by herbalists or healthcare providers based on individual health needs and the herb's strength.

Quality: Use high-quality, organic herbs sourced from reputable suppliers to ensure potency and purity in tinctures and extracts.

Storage: Store tinctures and extracts in dark glass bottles in a cool, dry place away from direct sunlight to preserve their medicinal properties.

Tinctures and extracts are potent herbal preparations valued for their concentrated medicinal benefits, ease of administration, and long shelf life. Barbara O'Neill's advocacy for tinctures and extracts underscores their role in supporting holistic health through the therapeutic properties of medicinal plants. By incorporating these preparations into wellness routines and understanding their specific benefits, individuals can enhance their natural healing practices and promote overall well-being effectively and sustainably.

3.8 Making Alcohol-Based and Glycerin Tinctures

Tinctures are concentrated herbal extracts made by steeping medicinal herbs in alcohol or glycerin to extract their active compounds. Barbara O'Neill promotes tinctures for their potency, versatility, and ease of use in supporting holistic health practices.

Alcohol-Based Tinctures

Selection of Herbs: Choosing the right herbs is crucial for preparing effective alcohol-based tinctures. Opt for dried herbs known for their medicinal properties and compatibility with alcohol extraction. Herbs like echinacea for immune support, valerian for relaxation, and hawthorn for cardiovascular health are popular choices.

Alcohol Selection: High-proof alcohol such as vodka or brandy is commonly used for alcohol-based tinctures due to its ability to effectively extract and preserve the active constituents of herbs. The alcohol concentration should typically be between 40% to 60% to ensure optimal extraction.

Preparation Process

Herb Preparation: Begin by finely chopping or grinding dried herbs to increase surface area and facilitate extraction.

Steeping: Place the prepared herbs into a clean glass jar and cover them completely with alcohol. Seal the jar tightly and shake it well to ensure all herbs are fully submerged.

Extraction: Store the sealed jar in a cool, dark place for 4 to 6 weeks, shaking it daily to facilitate the extraction process. The alcohol gradually extracts the medicinal compounds from the herbs, creating a potent herbal tincture.

Straining and Storage: After the steeping period, strain the liquid through a fine-mesh strainer or cheesecloth into a clean bowl or directly into dark glass bottles with dropper tops. Press the herbs to extract as much liquid as possible, ensuring the tincture is clear and free of debris.

Bottling: Transfer the strained tincture into dark glass bottles with dropper tops to protect it from light and maintain its potency. Label each bottle with the herb name, preparation date, and dosage instructions.

<u>Glycerin-Based Tinctures</u>

Glycerin-based tinctures are ideal for herbs with water-soluble constituents or for individuals sensitive to alcohol. Suitable herbs include marshmallow root for soothing mucous membranes and lemon balm for calming effects.

Preparation Process

Herb Preparation: Similar to alcohol-based tinctures, finely chop or grind dried herbs to increase their surface area for extraction.

Combining Ingredients: Place the prepared herbs into a glass jar and cover them completely with vegetable glycerin. Ensure all herbs are fully submerged in the glycerin.

Steeping: Seal the jar tightly and store it in a cool, dark place for 4 to 6 weeks, shaking it daily to facilitate the extraction process. Glycerin extracts the medicinal compounds from the herbs, creating a sweet-tasting herbal preparation.

Straining and Bottling: After the steeping period, strain the glycerin-extracted liquid through a fine-mesh strainer or cheesecloth into dark glass bottles with dropper tops. Press the herbs to extract as much liquid as possible, ensuring the glycerin tincture is clear and free of sediment.

Storage: Store glycerin-based tinctures in a cool, dark place away from direct sunlight to maintain their potency and shelf life. Properly stored glycerin tinctures can be kept for up to one year.

<u>Benefits and Considerations</u>

Both alcohol-based and glycerin-based tinctures deliver concentrated doses of medicinal compounds, offering potent therapeutic effects.

Tinctures can be taken directly under the tongue, diluted in water or juice, or added to teas, offering versatility in administration.

Properly stored tinctures maintain their potency for several years, making them a reliable option for long-term herbal support.

3.9 Using Herbal Extracts Effectively

Herbal extracts, including tinctures and glycerites, are potent preparations that provide concentrated doses of medicinal compounds extracted from herbs. Barbara O'Neill emphasizes the effective use of herbal extracts as versatile tools for promoting holistic health and addressing specific health concerns.

<u>Understanding Potency and Dosage</u>

1. Concentration Levels:

Alcohol-Based Tinctures: Typically have a higher concentration of medicinal compounds due to the alcohol extraction process. This makes them suitable for addressing acute conditions or providing strong therapeutic effects.

Glycerin-Based Extracts: Have a sweeter taste and are suitable for children or individuals sensitive to alcohol. They may have a lower concentration of active compounds compared to alcohol-based tinctures but still offer effective herbal support.

2. Dosage Considerations:

Follow dosage recommendations provided by herbalists, healthcare providers, or the guidelines on the tincture bottle.

Start with a lower dosage and gradually increase as needed, based on individual response and health goals.

Adjust dosages for children, elderly individuals, or those with specific health conditions to ensure safe and effective use of herbal extracts.

Methods of Administration

1. Sublingual Application:

Administer tinctures directly under the tongue (sublingually) for rapid absorption into the bloodstream.

Hold the tincture under the tongue for 30-60 seconds before swallowing to enhance absorption and effectiveness.

2. Dilution in Water or Juice:

Mix tinctures or glycerin extracts into a glass of water or juice to dilute the concentrated herbal preparation.

This method masks the strong taste of some tinctures and makes them more palatable for consumption.

3. Addition to Teas or Beverages:

Add herbal extracts to herbal teas or other beverages to enhance their therapeutic effects.

This method allows for customization of flavors and additional herbal support in everyday drinks.

Targeted Uses for Herbal Extracts

1. Immune Support:

Echinacea, elderberry, and astragalus tinctures are commonly used to support immune function and enhance resistance to infections.

Take at the onset of cold or flu symptoms or as a preventive measure during cold and flu season.

2. Digestive Health:

Peppermint, ginger, and chamomile tinctures help soothe digestive discomfort, relieve nausea, and support overall gastrointestinal health.

Take before or after meals to aid digestion or alleviate symptoms of indigestion.

3. Stress and Relaxation: Valerian, passionflower, and lemon balm tinctures are known for their calming and anxiety-relieving effects. Use during times of stress or before bedtime to promote relaxation and improve sleep quality.

4. Chronic Conditions:

Turmeric, milk thistle, and St. John's wort tinctures support management of chronic conditions such as inflammation, liver health, and mood disorders. Incorporate into daily routines to provide ongoing support for long-term health goals.

<u>Safety and Precautions</u>

1. Interaction with Medications:

Consult with a healthcare provider before using herbal extracts, especially if taking medications or managing chronic health conditions. Some herbs may interact with medications or exacerbate certain health conditions.

2. Quality and Sourcing:

Choose high-quality, organic herbs and reputable suppliers to ensure purity and potency of herbal extracts.

Proper storage in dark glass bottles away from light and heat preserves the effectiveness of herbal preparations.

Chapter 4: Top Herbs for Everyday Use

4.1 Chamomile

4.1.1 Benefits and Uses

Chamomile (*Matricaria chamomilla* or *Chamaemelum nobile*) is a versatile herb renowned for its soothing properties and gentle effectiveness in addressing various health concerns. Barbara O'Neill often recommends chamomile for its calming effects on the nervous system and its ability to promote relaxation and sleep. Here are some key benefits and uses of chamomile:

1. Promotes Relaxation: Chamomile is widely recognized for its calming effects, making it beneficial for reducing anxiety, stress, and promoting overall relaxation. It contains compounds like apigenin, which interact with neurotransmitters in the brain to induce relaxation.

2. Improves Sleep Quality: Due to its calming properties, chamomile tea or tinctures are often used to improve sleep quality and treat insomnia. Consuming chamomile before bedtime can help relax muscles and ease tension, promoting a more restful night's sleep.

3. Digestive Support: Chamomile has been traditionally used to soothe digestive issues such as indigestion, gas, bloating, and stomach cramps. It has anti-inflammatory properties that can help alleviate gastrointestinal discomfort and promote digestive health.

4. Anti-inflammatory and Antioxidant Properties: Chamomile contains flavonoids and other antioxidants that help reduce inflammation and protect against oxidative stress. This makes it beneficial for supporting immune function and overall health.

5. Skin Care: Chamomile's anti-inflammatory and antioxidant properties extend to skincare. It can soothe skin irritations, rashes, and sunburns when used topically in creams or infused in bathwater.

4.1.2 Preparation and Dosage

Chamomile can be prepared and consumed in various forms, including teas, tinctures, and topical applications. Barbara O'Neill suggests the following methods for preparing and dosing chamomile effectively:

1. Chamomile Tea:

   o Preparation: Steep 1-2 teaspoons of dried chamomile flowers in hot water for 5-10 minutes.

   o Dosage: Drink 1-2 cups of chamomile tea daily, preferably before bedtime for relaxation and sleep support. Adjust the strength of the tea based on individual preference and desired effects.

2. Chamomile Tincture:

- Preparation: Prepare a chamomile tincture using dried chamomile flowers and alcohol (such as vodka). Follow the guidelines for making alcohol-based tinctures mentioned earlier in Chapter 3.

- Dosage: Take 1-2 ml (approximately 20-40 drops) of chamomile tincture diluted in water, tea, or juice up to three times daily. Adjust the dosage based on individual response and health goals.

3. Topical Applications:

- Preparation: Create a chamomile-infused oil or cream for topical use to soothe skin irritations and promote healing.

- Dosage: Apply the chamomile-infused oil or cream to affected areas of the skin as needed, gently massaging until absorbed.

4.2 Echinacea

4.2.1 Immune-Boosting Properties

Echinacea, also known as purple coneflower, is a well-known herb celebrated for its potent immune-boosting properties. Barbara O'Neill often recommends echinacea for supporting the body's natural defenses against infections and enhancing overall immune function. Here are some key immune-boosting properties of echinacea:

1. Stimulates Immune Response: Echinacea contains active compounds such as alkamides, polysaccharides, and flavonoids that stimulate the activity of immune cells like macrophages and T-cells. This enhances the body's ability to defend against pathogens, including viruses and bacteria.

2. Antiviral and Antibacterial Effects: Echinacea has demonstrated antiviral and antibacterial properties in research studies. It can help prevent the onset of colds, flu, and other respiratory infections by inhibiting the growth and replication of viruses and bacteria.

3. Reduces Inflammation: Echinacea possesses anti-inflammatory properties that help reduce inflammation in the body. This can be beneficial for alleviating symptoms of inflammatory conditions and supporting overall immune health.

4. Antioxidant Activity: The antioxidants found in echinacea, such as flavonoids and phenolic compounds, help neutralize harmful free radicals and reduce oxidative stress. This contributes to overall health and supports immune function.

5. Adaptogenic Qualities: Echinacea is considered an adaptogen, which means it helps the body adapt to stress and strengthens resilience. Regular use of echinacea can support immune resilience during periods of physical or emotional stress.

4.2.2 How to Use Echinacea

Barbara O'Neill recommends several effective methods for using echinacea to maximize its immune-boosting benefits:

1. Echinacea Tea:

- Preparation: Steep 1-2 teaspoons of dried echinacea root or flowers in hot water for 10-15 minutes.

- Dosage: Drink 1-2 cups of echinacea tea daily during cold and flu season or at the onset of symptoms to support immune function. Adjust the strength of the tea based on individual tolerance.

2. Echinacea Tincture:

- Preparation: Prepare an echinacea tincture using dried echinacea root or aerial parts and alcohol (such as vodka or brandy). Follow the guidelines for making alcohol-based tinctures as discussed earlier in Chapter 3.

- Dosage: Take 1-2 ml (approximately 20-40 drops) of echinacea tincture diluted in water or juice up to three times daily. Increase the dosage at the onset of symptoms or during periods of increased immune challenge.

3. Echinacea Capsules or Tablets:

- Dosage: Follow the dosage recommendations provided on the product label or as recommended by a healthcare provider. Echinacea supplements are available in various forms and strengths for convenience.

4. Topical Applications:

- Preparation: Use echinacea-infused creams or ointments topically to support skin health and wound healing. Apply as needed to affected areas of the skin.

Echinacea is a valuable herb known for its immune-boosting properties and ability to enhance overall health. Barbara O'Neill's advocacy for echinacea highlights its role in supporting immune resilience and defending against infections naturally. By incorporating echinacea into daily routines through teas, tinctures, or supplements, individuals can harness its immune-boosting benefits effectively and promote long-term wellness.

4.3 Lavender

4.3.1 Calming and Healing Benefits

Lavender (*Lavandula angustifolia*) is a versatile herb renowned for its calming and healing properties. Barbara O'Neill often recommends lavender for its soothing effects on the nervous system, ability to promote relaxation, and its diverse applications in holistic health. Here are some key benefits of lavender:

1. Relaxation and Stress Reduction: Lavender is widely recognized for its ability to induce relaxation and reduce stress. It contains compounds like linalool and linalyl acetate that have sedative effects, calming the mind and promoting a sense of tranquility.

2. Sleep Aid: Due to its calming properties, lavender is used to improve sleep quality and treat insomnia. Aromatherapy with lavender essential oil or using lavender sachets near the bed can promote a restful night's sleep.

3. Pain Relief: Lavender has analgesic properties that can help alleviate headaches, muscle aches, and joint pain when applied topically or used in massage oils.

4. Skin Care: Lavender is beneficial for skin health, with antiseptic and anti-inflammatory properties that can soothe minor burns, insect bites, and skin irritations. It is commonly used in skincare products for its healing effects.

5. Antioxidant and Antimicrobial Properties: The antioxidants in lavender help protect cells from damage caused by free radicals, supporting overall health. It also has antimicrobial properties that can help fight bacteria and prevent infections.

4.3.2 Applications in Everyday Life

Barbara O'Neill recommends several practical ways to incorporate lavender into daily routines for its calming and healing benefits:

1. Aromatherapy: Use a few drops of lavender essential oil in a diffuser to fill the air with its soothing aroma. This promotes relaxation, reduces stress levels, and creates a calming atmosphere at home or work.

2. Lavender Tea: Steep dried lavender flowers in hot water to make a fragrant herbal tea. Lavender tea can help relax the mind and body, promote sleep, and support digestive health.

3. Topical Use: Apply diluted lavender essential oil topically to the skin to soothe minor burns, cuts, insect bites, or skin irritations. Mix lavender oil with a carrier oil like coconut or almond oil before applying.

4. Bath Additive: Add a few drops of lavender essential oil to a warm bath to create a relaxing and aromatic soak. This helps relieve muscle tension, promote relaxation, and enhance overall well-being.

5. Lavender Sachets: Place dried lavender flowers in fabric sachets and tuck them into drawers or closets. Lavender sachets impart a pleasant scent while also repelling moths and insects.

6. Massage Oil: Mix lavender essential oil with a carrier oil and use it for massage to relax muscles, reduce tension, and promote overall relaxation.

Lavender is a versatile herb valued for its calming, healing, and therapeutic properties in holistic health practices. Barbara O'Neill's advocacy for lavender underscores its effectiveness in promoting relaxation, reducing stress, and supporting overall well-being. By incorporating lavender into daily routines through aromatherapy, teas, topical applications, and other methods, individuals can harness its calming and healing benefits to enhance their holistic health and quality of life.

4.4 Other Essential Herbs

In addition to lavender, echinacea, and chamomile, Barbara O'Neill advocates for several other essential herbs known for their therapeutic benefits and versatile applications in natural healing. These herbs offer various health-promoting properties and can be incorporated into daily routines to support overall well-being. Here are some of the key essential herbs recommended by Barbara O'Neill.

1. Peppermint (*Mentha piperita*):
   o Digestive Support: Peppermint is valued for its ability to soothe digestive discomfort, relieve gas and bloating, and promote healthy digestion. It can be consumed as a tea or used in culinary dishes for its refreshing taste and digestive benefits.

2. Ginger (*Zingiber officinale*):

   o Anti-inflammatory: Ginger has potent anti-inflammatory properties that can help reduce inflammation, alleviate muscle soreness, and support joint health. It is commonly used in teas, soups, and stir-fries for its warming and healing effects.

3. Lemon Balm (*Melissa officinalis*):

   o Calming and Mood Support: Lemon balm is known for its calming effects on the nervous system, helping to reduce anxiety, promote relaxation, and improve mood. It can be consumed as a tea or used in aromatherapy for its soothing aroma.

4. Valerian (*Valeriana officinalis*):

   o Sleep Aid: Valerian is a powerful herb used to promote sleep and relieve insomnia. It has sedative properties that help calm the mind and body, making it beneficial for improving sleep quality and managing stress.

5. Turmeric (*Curcuma longa*):

   o Anti-inflammatory and Antioxidant: Turmeric contains curcumin, a compound known for its strong anti-inflammatory and antioxidant properties. It supports joint health, reduces inflammation, and promotes overall immune function when consumed regularly.

6. St. John's Wort (*Hypericum perforatum*):

   o Mood Support: St. John's Wort is traditionally used to alleviate symptoms of mild to moderate depression and anxiety. It has mood-stabilizing properties that promote emotional well-being and mental clarity.

7. Nettle (*Urtica dioica*):

   o Nutrient-Rich: Nettle is a nutrient-dense herb rich in vitamins, minerals, and antioxidants. It supports overall health and vitality, helps maintain healthy skin, and promotes detoxification when consumed as a tea or included in culinary dishes.

8. Holy Basil (Tulsi) (*Ocimum sanctum*):

   o Adaptogenic and Stress Relief: Holy Basil, or Tulsi, is an adaptogenic herb known for its ability to reduce stress, enhance resilience to stressors, and support immune function. It can be consumed as a tea or used in herbal formulations.

These essential herbs recommended by Barbara O'Neill offer a range of health benefits and therapeutic properties that support natural healing and holistic well-being. By incorporating these herbs into daily routines through teas, tinctures, culinary dishes, and topical applications, individuals can harness their healing potential and promote overall health effectively.

Chapter 5: Herbal Remedies for Common Ailments

5.1 Colds and Flu

Colds and flu, commonly caused by viruses, are seasonal ailments that affect the respiratory system. Barbara O'Neill emphasizes natural approaches to prevent and manage these illnesses, focusing on strengthening the immune system and supporting overall health.

Understanding Colds and Flu

Understanding the viral Nature of Colds and Flu: These illnesses are primarily transmitted through respiratory droplets or contact with contaminated surfaces. Common symptoms include coughing, sneezing, congestion, fever, and fatigue. This understanding is crucial for effective prevention and management.

Seasonal Variability: Both colds and flu exhibit seasonal peaks, typically during the fall and winter months. Cold symptoms are generally milder, while flu symptoms can be more severe and may lead to complications, especially in vulnerable populations. Being aware of these seasonal patterns can help you prepare and take necessary precautions.

Natural Remedies and Prevention Strategies

Boosting Immunity: Barbara O'Neill recommends strategies to enhance immune function, such as consuming immune-boosting herbs like echinacea and elderberry, maintaining a balanced diet rich in vitamins and minerals, and getting adequate rest and exercise.

Hydration and Nutrition: Staying hydrated with water, herbal teas, and broths helps maintain mucous membrane hydration and supports immune function. Nutrient-dense foods, including fruits, vegetables, and lean proteins, provide essential vitamins and minerals necessary for immune health.

Herbal Support: Herbal remedies such as ginger and garlic are valued for their anti-inflammatory and antimicrobial properties. They can help alleviate symptoms and support the body's natural defenses against viruses. Incorporating these natural remedies into your routine can provide additional support in managing colds and flu.

Rest and Recovery: Barbara O'Neill advocates for the importance of rest, a crucial aspect of healing and recovery. By prioritizing sleep and reducing stress, she ensures that your immune resilience is enhanced and recovery is faster, making you feel cared for.

Hygiene Practices: Practicing good hygiene, including frequent handwashing, covering coughs and sneezes, and avoiding close contact with sick individuals helps prevent the spread of viruses that cause colds and flu.

Holistic Approaches

Symptom Management: Natural remedies such as herbal teas with honey and lemon can soothe sore throats and coughs. Steam inhalation with eucalyptus oil or peppermint can ease congestion and promote respiratory comfort.

Long-Term Health Practices: Barbara O'Neill emphasizes lifestyle changes that promote overall health and immune resilience, including regular exercise, stress management techniques like meditation or yoga, and maintaining a healthy weight.

5.2 Herbal Treatments and Preventive Measures

<u>Herbal Treatments</u>

1. Echinacea and Elderberry:

    o   Immune Support: Echinacea and elderberry are renowned for their immune-boosting properties. Echinacea stimulates the immune system, enhancing the body's defense against infections. Elderberry is rich in antioxidants and has antiviral properties, particularly beneficial during cold and flu season.

2. Garlic and Ginger:

    o   Antimicrobial Effects: Garlic and ginger possess potent antimicrobial properties that help combat infections. Garlic is known for its ability to support cardiovascular health and lower blood pressure, while ginger aids digestion and reduces inflammation.

3. Turmeric and Boswellia:

    o   Anti-inflammatory Benefits: Turmeric and boswellia are effective in reducing inflammation and alleviating symptoms of arthritis and other inflammatory conditions. Turmeric contains curcumin, a powerful antioxidant with numerous health benefits, while boswellia helps improve joint function and mobility.

4. Lavender and Chamomile:

    o   Calming and Relaxation: Lavender and chamomile are prized for their calming effects on the nervous system. They promote relaxation, reduce stress, and improve sleep quality. Lavender also offers skin-healing properties, while chamomile aids digestion and soothes gastrointestinal discomfort.

<u>Preventive Measures</u>

1. Healthy Diet:

    o   Nutrient-Rich Foods: Consuming a diet rich in fruits, vegetables, whole grains, and lean proteins provides essential vitamins, minerals, and antioxidants necessary for immune function and overall health. Avoiding processed foods and excessive sugar supports immune resilience.

2. Hydration:

    o   Water and Herbal Teas: Staying hydrated with water and herbal teas supports optimal hydration levels and aids in flushing toxins from the body. Herbal teas like peppermint and nettle offer additional health benefits and can be enjoyed throughout the day.

3. Regular Exercise:

o Physical Activity: Engaging in regular exercise strengthens the immune system, improves circulation, and enhances overall well-being. Incorporate activities like walking, yoga, or swimming into daily routines to promote immune resilience and mental clarity.

4. Stress Management:

   o Mind-Body Practices: Practicing stress-reduction techniques such as meditation, deep breathing exercises, or aromatherapy with essential oils like lavender or eucalyptus helps manage stress levels and supports immune function.

5. Hygiene Practices:

   o Handwashing and Cleanliness: Practicing good hygiene, including frequent handwashing with soap and water, disinfecting surfaces, and avoiding close contact with sick individuals, reduces the risk of viral and bacterial infections.

5.3 Digestive Issues

Common Digestive Issues

1. Indigestion and Heartburn:

   o Indigestion, characterized by discomfort or pain in the upper abdomen, and heartburn, a burning sensation in the chest, often result from poor dietary choices, stress, or underlying health conditions. Herbal remedies like ginger and peppermint can help alleviate symptoms by promoting digestion and reducing inflammation.

2. Bloating and Gas:

   o Bloating and excessive gas can be caused by factors such as dietary intolerances, poor eating habits, or imbalances in gut bacteria. Barbara O'Neill recommends incorporating probiotic-rich foods like yogurt and fermented vegetables into the diet to support gut flora balance and improve digestion.

3. Constipation and Diarrhea:

   o Constipation, characterized by infrequent bowel movements or difficulty passing stool, and diarrhea, characterized by loose or watery stools, can disrupt digestive function. Fiber-rich foods, such as whole grains, fruits, and vegetables, along with adequate hydration, help regulate bowel movements and promote digestive regularity.

Holistic Approaches to Digestive Health

1. Dietary Adjustments:

   o Balanced Diet: Consuming a balanced diet that includes fiber-rich foods, lean proteins, healthy fats, and probiotic-rich foods supports digestive health. Avoiding processed foods, excessive sugar, and alcohol helps maintain gut integrity and reduces inflammation.

2. Herbal Remedies:

   o Digestive Herbs: Herbs like ginger, peppermint, chamomile, and fennel have digestive benefits. Ginger aids digestion and alleviates nausea, while peppermint soothes digestive spasms and reduces bloating. Chamomile and fennel help calm digestive discomfort and promote gastrointestinal health.

3. Probiotics and Prebiotics:

   o Gut Flora Support: Probiotics are beneficial bacteria that promote gut health and aid digestion. Foods like yogurt, kefir, sauerkraut, and kimchi contain probiotics. Prebiotics, found in foods like garlic, onions, and bananas, nourish beneficial gut bacteria and support digestive balance.

4. Lifestyle Practices:

   o Stress Management: Stress can impact digestive function. Practicing relaxation techniques such as meditation, deep breathing exercises, or yoga helps reduce stress levels and support optimal digestion.

5. Hydration and Regular Exercise:

   o Hydration: Drinking an adequate amount of water throughout the day supports digestion and helps prevent constipation. Herbal teas like chamomile or ginger tea can also aid digestion.

6. Identifying Food Triggers: Keeping a food diary can help identify triggers for digestive discomfort or symptoms. Avoiding foods that trigger digestive issues, such as spicy foods or certain allergens, supports digestive health.

5.4 Stress and Anxiety

Stress is the body's natural response to perceived threats or challenges, triggering a cascade of physiological responses known as the fight-or-flight response. Chronic stress can lead to anxiety disorders, affecting mood, sleep, digestion, and overall health.

Symptoms of stress and anxiety may include increased heart rate, muscle tension, irritability, restlessness, difficulty concentrating, and sleep disturbances. Prolonged exposure to stress can weaken the immune system and contribute to various health problems.

5.4.1 Holistic Approaches to Managing Stress and Anxiety

1. Mind-Body Techniques:

   o Meditation and Mindfulness: Practicing meditation, mindfulness, and deep breathing exercises promotes relaxation, reduces stress hormone levels (e.g., cortisol), and enhances emotional resilience. These techniques help cultivate present-moment awareness and foster a sense of calm.

2. Herbal Remedies:

   o Adaptogenic Herbs: Adaptogens like ashwagandha, holy basil (tulsi), and rhodiola help the body adapt to stress and support adrenal function. They promote a balanced stress response and enhance overall resilience to stressors.

3. Nutritional Support:

- o Balanced Diet: Consuming a nutrient-rich diet that includes whole grains, lean proteins, fruits, vegetables, and healthy fats supports brain health and mood stability. Avoiding excessive caffeine, sugar, and processed foods helps maintain stable blood sugar levels and supports emotional well-being.

4. Physical Activity:

- o Exercise and Movement: Regular physical activity, such as walking, jogging, yoga, or dancing, releases endorphins (feel-good hormones) and reduces levels of stress hormones. Exercise promotes relaxation, improves mood, and enhances overall well-being.

5. Sleep Hygiene:

- o Quality Sleep: Establishing a consistent sleep schedule and practicing good sleep hygiene supports mental health and reduces stress. Avoiding electronic devices before bedtime, creating a relaxing bedtime routine, and ensuring a comfortable sleep environment promote restful sleep.

6. Social Support and Connection:

- o Emotional Well-being: Maintaining strong social connections and seeking support from friends, family, or support groups can reduce feelings of isolation, enhance emotional resilience, and provide a sense of belonging.

5.5 Herbal Remedies for Acne, Eczema, and Rashes

These conditions can be distressing and affect both physical comfort and self-esteem. Barbara O'Neill advocates for natural treatments that support skin health and promote healing without the side effects associated with conventional treatments.

Acne

1. Tea Tree Oil:

- o Tea tree oil has antibacterial and anti-inflammatory properties that help reduce acne-causing bacteria on the skin. It can be applied topically in diluted form to affected areas to reduce inflammation and promote healing.

2. Aloe Vera:

- o Aloe vera gel soothes inflamed skin and helps heal acne lesions. It has antimicrobial properties that can reduce acne-causing bacteria and promote skin regeneration. Apply aloe vera gel directly to clean skin or use skincare products containing aloe vera.

3. Turmeric:

- o Turmeric contains curcumin, a compound with anti-inflammatory and antioxidant properties. It helps reduce inflammation and can be used topically as a paste or taken internally to support overall skin health.

Eczema

1. Calendula:

   o Calendula has anti-inflammatory, antifungal, and antibacterial properties that soothe irritated skin and promote healing. Calendula creams or ointments can be applied to eczema-prone areas to relieve itching and inflammation.

2. Oatmeal Baths:

   o Colloidal oatmeal baths help soothe eczema symptoms by moisturizing the skin and reducing itchiness. Adding finely ground oatmeal to lukewarm bathwater and soaking for 10-15 minutes can provide relief.

3. Chamomile:

   o Chamomile has calming and anti-inflammatory properties that help reduce itching and irritation associated with eczema. It can be used in the form of chamomile tea compresses or added to bathwater for soothing effects.

Rashes

1. Lavender:

   o Lavender essential oil has soothing and anti-inflammatory properties that help calm skin irritation and reduce redness associated with rashes. Dilute lavender oil with a carrier oil like coconut oil and apply gently to affected areas.

2. Licorice Root:

   o Licorice root extract has anti-inflammatory and skin-soothing properties that help alleviate itching and irritation caused by rashes. It can be applied topically in cream or gel form to reduce inflammation and promote healing.

3. Neem:

   o Neem oil has antibacterial, antifungal, and anti-inflammatory properties that help treat various skin conditions, including rashes. Apply diluted neem oil to affected areas to soothe irritation and support skin health.

Application and Considerations

- Patch Test: Before using any herbal remedy, perform a patch test to check for potential allergic reactions or skin sensitivity.

- Consistency: Consistent use of herbal remedies is key to achieving desired results. Incorporate them into daily skincare routines for optimal effectiveness.

- Consultation: For severe or persistent skin conditions, consult a healthcare professional or dermatologist before starting any new treatment regimen.

Book 6: Advanced Herbal Therapies

Innovative Approaches for Maximizing the Healing Power of Plants

Chapter 1: Herbal Salves and Balms

Herbal salves and balms are topical formulations that utilize the healing properties of various herbs to treat skin conditions, soothe inflammation, and promote overall skin health. These preparations are easy to make at home and can be customized to address specific needs, making them a staple in natural healing practices advocated by Barbara O'Neill.

1. **Components:**

   o **Base Ingredients:** The foundation of any salve or balm is a combination of oils and waxes. Commonly used oils include olive oil, coconut oil, and almond oil, which act as carriers for the herbal extracts. Beeswax or plant-based waxes like candelilla wax are added to give the mixture a solid consistency.

   o **Herbal Infusions:** Herbs are infused into the carrier oils to extract their beneficial properties. This can be done by gently heating the herbs and oil together for several hours or by allowing the mixture to steep at room temperature for several weeks.

2. **Herbal Choices:**

   o **Calendula:** Known for its anti-inflammatory and skin-healing properties, calendula is excellent for treating minor cuts, scrapes, and burns.

   o **Comfrey:** Often referred to as "knitbone," comfrey promotes cell regeneration and is used for bruises, sprains, and fractures.

   o **Arnica:** Renowned for its ability to reduce swelling and bruising, arnica is effective in soothing sore muscles and joint pain.

   o **Lavender:** With its calming scent and antibacterial properties, lavender is great for general skin health and can help treat minor burns and insect bites.

3. **Preparation:**

   o **Infusing the Oil:** Start by drying the chosen herbs to prevent moisture from causing mold. Place the dried herbs in a clean, dry jar and cover them with the carrier oil. Seal the jar and let it sit in a warm, sunny spot for 4-6 weeks, shaking it occasionally. Alternatively, heat the oil and herbs in a double boiler on low heat for 2-3 hours.

   o **Straining:** Once the herbs have infused, strain the oil through a fine mesh strainer or cheesecloth to remove the plant material, leaving behind a rich, herbal-infused oil.

   o **Combining with Wax:** Gently heat the infused oil and beeswax in a double boiler until the wax melts completely. The typical ratio is 1 cup of infused oil to 1 ounce of beeswax, but this can be adjusted for a softer or firmer consistency.

   o **Pouring and Setting:** Pour the warm mixture into clean, sterilized jars or tins. Allow it to cool and harden completely before sealing and labeling.

4. **Applications:**

- o **Skin Healing:** Apply herbal salves to cuts, scrapes, burns, and rashes to promote healing and reduce inflammation.

- o **Pain Relief:** Use balms with arnica or comfrey on sore muscles, bruises, and joint pain to alleviate discomfort.

- o **Moisturizing:** Herbal salves can also serve as natural moisturizers for dry or chapped skin, providing soothing hydration.

Herbal salves and balms are versatile, natural remedies that harness the therapeutic properties of plants to support skin health and healing. By incorporating these preparations into daily skincare routines, individuals can enjoy the benefits of herbs in a convenient, topical form. Barbara O'Neill's emphasis on natural healing underscores the importance of these traditional remedies in achieving holistic wellness and maintaining healthy skin naturally.

1.1 Making Healing Ointments

Healing ointments are potent, concentrated topical formulations designed to address a variety of skin issues, from minor cuts and scrapes to chronic conditions like eczema and psoriasis. These ointments leverage the medicinal properties of herbs and essential oils to promote skin healing, reduce inflammation, and provide a protective barrier. Barbara O'Neill's approach to making healing ointments emphasizes simplicity, natural ingredients, and the power of herbal medicine.

1. **Base Ingredients:**

   - o **Carrier Oils:** The foundation of any healing ointment is a carrier oil, which helps deliver the medicinal properties of herbs to the skin. Common choices include olive oil, coconut oil, jojoba oil, and sweet almond oil. These oils not only carry the herbal extracts but also nourish and moisturize the skin.

   - o **Beeswax:** Beeswax is added to provide the ointment with a thick, spreadable consistency. It also acts as a natural barrier, protecting the skin from environmental elements while allowing it to breathe. For a vegan alternative, candelilla wax can be used.

   - o **Essential Oils:** Essential oils are concentrated plant extracts that add therapeutic properties and fragrance to the ointment. Lavender, tea tree, and chamomile essential oils are popular choices for their soothing and healing effects.

2. **Herbal Infusions:**

   - o **Herb Selection:** Choose herbs known for their skin-healing properties. Calendula, comfrey, plantain, and St. John's wort are excellent options. These herbs can help reduce inflammation, promote cell regeneration, and fight infections.

   - o **Infusion Process:** To extract the beneficial compounds from herbs, infuse them in a carrier oil. This can be done using a cold infusion method (letting the herbs steep in oil for several weeks in a sunny spot) or a hot infusion method (gently heating the herbs and oil in a double boiler for a few hours).

3. **Preparation:**

- o **Straining the Oil:** Once the herbs have infused into the oil, strain the mixture through a fine mesh strainer or cheesecloth to remove the plant material, leaving behind a nutrient-rich, herbal-infused oil.

- o **Melting the Beeswax:** In a double boiler, combine the herbal-infused oil with beeswax. Heat gently until the beeswax is completely melted. The general ratio is 1 ounce of beeswax to 1 cup of infused oil, but this can be adjusted for desired consistency.

- o **Adding Essential Oils:** Once the beeswax is melted, remove the mixture from heat and allow it to cool slightly before adding essential oils. Typically, add 10-20 drops of essential oil per cup of infused oil, depending on the desired potency.

4. **Pouring and Storing:**

- o **Container Selection:** Pour the warm mixture into clean, sterilized jars or tins. Allow the ointment to cool and harden completely before sealing with a lid.

- o **Labeling:** Clearly label the containers with the ingredients and date of preparation. Store the ointments in a cool, dark place to preserve their potency.

5. **Applications:**

- o **Minor Cuts and Scrapes:** Apply healing ointments to clean wounds to promote faster healing and prevent infection.

- o **Dry, Chapped Skin:** Use on areas of dry, cracked, or chapped skin to moisturize and protect.

- o **Inflammatory Skin Conditions:** Apply to eczema, psoriasis, and other inflammatory skin conditions to soothe irritation and reduce inflammation.

Making healing ointments is a practical and effective way to harness the power of natural ingredients for skin health. Barbara O'Neill's method emphasizes the use of high-quality, natural components and simple techniques to create powerful, healing topical remedies. By incorporating these ointments into your skincare routine, you can naturally support skin healing, reduce inflammation, and protect against environmental damage, promoting overall skin health and well-being.

1.2 Herbal Syrups and Honeys

Herbal syrups and honeys are delightful and effective ways to harness the healing properties of herbs. These natural remedies, often used to soothe sore throats, ease coughs, and support the immune system, combine the medicinal benefits of herbs with the soothing qualities of honey. Barbara O'Neill's approach to making herbal syrups and honeys emphasizes simplicity, natural ingredients, and the therapeutic power of herbs.

Understanding Herbal Syrups and Honeys:

1. **Base Ingredients:**

- o **Herbs:** Choose herbs based on the desired therapeutic effect. Common herbs used in syrups and honeys include elderberry, echinacea, ginger, thyme, and marshmallow root. These herbs are known for their immune-boosting, anti-inflammatory, and soothing properties.

- o **Honey:** Raw, unpasteurized honey is preferred for its natural antimicrobial and soothing properties. Honey acts as a natural preservative, enhances the taste, and adds its own health benefits to the remedy.

- o **Water:** Used to extract the medicinal compounds from the herbs. Distilled or filtered water is recommended to ensure purity.

2. **Preparation of Herbal Syrups:**

- o **Infusion:** Begin by making a strong herbal infusion or decoction. For delicate herbs like flowers and leaves, steep them in hot water for about 30 minutes. For tougher herbs like roots and bark, simmer them gently for 20-30 minutes to extract their medicinal properties.

- o **Straining:** After the infusion or decoction is complete, strain the liquid through a fine mesh strainer or cheesecloth to remove the plant material.

- o **Combining with Honey:** Measure the strained herbal liquid and combine it with an equal amount of honey. For a thicker syrup, you can use a 2:1 ratio of honey to herbal liquid. Warm the mixture gently, stirring until the honey is fully dissolved, but avoid boiling to preserve the beneficial properties of the honey.

- o **Bottling and Storing:** Pour the syrup into clean, sterilized glass bottles or jars. Label the containers with the ingredients and date of preparation. Store in the refrigerator, where it can last for several months.

3. **Preparation of Herbal Honeys:**

- o **Herb Selection:** Choose fresh or dried herbs based on the desired effect. Popular choices include thyme, sage, lavender, and chamomile.

- o **Infusion:** Fill a clean jar about halfway with the chosen herbs. Pour raw honey over the herbs, ensuring they are fully submerged. Stir to remove air bubbles and seal the jar tightly.

- o **Steeping:** Allow the mixture to steep in a warm, sunny spot for 2-4 weeks. Shake the jar occasionally to ensure even infusion.

- o **Straining (Optional):** After steeping, you can strain the honey to remove the herbs or leave them in for continued infusion.

- o **Storage:** Store the herbal honey in a cool, dark place. It can last indefinitely due to the preservative nature of honey.

4. **Applications and Benefits:**

- o **Cough and Cold Relief:** Herbal syrups with ingredients like elderberry and ginger are excellent for soothing coughs, reducing mucus, and boosting the immune system. A teaspoon taken several times a day can provide relief.

- o **Digestive Support:** Herbal honeys with ginger, fennel, or chamomile can be taken to soothe digestive issues such as indigestion, gas, and bloating. A spoonful before or after meals aids digestion.

- o **Immune Boosting:** Echinacea and elderberry syrups are known for their immune-boosting properties. Regular consumption, especially during cold and flu season, can help strengthen the immune system.

- **Sore Throat Relief:** Herbal honeys with thyme or sage can be used to soothe sore throats. Adding a spoonful to warm tea or taking it directly provides relief from throat irritation and inflammation.

Herbal syrups and honeys are not only effective remedies but also delightful ways to incorporate the healing power of herbs into daily life. Barbara O'Neill's approach to these preparations emphasizes the use of natural, high-quality ingredients and simple methods to create potent, soothing remedies. By adding herbal syrups and honeys to your natural healing toolkit, you can enjoy the benefits of herbs in a delicious and therapeutic form, supporting overall health and well-being naturally.

1.3 Preparing Medicinal Syrups

Medicinal syrups are a cornerstone of natural remedies, offering a palatable way to deliver the healing properties of herbs, especially for respiratory issues, digestive disturbances, and immune support. These syrups are particularly beneficial because they combine the therapeutic effects of herbs with the soothing, preservative qualities of honey or sugar. Barbara O'Neill's method of preparing medicinal syrups emphasizes simplicity, efficacy, and the use of natural ingredients.

Understanding Medicinal Syrups:

1. **Choosing the Right Herbs:**

   - **Herbs for Respiratory Health:** Common choices include elderberry, thyme, and licorice root. These herbs are known for their ability to soothe coughs, reduce inflammation, and support lung function.

   - **Herbs for Immune Support:** Echinacea, elderberry, and astragalus are popular for their immune-boosting properties, helping to fend off colds and flu.

   - **Herbs for Digestive Health:** Ginger, fennel, and chamomile can alleviate digestive issues such as nausea, indigestion, and bloating.

2. **Basic Ingredients:**

   - **Herbal Infusion or Decoction:** The foundation of a medicinal syrup is a strong herbal tea. Infusions are made by steeping leaves, flowers, or delicate parts of herbs in hot water, while decoctions involve simmering tougher parts like roots or bark.

   - **Sweetener:** Raw honey is preferred for its additional health benefits, but organic cane sugar or maple syrup can also be used. The sweetener not only improves the taste but acts as a preservative.

3. **Preparation Steps:**

   - **Making the Herbal Infusion or Decoction:** Begin by measuring out the herbs. A common ratio is 1 ounce of dried herbs (or 2 ounces of fresh herbs) to 1 quart of water. For infusions, pour boiling water over the herbs, cover, and steep for 30-60 minutes. For decoctions, add herbs to cold water, bring to a boil, then simmer for 20-40 minutes.

   - **Straining the Liquid:** Once the infusion or decoction is complete, strain the liquid through a fine mesh strainer or cheesecloth to remove the plant material. This leaves you with a concentrated herbal liquid.

- Combining with Sweetener: Measure the strained liquid and pour it back into a clean pot. Add an equal amount of honey or sugar. For example, if you have 2 cups of herbal liquid, add 2 cups of honey or sugar. Warm the mixture gently over low heat, stirring continuously until the sweetener is fully dissolved. Avoid boiling to preserve the beneficial properties of the herbs and honey.

4. **Finalizing the Syrup:**

   - **Optional Additions:** Essential oils or tinctures can be added at this stage to enhance the medicinal properties. For instance, adding a few drops of peppermint essential oil can boost respiratory relief.

   - **Bottling and Storage:** Pour the warm syrup into sterilized glass bottles or jars. Seal tightly and label with the date and ingredients. Store the syrup in the refrigerator, where it can last for several months due to the preservative action of the honey or sugar.

5. **Using Medicinal Syrups:**

   - **Dosage:** For general wellness or to address specific ailments, the typical dosage is 1-2 teaspoons of syrup taken several times a day. For children, the dose is usually halved.

   - **Applications:** Medicinal syrups can be taken directly by the spoonful, added to hot water or tea, or mixed with other beverages. They are particularly effective for soothing sore throats, alleviating coughs, and boosting the immune system during cold and flu season.

Chapter 2: Integrating Herbal Remedies into Daily Life

2.1 Creating a Home Apothecary

Creating a home apothecary is a foundational step in embracing a natural and holistic approach to health and wellness. A home apothecary serves as a personal pharmacy, stocked with herbs, essential oils, and natural remedies tailored to your family's needs. Barbara O'Neill's philosophy emphasizes the importance of self-sufficiency, knowledge, and the use of natural ingredients to maintain health and treat common ailments. This section outlines the essential components, organization, and maintenance of a home apothecary.

Essential Components of a Home Apothecary:

1. **Herbs:**

    o **Dried Herbs:** Stock a variety of dried herbs known for their medicinal properties, such as chamomile, echinacea, peppermint, elderberry, and calendula. These can be used for making teas, infusions, decoctions, and topical preparations.

    o **Fresh Herbs:** If possible, grow fresh herbs like basil, thyme, rosemary, and mint in a garden or indoor pots. Fresh herbs can be used in cooking, teas, and poultices.

2. **Essential Oils:**

    o Essential oils are concentrated plant extracts that provide therapeutic benefits. Commonly used oils include lavender, tea tree, eucalyptus, peppermint, and chamomile. They can be used in diffusers, massage oils, balms, and bath products.

3. **Carrier Oils:**

    o Carrier oils are used to dilute essential oils and make herbal infusions. Popular choices include olive oil, coconut oil, jojoba oil, and sweet almond oil. These oils are also excellent for skin care preparations.

4. **Tinctures and Extracts:**

    o Tinctures are concentrated herbal extracts made using alcohol or glycerin. They are used for internal consumption to address various health issues. Common tinctures include echinacea for immune support and valerian for relaxation.

5. **Salves and Balms:**

    o Prepared herbal salves and balms can be used for skin conditions, muscle pain, and wound healing. Having a few ready-made or homemade options on hand ensures you can quickly address minor injuries and skin issues.

6. **Herbal Teas and Infusions:**

o   Keep a selection of herbal teas and infusion blends for various purposes, such as calming, digestive support, and immune boosting. Pre-made tea bags or loose-leaf blends can be stored in airtight containers.

7. **Miscellaneous Supplies:**

o   Additional items such as beeswax, natural clays, apple cider vinegar, and honey are useful for creating a variety of natural remedies and personal care products.

Organization and Storage:

1. **Storage Containers:**

o   Use airtight glass jars or containers to store dried herbs, powders, and teas. Glass containers prevent moisture and air from degrading the herbs' potency.

o   Essential oils should be stored in dark glass bottles to protect them from light and maintain their efficacy.

2. **Labeling:**

o   Clearly label all containers with the name of the herb or product, date of purchase or preparation, and any relevant usage instructions. This helps in easy identification and ensures the use of fresh ingredients.

3. **Storage Area:**

o   Designate a cool, dry, and dark area for your home apothecary. A dedicated cupboard, shelf, or pantry is ideal. Avoid areas with fluctuating temperatures or high humidity, such as kitchens and bathrooms.

4. **Herb Drying and Preparation Area:**

o   If you grow your own herbs, set up a space for drying and processing them. A drying rack or hanging bundles in a well-ventilated area ensures herbs are properly dried before storage.

Maintenance:

1. **Regular Inventory Check:**

o   Periodically check your stock to ensure you have adequate supplies and that none of the herbs or oils have expired. Rotate your stock to use older items first.

2. **Cleaning:**

o   Keep your storage area clean and organized. Wipe down shelves and containers regularly to prevent dust and contamination.

3. **Restocking:**

o   Keep a list of herbs and supplies you frequently use and restock them as needed. This ensures you are always prepared to create remedies without delay.

4. **Education and Reference:**

o   Maintain a collection of reference books, guides, and notes on herbal medicine. Continued education helps you stay informed about new remedies and practices.

2.2 Daily Herbal Practices for Health Maintenance

Incorporating daily herbal practices into your routine is a powerful way to maintain and enhance overall health. Barbara O'Neill's approach to natural healing emphasizes the consistent, everyday use of herbs to support the body's systems, prevent illness, and promote well-being. Daily herbal practices can be simple, enjoyable, and highly effective, providing both immediate benefits and long-term health improvements.

Morning Rituals:

1. **Herbal Teas:**

   o Start your day with a cup of herbal tea to wake up your senses and support your health. Options like ginger tea can boost digestion and circulation, while green tea offers antioxidants to kickstart your day.

   o For a calming start, chamomile or lemon balm tea can help set a peaceful tone.

2. **Herbal Infused Water:**

   o Prepare a jug of herbal-infused water to sip throughout the day. Add herbs like mint, basil, or rosemary to your water for a refreshing and hydrating boost. Herbal-infused water not only keeps you hydrated but also delivers subtle therapeutic benefits.

3. **Herbal Supplements:**

   o Consider taking herbal supplements or tinctures as part of your morning routine. Echinacea or elderberry tinctures can support immune function, while adaptogens like ashwagandha can help manage stress.

Midday Practices:

1. **Herbal Snacks:**

   o Incorporate herbs into your meals and snacks. Sprinkle fresh herbs like parsley, cilantro, or dill on your salads, soups, or sandwiches. These herbs add flavor and provide vital nutrients and antioxidants.

2. **Herbal Smoothies:**

   o Blend a handful of greens such as kale or spinach with fruits, and add herbal powders like spirulina or moringa. These nutrient-dense smoothies provide a midday energy boost and support overall health.

3. **Digestive Support:**

   o After lunch, consider drinking a cup of peppermint or fennel tea to aid digestion. These herbs can help alleviate bloating and discomfort, ensuring that your digestive system functions smoothly.

Evening Practices:

1. **Relaxing Herbal Teas:**

- o As the day winds down, drink a calming herbal tea such as chamomile, lavender, or valerian root. These herbs help relax the mind and body, promoting restful sleep.

2. **Herbal Baths:**

   - o Enjoy an herbal bath to relax and soothe your muscles. Add a sachet of dried herbs like lavender, rosemary, or calendula to your bathwater. The warm water helps release the herbs' beneficial compounds, creating a soothing and therapeutic experience.

3. **Herbal Skincare:**

   - o Integrate herbs into your skincare routine. Use products infused with aloe vera, calendula, or tea tree oil to cleanse and nourish your skin. A nightly facial steam with chamomile or rose petals can open pores and refresh your complexion.

Weekly and Seasonal Practices:

1. **Herbal Steams and Inhalations:**

   - o Once a week, treat yourself to an herbal steam. Boil water with herbs like eucalyptus, thyme, or peppermint, and inhale the steam to clear respiratory passages and support sinus health.

2. **Seasonal Detox:**

   - o At the change of seasons, consider a gentle herbal detox. Use herbs like dandelion, burdock, and milk thistle to support liver function and cleanse the body. This can be done through teas, tinctures, or incorporating these herbs into meals.

Creating a Balanced Routine:

1. **Personalized Herbal Blends:**

   - o Create personalized herbal blends tailored to your specific health needs. For example, if you need more energy, combine ginseng, licorice, and ginger. If you seek stress relief, blend chamomile, lavender, and lemon balm.

2. **Mindful Consumption:**

   - o Practice mindfulness when consuming herbal remedies. Pay attention to how your body responds to different herbs and adjust your routine accordingly. This helps you understand what works best for you and ensures optimal benefits.

3. **Consistency and Patience:**

   - o Consistency is key in herbal practice. The benefits of herbs often build over time, so make herbal practices a regular part of your lifestyle. Be patient and give your body time to adjust and respond.

Daily herbal practices are an integral part of maintaining health and preventing illness. By incorporating simple, enjoyable herbal rituals into your routine, you can support your body's systems, enhance your well-being, and cultivate a deeper connection with nature's healing resources. Barbara O'Neill's holistic approach emphasizes the importance of consistency, mindfulness, and the therapeutic power of herbs, offering a natural path to sustained health and vitality.

2.3 Seasonal Herbal Practices

Seasonal herbal practices are a vital component of maintaining balance and health throughout the year. Barbara O'Neill's approach emphasizes adapting herbal routines to the changing seasons, ensuring that the body remains in harmony with nature's cycles. By aligning herbal practices with seasonal shifts, you can address specific health needs, support the body's natural rhythms, and optimize overall well-being.

Spring: Renewal and Detoxification

1. **Focus on Cleansing:**

   o Spring is the ideal time for detoxification, helping the body shed accumulated toxins from the winter months. Incorporate herbs like dandelion, burdock root, and milk thistle into your routine. These herbs support liver function and promote gentle cleansing.

   o Consider a detox tea blend made from nettle, cleavers, and lemon balm to support lymphatic drainage and overall detoxification.

2. **Allergy Support:**

   o Spring allergies can be managed with herbs that support the respiratory system and reduce inflammation. Stinging nettle, butterbur, and quercetin-rich herbs can help alleviate allergy symptoms.

   o Herbal steams with eucalyptus, peppermint, and thyme can clear nasal passages and provide relief from congestion.

3. **Energizing Herbal Practices:**

   o As the days get longer, incorporate energizing herbs to boost vitality and shake off winter lethargy. Ginseng, rhodiola, and ashwagandha are excellent adaptogens that enhance energy levels and resilience.

Summer: Cooling and Hydrating

1. **Hydration and Cooling:**

   o The heat of summer calls for herbs that cool and hydrate the body. Peppermint, hibiscus, and cucumber are refreshing choices that can be infused in water or teas to keep you cool and hydrated.

   o Aloe vera juice is another excellent option for its cooling and soothing properties, especially if you've spent time in the sun.

2. **Skin Protection and Care:**

   o Summer sun exposure requires herbs that protect and nourish the skin. Calendula, chamomile, and lavender can be used in homemade sunscreens and soothing after-sun balms.

   o Herbal baths with rose petals, lavender, and chamomile can soothe sunburned skin and provide relaxation.

3. **Digestive Health:**

   o The heat can sometimes lead to digestive discomfort. Ginger, mint, and fennel can be added to your diet to support digestion and alleviate bloating or nausea.

o   Consider drinking a cooling digestive tea made from peppermint and ginger after meals.

Autumn: Immune Support and Grounding

1. **Boosting Immunity:**

    o   As the weather cools and the immune system becomes more vulnerable, focus on herbs that enhance immune function. Echinacea, elderberry, and astragalus are excellent choices for immune support.

    o   Prepare immune-boosting syrups and tinctures with elderberries and echinacea to take regularly as a preventive measure.

2. **Grounding and Nourishing:**

    o   Autumn is a time to ground and nourish the body in preparation for the colder months. Use warming, grounding herbs like ginger, turmeric, and cinnamon in your cooking and teas.

    o   Root vegetables and herbs like carrots, sweet potatoes, and burdock root can be incorporated into meals to provide warmth and nourishment.

3. **Respiratory Health:**

    o   With the onset of cold and flu season, focus on herbs that support respiratory health. Thyme, oregano, and mullein can be used in teas, steams, and syrups to keep the respiratory system clear and healthy.

Winter: Warming and Restorative

1. **Warming Herbs:**

    o   The cold of winter requires warming herbs to maintain internal heat and circulation. Ginger, cinnamon, and clove can be added to teas, broths, and meals for their warming properties.

    o   A daily cup of chai tea with these warming spices can boost circulation and keep you cozy.

2. **Support for the Immune System:**

    o   Continue supporting the immune system with herbs like elderberry, garlic, and reishi mushrooms. These can be incorporated into soups, stews, and herbal teas.

    o   Bone broths infused with immune-boosting herbs provide nourishment and help stave off winter illnesses.

3. **Rest and Restoration:**

    o   Winter is a time for rest and restoration. Incorporate calming herbs like chamomile, valerian, and passionflower into your evening routine to promote restful sleep.

    o   Herbal baths with lavender, rose, and cedarwood can help relax the body and mind, aiding in deep, restorative sleep.

Chapter 3: Safety and Ethical Considerations

3.1 Safe Usage of Herbal Remedies

The safe usage of herbal remedies is paramount for maximizing their benefits while minimizing potential risks. Barbara O'Neill's approach to natural healing emphasizes the importance of understanding and respecting the potency of herbs. While herbs offer numerous health benefits, it is crucial to use them responsibly and knowledgeably. This section outlines key principles and practices for the safe and effective use of herbal remedies.

1. **Respecting Dosages:**

   o   Herbs, like pharmaceutical medications, have specific dosages that should be adhered to. Overuse or misuse can lead to adverse effects. Always follow recommended dosages provided by reliable sources or a qualified herbalist.

2. **Start with Small Amounts:**

   o   When using a new herb, start with a small amount to see how your body reacts. Gradually increase the dosage if no adverse reactions occur. This approach helps in identifying any potential allergies or sensitivities.

3. **Consider Individual Differences:**

   o   Factors such as age, weight, health status, and individual sensitivity can influence how an herb affects you. Tailor dosages and usage according to your personal needs and consult a healthcare provider if necessary.

Quality and Sourcing of Herbs:

1. **Choose High-Quality Products:**

   o   Use herbs from reputable sources to ensure they are free from contaminants, pesticides, and adulterants. Organic and wild-crafted herbs are often of higher quality and provide better therapeutic benefits.

2. **Proper Identification:**

   o   Ensure correct identification of herbs, especially if foraging. Misidentification can lead to the use of toxic plants. Use reliable resources or consult an experienced herbalist for accurate identification.

3. **Avoid Contaminated Herbs:**

   o   Be cautious of herbs grown in polluted areas or those that may have been exposed to heavy metals and other contaminants. Choose suppliers that provide transparency about their sourcing practices.

Preparation and Storage:

1. **Proper Preparation:**

   o Different herbs require different methods of preparation to release their medicinal properties effectively. Follow correct procedures for making teas, tinctures, infusions, decoctions, and other preparations.

   o Avoid using aluminum or non-food grade plastic containers for preparing and storing herbal remedies as they can leach harmful substances.

2. **Appropriate Storage:**

   o Store herbs in a cool, dry, and dark place to preserve their potency. Use airtight containers to protect them from moisture, light, and air exposure. Proper storage extends the shelf life and effectiveness of herbal remedies.

3. **Shelf Life Awareness:**

   o Be aware of the shelf life of your herbal preparations. Dried herbs typically last for about one year, while tinctures and essential oils may last longer if stored properly. Discard any herbs or preparations that show signs of mold, spoilage, or significant degradation.

Interactions and Contraindications:

1. **Potential Interactions:**

   o Herbs can interact with medications, other herbs, and supplements. These interactions can either enhance or diminish their effects, or lead to adverse reactions. Always consult with a healthcare provider before combining herbal remedies with other treatments.

2. **Contraindications:**

   o Some herbs are not suitable for certain individuals, such as pregnant or breastfeeding women, children, or those with specific health conditions. Research or consult a qualified herbalist to understand any contraindications associated with the herbs you plan to use.

3. **Allergies and Sensitivities:**

   o Monitor for allergic reactions or sensitivities, which can manifest as skin rashes, digestive issues, or respiratory symptoms. Discontinue use immediately if any adverse reactions occur and seek medical advice.

Education and Consultation:

1. **Continual Learning:**

   o Stay informed about the herbs you use through books, courses, and reputable online resources. Understanding the properties, uses, and safety considerations of each herb is crucial for safe and effective use.

2. **Consultation with Experts:**

   o When in doubt, consult a qualified herbalist or healthcare provider, especially if you have underlying health conditions or are on medication. Professional guidance ensures that herbal remedies are used safely and effectively.

3. **Reliable Resources:**

o   Use reliable resources for information about herbs. Books by reputable herbalists, peer-reviewed studies, and professional herbal organizations provide accurate and up-to-date information.

The safe usage of herbal remedies is a fundamental aspect of natural healing practices. By understanding dosages, sourcing high-quality herbs, preparing and storing them properly, and being aware of potential interactions and contraindications, you can harness the benefits of herbal medicine while minimizing risks. Barbara O'Neill's approach underscores the importance of education, respect for herb potency, and professional guidance, ensuring that herbal remedies are used in a manner that promotes health and well-being effectively and safely.

3.2 Understanding Potential Interactions and Side Effects

Understanding potential interactions and side effects is crucial for the safe and effective use of herbal remedies. While herbs offer a natural way to support health, they are potent substances that can interact with medications, other herbs, and certain health conditions. Being aware of these interactions and side effects ensures that herbal treatments complement your overall health regimen without causing harm.

Herb-Drug Interactions:

1. **Enhancing or Diminishing Effects:**

   o   Some herbs can enhance or diminish the effects of pharmaceutical drugs. For instance, St. John's Wort is known to interfere with medications such as antidepressants, birth control pills, and blood thinners, potentially reducing their efficacy.

2. **Altered Absorption and Metabolism:**

   o   Herbs like ginseng and gingko biloba can affect how the body absorbs and metabolizes medications. Ginseng, for example, can increase blood pressure and interact with anticoagulants, while gingko biloba can increase the risk of bleeding when taken with blood thinners.

3. **Impact on Liver Enzymes:**

   o   Certain herbs can influence liver enzymes that metabolize drugs, leading to increased or decreased drug levels in the bloodstream. Milk thistle, while protective of the liver, can alter the metabolism of drugs processed by the liver, necessitating adjustments in medication dosages.

Herb-Herb Interactions:

1. **Synergistic Effects:**

   o   While some herbs can work synergistically to enhance therapeutic effects, others can lead to adverse reactions when combined. For instance, combining sedative herbs like valerian with other calming herbs such as kava kava can lead to excessive drowsiness and impaired motor function.

2. **Antagonistic Effects:**

   o   Some herbs may counteract each other's effects. For example, using an adaptogenic herb like ginseng, which can increase energy levels, alongside a calming herb like chamomile might reduce the overall effectiveness of both.

Herb-Supplement Interactions:

1. **Nutrient Absorption:**

   o   Certain herbs can affect the absorption of vitamins and minerals. For example, tannin-rich herbs like green tea can inhibit the absorption of iron from plant-based sources, which is important for individuals with iron-deficiency anemia to consider.

2. **Combined Effects:**

   o   Combining herbal supplements with other dietary supplements requires caution. High doses of vitamin E with ginkgo biloba, for example, can increase the risk of bleeding due to their anticoagulant properties.

Health Condition Interactions:

1. **Chronic Conditions:**

   o   Individuals with chronic conditions such as diabetes, hypertension, or autoimmune disorders need to be particularly cautious. Herbs like licorice can raise blood pressure, while fenugreek can lower blood sugar levels, potentially interfering with diabetes management.

2. **Pregnancy and Lactation:**

   o   Pregnant or breastfeeding women should be cautious with herbs, as some can affect fetal development or milk production. Herbs like pennyroyal and blue cohosh can induce contractions and should be avoided during pregnancy.

Recognizing Side Effects:

1. **Common Side Effects:**

   o   Like conventional medications, herbs can cause side effects. Common side effects include digestive issues (nausea, vomiting, diarrhea), allergic reactions (rashes, itching), and headaches. These can often be mitigated by adjusting the dosage or discontinuing use.

2. **Severe Reactions:**

   o   Severe reactions, although rare, require immediate attention. Signs of anaphylaxis (difficulty breathing, swelling of the face and throat) after taking an herb necessitate urgent medical intervention. Liver toxicity, characterized by jaundice and abdominal pain, can occur with misuse of certain herbs like kava kava.

3. **Monitoring and Reporting:**

   o   Regular monitoring of your body's response to herbal remedies is essential. Keep a journal of any new symptoms or side effects. Reporting adverse effects to a healthcare provider helps in adjusting the regimen and ensuring safety.

Education and Professional Guidance:

1. **Consultation with Healthcare Providers:**

   o   Before starting any herbal remedy, consult with a healthcare provider, especially if you are taking medications or have underlying health conditions. Professional guidance ensures that herbal remedies are safe and appropriate for your specific health needs.

2. **Using Reliable Sources:**

o   Educate yourself using reliable sources such as scientific journals, books by reputable herbalists, and trusted websites. Understanding the properties, benefits, and risks associated with each herb enhances safe usage.

3. **Qualified Herbalists:**

o   Work with qualified herbalists who can provide personalized advice and monitor your progress. Herbalists can help identify potential interactions, suggest suitable herbs, and adjust dosages as needed.

Here you can access the 20+ Hour BONUS VIDEO

Scan this **QR code** using your phone's camera or click this **LINK** to access your **VIDEO BONUS** content now:

SCAN THE QR CODE BELOW AND FOLLOW THE ISTRUCTIONS:

You will access to 20+ Hour BONUS VIDEO of BARBARA O'NEILL

Book 7: Setting up Your Herbal Apothecary

A Step-by-Step Guide to Creating Your Own Natural Pharmacy

Chapter 1: Essential tools and equipment

When embarking on the journey of herbal remedies, having the right tools and equipment is essential for effectively preparing, storing, and administering herbal treatments. These tools ensure the quality and potency of herbal remedies and contribute to a safe and organized herbal practice. Here are the key categories of essential tools and equipment every herbalist should consider:

Preparation Tools

Preparing herbal remedies involves various processes such as harvesting, drying, grinding, and extracting. The proper preparation tools ensure that herbs are processed effectively while preserving their medicinal properties.

Harvesting Tools: Sharp pruning shears or scissors are essential for harvesting herbs at the right time to maximize their potency. Harvesting baskets or trays are also useful for collecting herbs without damaging them.

Drying Equipment: Proper drying is crucial to prevent mold and preserve the quality of herbs. Herb drying racks or screens allow for adequate airflow, while dehydrators offer a controlled environment for faster drying.

Grinding and Milling: Mortar and pestle sets or electric herb grinders grind dried herbs into powder or smaller pieces for teas, capsules, or tinctures. This ensures consistent particle size and enhances extraction efficiency.

Extraction Tools: For making herbal extracts like tinctures or infused oils, glass jars, bottles, and straining cloths or fine mesh sieves are necessary. Some herbalists also use equipment like a double boiler or slow cooker for the gentle extraction of active compounds.

Storage and Preservation Tools

Proper storage and preservation of herbs and herbal preparations are essential to maintain their potency and freshness.

Glass Jars and Containers: Dark-colored glass jars or amber glass bottles are preferred for storing dried herbs, tinctures, and oils. They protect against light exposure, which can degrade herbal compounds.

Labeling Materials: Labels and markers are indispensable for accurately identifying herbs and noting essential details such as harvest date, botanical name, and preparation method. Clear labeling ensures safe and organized storage.

Storage Solutions: Shelving units or cabinets with adjustable shelves provide a dedicated space for storing herbs and herbal products. Proper organization by herb type or preparation method makes it easy to access and rotate stock.

Administration and Application Tools

Administering herbal remedies involves various methods, from brewing teas to applying topical treatments. Having the appropriate tools ensures accurate dosing and effective application.

Tea Making Equipment: Tea infusers, teapots, or stainless-steel tea balls are used to brew herbal teas. These tools allow for the proper extraction of medicinal compounds and convenient preparation of single servings or larger batches.

Capsule Filling Devices: For individuals preferring capsules, capsule machines or hand-held capsule fillers enable efficient filling of empty capsules with powdered herbs. This ensures consistent dosage and easy consumption.

Topical Application Tools: Cotton balls, gauze pads, or soft brushes apply herbal poultices, compresses, or salves to the skin. These tools help deliver herbal benefits directly to affected areas.

Having the right tools and equipment is crucial for anyone practicing herbal remedies. These tools facilitate the preparation, storage, and administration of herbal treatments and ensure safety, efficacy, and consistency in herbal practice. Whether harvesting fresh herbs, preparing tinctures, or administering herbal teas, investing in quality tools appropriate for your needs will enhance your herbal practice and promote successful outcomes in natural healthcare.

Chapter 2: Sourcing and selecting herbs

Understanding the process of sourcing and selecting herbs is a powerful tool in your herbal practice. It gives you control over the quality, potency, and safety of your herbal remedies. Whether you're harvesting from your garden, buying from trusted suppliers, or wildcrafting, this knowledge empowers you to choose herbs that align with your health goals and ethical standards.

2.1 Cultivation and Harvesting Practices

1) Cultivating Herbs

Growing herbs in your garden or on a small farm provides control over cultivation practices. Organic methods, free from synthetic pesticides and herbicides, ensure herbs are free from chemical residues that can compromise their medicinal properties. Maintaining soil fertility through composting and natural fertilizers supports healthy plant growth and robust medicinal compounds.

2) Harvesting Techniques

Proper timing and technique are crucial for harvesting herbs to maximize potency. Harvest herbs in the morning after the dew has evaporated but before the sun is too intense to preserve essential oils. Use sharp scissors or pruning shears to avoid damaging plants. Harvest only what is needed, allowing the plant to regenerate and continue producing throughout the season.

2.2 Selecting Quality Herbs

1) Quality Indicators

When purchasing herbs, whether dried or fresh, several indicators can help assess their quality:

Appearance: Herbs should have vibrant colors, indicating freshness and vitality. Avoid herbs that are discolored, moldy, or wilted.

Aroma: Many herbs have distinctive aromas due to their essential oils. A strong, fresh aroma often indicates high potency.

Texture: Dried herbs should be crisp and break easily. They should not feel damp or excessively brittle.

Storage Conditions: Herbs should be stored in proper containers away from light and moisture to maintain quality.

2) Certifications and Testing

Look for suppliers who provide transparency regarding their sourcing practices. Certifications such as USDA Organic or Good Manufacturing Practice (GMP) ensure herbs meet stringent quality standards. Suppliers may also conduct testing for purity, potency, and absence of contaminants like heavy metals or pesticides.

2.3 Wildcrafting Ethics and Safety

Wildcrafting, the practice of harvesting herbs from their natural habitat, is a privilege that comes with great responsibility. It's crucial to follow ethical guidelines to ensure the long-term health of wild plant populations. This respect for nature is a fundamental aspect of herbal practice.

Responsible Harvesting: Harvest only from abundant populations, leaving enough plants to regenerate. Over-harvesting can lead to the depletion of plant populations and disrupt the ecosystem. Avoid harvesting endangered or protected species.

Permission: Obtain permission from landowners or authorities before wildcrafting on private or protected lands. Failure to do so can result in legal consequences and damage relationships with the community.

Harvesting Practices: Use sustainable harvesting techniques, such as selective harvesting (only taking a portion of the plant, allowing the rest to continue growing) and avoiding habitat damage (not trampling other plants or disturbing the soil).

When wildcrafting, be aware of potential contaminants, such as pollutants or pesticides, from nearby areas. Proper plant identification is crucial to avoid harvesting toxic look-alikes. Consult local field guides or seek guidance from experienced herbalists.

2.4 Storage and Preservation

Once you've harvested or purchased your herbs, knowing how to store them properly provides a sense of security. It ensures that their potency is maintained over time. Whether you're drying, freezing, or making tinctures and extracts, these techniques give you confidence in the longevity of your herbs.

Drying: Most herbs are dried for long-term storage. Drying racks or dehydrators are used to remove moisture thoroughly. Store dried herbs in airtight containers away from light and heat.

Freezing: Some herbs, like basil or parsley, can be frozen for longer preservation. Blanching before freezing helps retain color and flavor.

Tinctures and Extracts: Store tinctures and herbal extracts in dark glass bottles away from light and heat to prevent the degradation of active compounds.

Sourcing and selecting herbs is a foundational skill in herbal practice, influencing the effectiveness and safety of herbal remedies. Whether cultivating in your garden, purchasing from trusted suppliers, or wildcrafting responsibly, understanding quality indicators, ethical considerations, and proper storage practices ensures access to potent and safe herbs. By integrating these principles into your herbal practice, you can confidently harness the healing power of herbs to support health and well-being naturally.

Chapter 3: Safe storage and preservation methods

Safe storage and preservation of herbs are essential to maintaining their potency, flavor, and efficacy. Whether you store freshly harvested herbs from your garden or purchased herbs, proper methods ensure that they retain their medicinal properties and remain safe for consumption. Here's a guide to secure storage and preservation methods for herbs:

<u>Drying Herbs</u>

Drying herbs is one of the most common methods to preserve them for long-term storage. Proper drying prevents mold and degradation of essential oils, preserving the flavor and medicinal compounds of the herbs.

Harvesting: Harvest herbs in the morning after the dew has evaporated but before the sun is too intense. Use sharp scissors or pruning shears to cut herbs, avoiding damage to the plant.

Cleaning: Remove any dirt, insects, or damaged parts from the herbs. Rinse lightly under cold water and pat dry with a clean cloth or paper towel.

Air Drying: Tie small bunches of herbs with twine and hang them upside down in a well-ventilated, dry area away from direct sunlight. Ensure good airflow around the herbs to prevent mold.

Drying Racks: Use drying racks or screens for larger quantities of herbs. Arrange herbs in a single layer on the racks and place them in a dry, airy location. Turn herbs occasionally to ensure even drying.

Dehydrator: Electric dehydrators offer a controlled environment for drying herbs quickly and efficiently. Follow the manufacturer's instructions for temperature and drying times suitable for herbs.

<u>Storing Dried Herbs</u>

Once herbs are dried, proper storage is crucial to maintain their quality and potency:

Containers: Store dried herbs in clean, airtight containers made of glass or ceramic. Avoid plastic containers, as they may not provide adequate protection from moisture and light.

Labeling: Label containers with the herb's name, harvest date, and other relevant information. Clear labeling prevents confusion and ensures you use herbs before their potency diminishes.

Location: Store herb containers in a cool, dark place such as a pantry or cupboard. Exposure to light and heat can degrade the herbs' medicinal compounds and flavor.

Avoid Moisture: Ensure herbs are completely dry before storing to prevent mold growth. Use silica gel packets or rice grains at the bottom of containers to absorb any residual moisture.

<u>Freezing Herbs</u>

Freezing herbs is another effective method for preserving their freshness and flavor, especially for herbs that are sensitive to drying:

Blanching: Blanch herbs like basil or parsley by briefly immersing them in boiling water for 10-30 seconds, then immediately transferring them to ice water to halt cooking. Blanching helps preserve color and flavor.

Drying: Pat blanched herbs dry with a clean cloth or paper towel to remove excess moisture before freezing.

Packaging: Place blanched herbs in airtight containers or freezer bags. Squeeze out excess air to minimize freezer burn and maintain freshness.

Labeling: Label containers with the herb's name and date of freezing. Use within 6-12 months for optimal flavor and potency.

Making Herbal Extracts

Herbal extracts such as tinctures and infused oils preserve medicinal compounds in a concentrated form. Proper storage ensures their effectiveness and safety:

Dark Glass Bottles: Store tinctures and infused oils in dark glass bottles to protect them from light, which can degrade their potency. Amber or cobalt blue bottles are ideal.

Cool, Dark Location: Store bottles in a cool, dark place such as a pantry or refrigerator. Avoid storing near heat sources or in direct sunlight.

Labeling: Label bottles with the herb used, extraction method, and date of preparation. Proper labeling ensures you use extracts within their recommended shelf life.

Checking for Spoilage: Inspect tinctures and oils regularly for any signs of spoilage, such as changes in color, odor, or taste. Discard any extracts that appear contaminated or have an unusual smell.

Herbal Vinegar and Syrups

Herbal vinegars and syrups are flavorful ways to preserve herbs while extracting their medicinal properties. Proper storage maintains their quality:

Glass Bottles: Use glass bottles or jars with non-metallic lids to prevent corrosion. Ensure bottles are clean and dry before filling.

Storage: Store herbal vinegar and syrups in a cool, dark place. Refrigerate after opening to prolong shelf life and maintain flavor.

Labeling: Label bottles with the herb used, preparation date, and suggested uses. Proper labeling helps identify contents and expiration dates. Implementing safe storage and preservation methods is essential for maintaining the potency, flavor, and safety of herbs used in herbal remedies. Whether drying herbs for tea and culinary uses or preparing extracts for medicinal purposes, proper techniques ensure herbs retain their beneficial properties over time.

Chapter 4: Creation of herb inventory

Creating a comprehensive herb inventory is not just a step, but a crucial foundation for herbalists and enthusiasts. It paves the way for organized storage, efficient use, and informed decision-making in herbal practice. Whether managing a personal collection or inventory for a professional herbal business, this task involves careful planning, documentation, and maintenance to ensure herbs remain accessible and their qualities preserved.

4.1 Planning and Organization

1) Assessment of Needs

Begin by meticulously assessing your needs and goals for the herb inventory. Consider factors such as the types of herbs you use most frequently, the quantities needed for various preparations, and storage requirements based on your space and resources. This careful planning is the cornerstone of a successful herb inventory.

2) Inventory Categories

Organize herbs into categories based on their medicinal properties, culinary uses, or preparation methods. This systematic approach not only streamlines inventory management but also facilitates quick access when preparing herbal remedies, bringing a sense of order and ease to the process.

3) Storage Solutions

Determine appropriate storage solutions based on the types of herbs and their forms (dried, fresh, extracts). Choose containers that protect from light, moisture, and pests while maintaining the herbs' potency and freshness.

4.2 Documentation and Tracking

1) Detailed Records

Maintain detailed records of your herb inventory, including the botanical name, common name, source, harvest or purchase date, quantity, and relevant notes (e.g., medicinal uses, preparation methods). This information ensures traceability and supports informed decision-making in herb selection.

2) Inventory Management Tools

Utilize inventory management tools such as spreadsheets, database software, or herbal inventory apps to track herbs effectively. These tools can automate inventory updates, track usage, and generate reports for inventory assessment and planning.

3) Regular Updates

Update your herb inventory records regularly to reflect additions, usage, and changes in stock levels. Conduct periodic audits to verify inventory accuracy and identify herbs needing replenishment or preservation.

4.3 Preservation Techniques

a) Drying and Storage

For herbs harvested from your garden or purchased fresh, employ proper drying and storage techniques to maintain their quality. Ensure herbs are dehydrated before storage to prevent mold and degradation of medicinal compounds.

b) Freezing and Refrigeration

Some herbs, especially those used fresh or in culinary applications, can be preserved by freezing or refrigeration. Follow appropriate methods such as blanching, freezing in airtight containers, or storing in moisture-proof bags.

c) Herbal Extracts

To preserve herbs in concentrated forms, prepare herbal extracts such as tinctures, infused oils, or vinegars. Store these extracts in dark glass bottles in cool, dark environments to protect their potency from light and heat.

4.4 Inventory Maintenance and Rotation

First-In-First-Out (FIFO) Method: Implement the FIFO method to ensure older herbs are used first, reducing the risk of spoilage and maintaining freshness. Label containers with harvest or purchase dates for easy identification.

Quality Assurance: Regularly inspect herbs for signs of degradation, such as discoloration, loss of aroma, or pest infestation. Dispose of any herbs that show signs of spoilage to prevent contamination of the entire inventory.

Monitoring Shelf Life: Monitor the shelf life of herbs and herbal preparations based on their type and storage conditions. Rotate inventory accordingly to use herbs before their potency diminishes or before they exceed their optimal storage period.

Creating and maintaining an herb inventory is a vital aspect of herbal practice. It ensures herbs are readily available, properly preserved, and used effectively in herbal remedies. By implementing careful planning, documentation, and preservation techniques, herbalists can optimize their herb inventory management for personal and professional use. A well-managed herb inventory supports the sustainability of herbal practices, enhances the quality of herbal preparations, and contributes to the overall success of natural health and wellness efforts.

Chapter 5: Safety and hygiene

Safety and hygiene are paramount in herbal practice to ensure herbal remedies' effectiveness, quality, and safety. Whether preparing herbal teas, making tinctures, or handling fresh herbs, following proper safety protocols and maintaining hygiene standards is essential for both personal and professional herbalists. Here's a comprehensive guide to safety and hygiene practices in herbal practice.

5.1 Personal Safety Practices

1) Knowledge and Training

Before engaging in herbal practice, obtain adequate knowledge and training in herb identification, preparation methods, and safety precautions. Attend workshops or courses or seek guidance from experienced herbalists to deepen your understanding.

2) Use of Protective Gear

Wear protective gear such as gloves and masks when handling herbs, incredibly potent or potentially allergenic herbs. Protective gear helps prevent skin irritation, allergic reactions, and inhalation of herb particles.

3) Handling Toxic Herbs

Exercise caution when handling toxic herbs, such as belladonna or foxglove. Use gloves and avoid direct contact with skin. Follow specific guidelines for safe handling, preparation, and disposal of toxic herbs to minimize risks.

5.2 Hygiene Practices

Cleanliness

Maintain cleanliness in your workspace, utensils, and equipment to prevent contamination of herbs and herbal preparations. Wash hands thoroughly before and after handling herbs, especially when preparing fresh herbs or herbal remedies.

Sanitization of Equipment

Regularly sanitize equipment and utensils used for herb preparation, such as mortar and pestle, cutting boards, and drying racks. Use non-toxic sanitizers or natural cleaning agents to avoid residues affecting herb quality.

Storage Hygiene

Store herbs and herbal preparations in clean, dry containers to prevent mold growth and contamination. Labeling containers with herb names and dates helps maintain hygiene and traceability.

5.3 Herbal Preparation Safety

Follow recommended dosage guidelines for herbs to avoid potential adverse effects or toxicity. When trying new herbs or formulations, start with small amounts, especially for individuals with sensitivities or medical conditions.

Be aware of potential allergens among herbs and disclose allergen information to clients or users. Monitor for allergic reactions and discontinue use if adverse symptoms occur.

Properly label herbal preparations with ingredients, dosage instructions, and precautions for safe use. Use clear and concise labeling to ensure users understand how to administer and store herbal remedies safely.

5.4 Storage and Disposal

Store herbs in appropriate conditions, such as cool, dry environments away from direct sunlight and moisture. To maintain potency and freshness, use airtight containers for dried herbs and dark glass bottles for herbal extracts.

Properly dispose of expired herbs or herbal preparations to prevent accidental ingestion or environmental contamination. Follow local regulations to dispose of organic materials and hazardous waste, especially for toxic herbs or unused preparations.

5.5 Adherence to Regulations

Familiarize yourself with local regulations and guidelines governing herbal practice, including cultivation, preparation, labeling, and distribution of herbal products. Ensure compliance to uphold safety standards and legal obligations. Implement quality control measures to monitor the quality and purity of herbs and herbal preparations. Conduct periodic testing for contaminants such as heavy metals, pesticides, and microbial growth to ensure safety and efficacy.

Stay updated on advances in herbal research, safety protocols, and industry standards through professional organizations, publications, and continuing education programs. Incorporate new knowledge and best practices into your herbal practice to enhance safety and effectiveness.

Consult with qualified herbalists, healthcare professionals, or regulatory authorities for guidance on specific safety concerns or herbal interactions. Collaboration promotes safe practices and ensures informed decision-making in herbal practice.

Safety and hygiene practices are fundamental to the integrity and success of herbal practice, whether for personal use or professional application. By prioritizing personal safety, maintaining high hygiene standards, adhering to dosage guidelines, and complying with regulations, herbalists can ensure herbal remedies' quality, efficacy, and safety. These practices protect the herbalist and promote trust and confidence among clients and users seeking natural health solutions. Embracing a commitment to safety and hygiene underscores the responsible and professional approach to herbal practice, supporting the holistic well-being of individuals and communities alike.

Book 8: Common Herbs and their Uses

Unlocking the Benefits of Nature's Medicine Cabinet

Chapter 1: Introduction to key herbs

Understanding essential herbs is fundamental in exploring their diverse medicinal properties and applications in herbal practice. Each herb offers unique therapeutic benefits, whether supporting immune function, promoting relaxation, aiding digestion, or enhancing cognitive function. Herbs have been integral to traditional medicine systems worldwide for centuries, valued for their natural healing compounds and holistic approach to wellness.

Herbs are typically derived from various plant parts, including leaves, flowers, roots, seeds, and bark. Each contains potent bioactive compounds such as alkaloids, flavonoids, terpenes, and essential oils. These compounds contribute to the herbs' pharmacological effects, influencing physiological processes in the body to promote health and alleviate symptoms of illness.

In herbal practice, herbs are often prepared in different forms to maximize their efficacy and convenience. Common preparations include teas, tinctures, extracts, capsules, and topical applications such as ointments or poultices. Each method of preparation extracts and preserves specific constituents of the herb, allowing practitioners and individuals to tailor treatments to specific health concerns or preferences.

Moreover, the cultivation and harvesting of herbs play a crucial role in their quality and potency. Many herbs thrive in specific climates and soil conditions, requiring careful cultivation practices to ensure optimal growth and therapeutic properties. Harvesting at the right time of year and employing proper drying and storage techniques further preserve the herbs' medicinal qualities.

As individuals increasingly seek natural and sustainable approaches to health and wellness, the popularity of herbal medicine continues to grow. Scientific research continues to validate many traditional uses of herbs, uncovering new potential applications and refining our understanding of their mechanisms of action. Integrating key herbs into daily routines or professional practices offers a holistic approach to maintaining health, preventing illness, and supporting overall well-being.

By exploring the detailed profiles of essential herbs, including their uses, benefits, and considerations, herbal practitioners and enthusiasts can effectively harness these natural remedies' therapeutic potential. Whether addressing specific health concerns or promoting general wellness, herbs' versatility, and potency provide valuable tools for achieving optimal health outcomes naturally and sustainably.

Chapter 2: Detailed herb profiles

Lavender (Lavandula angustifolia)

Lavender is a fragrant herb known for its calming aroma and versatile uses. It has narrow, aromatic leaves and small purple-blue flowers that bloom in spikes.

Uses and Benefits:

- Relaxation: Lavender is renowned for its calming properties, making it a popular choice for promoting relaxation and reducing stress and anxiety.

- Sleep Aid: Used in herbal teas or pillow sachets, lavender can improve sleep quality and alleviate insomnia.

- Skin Care: Lavender essential oil is prized for its skincare benefits, including soothing minor burns, insect bites, and skin irritations.

Echinacea (Echinacea purpurea)

Echinacea, also known as purple coneflower, is a native North American herb with striking pink-purple petals and a spiky orange-brown central cone.

Uses and Benefits:

- Immune Support: Echinacea is widely used to stimulate the immune system and shorten the duration of colds and respiratory infections.

- Anti-inflammatory: It possesses anti-inflammatory properties that can help reduce inflammation and alleviate symptoms of conditions like arthritis.

- Wound Healing: Echinacea ointments or tinctures are applied topically to promote wound healing and reduce infection.

Ginger (Zingiber officinale)

Ginger is a rhizomatous herb with thick, knobby roots and long, green shoots with narrow leaves. It has a spicy, pungent flavor and is widely used in culinary and medicinal applications.

Uses and Benefits:

- Digestive Aid: Ginger is prized for its ability to alleviate nausea, indigestion, and motion sickness. It stimulates digestion and helps relieve gas and bloating.

- Anti-inflammatory: It has potent anti-inflammatory effects, beneficial for reducing inflammation associated with arthritis and other inflammatory conditions.

- Antioxidant: Ginger contains antioxidants that help combat oxidative stress and protect against cell damage.

Chamomile (Matricaria chamomilla)

Chamomile is a daisy-like herb with white petals and a yellow central disc. It has a mild, apple-like aroma and is commonly used in teas and herbal preparations.

Uses and Benefits:

- Calming Agent: Chamomile is renowned for its calming and soothing effects, promoting relaxation and reducing anxiety and insomnia.

- Digestive Support: It helps alleviate digestive discomfort, including gas, bloating, and stomach cramps.

- Skin Care: Chamomile's anti-inflammatory and antiseptic properties make it beneficial for

- treating skin conditions such as eczema and minor wounds.

Peppermint (Mentha piperita)

Peppermint is a hybrid mint with dark green leaves and purple-tinged stems. It has a refreshing, minty aroma and flavor, making it a popular herb in teas and culinary dishes.

Uses and Benefits:

- Digestive Health: Peppermint is effective in relieving digestive issues such as indigestion, gas, and irritable bowel syndrome (IBS).

- Headache Relief: It has analgesic properties that can help alleviate tension headaches and migraines when applied topically or inhaled.

- Respiratory Support: Peppermint's menthol content helps clear nasal congestion and soothe sore throats.

Turmeric (Curcuma longa)

Turmeric is a rhizomatous herbaceous perennial plant with bright yellow-orange roots. It has a warm, bitter taste and is commonly used in curry dishes and herbal remedies.

Uses and Benefits:

- Anti-inflammatory: Turmeric is renowned for its powerful anti-inflammatory properties, beneficial for reducing inflammation in arthritis and other inflammatory conditions.

- Antioxidant: It contains curcuminoids, potent antioxidants that protect against oxidative damage and support overall health.

- Digestive Aid: Turmeric aids digestion, stimulates bile production, and helps alleviate symptoms of indigestion and bloating.

St. John's Wort (Hypericum perforatum)

St. John's Wort is a perennial herb with clusters of bright yellow flowers and translucent dots that resemble perforations on its leaves.

Uses and Benefits:

- Mood Support: St. John's Wort is used to alleviate symptoms of mild to moderate depression and anxiety disorders.

- Nerve Health: It has nerve-calming properties that can help relieve nerve pain and inflammation associated with conditions like sciatica.

- Topical Use: St. John's Wort oil is applied topically to promote wound healing, reduce inflammation, and soothe nerve pain.

Valerian (Valeriana officinalis)

Valerian is a perennial herb with clusters of small, fragrant white or pink flowers and fern-like foliage. Its roots emit a strong, earthy odor.

Uses and Benefits:

- Sleep Aid: Valerian is renowned for its sedative effects, promoting relaxation and improving sleep quality without causing morning grogginess.

- Anxiety Relief: It helps alleviate symptoms of anxiety and nervous tension, making it useful for managing stress-related disorders.

- Muscle Relaxant: Valerian can reduce muscle tension and spasms, making it beneficial for conditions like menstrual cramps and muscle pain.

Exploring key herbs in herbal practice provides insight into their diverse uses, benefits, and contributions to natural health and wellness. From calming lavender and immune-boosting echinacea to digestive aids like ginger and peppermint, each herb offers unique therapeutic properties that can be harnessed through teas, tinctures, or topical applications. By incorporating these herbs into daily routines or professional practices, individuals can enhance their well-being naturally and embrace the holistic benefits of herbal medicine.

Garlic (Allium sativum)

Description: aroma and flavor, making it a staple in culinary dishes and herbal remedies.

Uses and Benefits:

- Immune Support: Garlic has antimicrobial and immune-boosting properties, aiding in fighting infections and supporting overall immune health.

- Cardiovascular Health: It helps lower cholesterol levels, regulate blood pressure, and improve circulation, reducing the risk of heart disease.

- Antioxidant: Garlic contains sulfur compounds like allicin, which act as antioxidants, protecting cells from oxidative damage.

Ginkgo (Ginkgo biloba)

Ginkgo is a deciduous tree with fan-shaped leaves and distinctive yellow fruit. Its leaves are used in herbal preparations for their medicinal properties.

Uses and Benefits:

- Cognitive Function: Ginkgo improves memory, concentration, and cognitive function by enhancing blood flow to the brain and protecting neurons from damage.

- Peripheral Circulation: It supports circulation to the extremities, alleviating symptoms of poor circulation such as cold hands and feet.

- Antioxidant: Ginkgo leaf extracts contain flavonoids and terpenoids that act as antioxidants, neutralizing free radicals and reducing oxidative stress.

Holy Basil (Ocimum sanctum)

Holy Basil, also known as Tulsi, is an aromatic herb with green or purple leaves and small purple flowers. It is revered in Ayurvedic medicine for its spiritual and medicinal properties.

Uses and Benefits:

- Adaptogen: Holy Basil helps the body adapt to stress and balance cortisol levels, promoting resilience and overall well-being.

- Antimicrobial: It has antimicrobial properties that help combat infections, bacteria, and fungi, supporting immune health.

- Anti-inflammatory: Holy Basil reduces inflammation and swelling, benefiting conditions like arthritis and respiratory ailments.

Ashwagandha (Withania somnifera)

Ashwagandha is a small shrub with yellow flowers and red fruit, native to India and North Africa. Its roots and leaves are used in herbal medicine.

Uses and Benefits:

- Stress Relief: Ashwagandha is an adaptogenic herb that helps reduce stress, anxiety, and cortisol levels, promoting relaxation and mental clarity.

- Energy and Stamina: It enhances vitality, endurance, and physical performance by improving energy metabolism and reducing fatigue.

- Hormonal Balance: Ashwagandha supports hormonal balance, particularly in women, by regulating cortisol and promoting thyroid function.

Milk Thistle (Silybum marianum)

Milk Thistle is a tall herbaceous plant with prickly leaves and purple flowers. Its seeds are used in herbal medicine for liver support and detoxification.

Uses and Benefits:

- Liver Health: Milk Thistle protects and supports liver function by promoting regeneration of liver cells and enhancing detoxification pathways.

- Antioxidant: It contains flavonoids and silymarin, potent antioxidants that protect liver cells from damage caused by toxins and free radicals.

- Digestive Support: Milk Thistle aids digestion, relieves indigestion, and supports gastrointestinal health by stimulating bile production.

Nettle (Urtica dioica)

Nettle is a perennial herb with serrated leaves and tiny, inconspicuous flowers. Despite its stinging hairs, nettle is valued for its medicinal properties.

Uses and Benefits:

- Allergy Relief: Nettle reduces symptoms of seasonal allergies, such as sneezing and itching, by inhibiting histamine release and inflammation.

- Nutrient-Rich: It is rich in vitamins (A, C, K) and minerals (iron, calcium, magnesium), supporting overall health and vitality.

- Diuretic: Nettle acts as a gentle diuretic, promoting kidney function and reducing fluid retention.

Hawthorn (Crataegus spp.)

Hawthorn is a thorny shrub or small tree with clusters of white or pink flowers and red berries. Its leaves, flowers, and berries are used in herbal medicine.

Uses and Benefits:

- Cardiovascular Support: Hawthorn strengthens the heart muscle, regulates blood pressure, and improves circulation, promoting cardiovascular health.

- Antioxidant: It contains flavonoids and oligomeric procyanidins (OPCs) that protect blood vessels from oxidative damage and support blood flow.

- Mild Sedative: Hawthorn has calming effects on the nervous system, reducing anxiety and promoting relaxation.

Calendula (Calendula officinalis)

Calendula, also known as marigold, is a bright, cheerful herb with yellow or orange petals. It is prized for its medicinal and cosmetic uses.

Uses and Benefits:

- Skin Care: Calendula promotes skin healing and reduces inflammation, making it ideal for treating cuts, wounds, burns, and skin irritations.

- Antimicrobial: It has antimicrobial properties that help fight infections and support wound healing without disrupting the skin's natural microbiome.

- Digestive Aid: Calendula tea or tincture can soothe gastrointestinal inflammation and relieve symptoms of gastritis and ulcers.

Sage (Salvia officinalis)

Sage is a woody perennial herb with gray-green leaves and blue to purplish flowers. It has a strong, aromatic flavor and is used in culinary and medicinal preparations.

Uses and Benefits:

- Cognitive Function: Sage enhances memory, concentration, and cognitive function by improving acetylcholine levels in the brain.

- Digestive Health: It stimulates digestion, relieves indigestion, and reduces gas and bloating after meals.

- Antioxidant: Sage contains rosmarinic acid and other antioxidants that protect cells from oxidative stress and inflammation.

Licorice Root (Glycyrrhiza glabra)

Licorice root is derived from the perennial Glycyrrhiza glabra plant, which features purple to blue flowers and grows in parts of Asia and Europe. It has been used in traditional medicine for centuries.

Uses and Benefits:

- Respiratory Health: Licorice root is known for its expectorant properties, making it effective in easing coughs and sore throats.

- Digestive Aid: It helps soothe gastrointestinal issues such as acid reflux, indigestion, and stomach ulcers.

- Adrenal Support: Licorice root can support adrenal gland function, helping the body cope with stress and promoting hormone balance.

Ginseng (Panax ginseng)

Ginseng is a perennial plant with fleshy roots that resembles the human body. It grows primarily in Asia and North America and is prized for its medicinal properties.

Uses and Benefits:

- Energy and Stamina: Ginseng is known as an adaptogen, helping the body cope with physical and mental stress while enhancing stamina and energy levels.

- Cognitive Function: It improves cognitive performance, memory, and concentration by supporting brain function and reducing mental fatigue.

- Immune Support: Ginseng boosts the immune system, enhancing resistance to infections and promoting overall health.

Astragalus (Astragalus membranaceus)

Astragalus is a perennial herb native to China and Mongolia, featuring small yellow flowers and hairy stems. Its roots are used in traditional Chinese medicine.

Uses and Benefits:

- Immune Modulation: Astragalus enhances immune function by stimulating the production of white blood cells and antibodies.

- Anti-inflammatory: It reduces inflammation, making it beneficial for conditions like arthritis and autoimmune disorders.

- Adaptogenic Properties: Astragalus helps the body adapt to stress, supporting adrenal gland function and promoting resilience.

Lemon Balm (Melissa officinalis)

Lemon balm is a perennial herb in the mint family with a lemony aroma and small white or yellow flowers. It is native to Europe, North Africa, and West Asia.

Uses and Benefits:

- Calming and Relaxation: Lemon balm has mild sedative properties, promoting relaxation, reducing anxiety, and improving sleep quality.

- Digestive Aid: It helps alleviate gastrointestinal discomfort, including gas, bloating, and indigestion.

- Antiviral: Lemon balm has antiviral properties, aiding in the treatment of cold sores caused by the herpes simplex virus.

Rosemary (Rosmarinus officinalis)

Rosemary is an evergreen shrub with needle-like leaves and small, pale blue flowers. It is native to the Mediterranean region and widely used in culinary and medicinal applications.

Uses and Benefits:

- Cognitive Enhancement: Rosemary improves memory, concentration, and mental clarity by enhancing blood flow to the brain.

- Digestive Health: It stimulates digestion, relieves intestinal gas, and supports liver and gallbladder function.

- Antioxidant: Rosemary contains rosmarinic acid and other antioxidants that protect cells from oxidative stress and inflammation.

Ashwagandha (Withania somnifera)

Ashwagandha, also known as Indian ginseng or winter cherry, is a small shrub native to India, the Middle East, and parts of Africa. It has oval leaves and small green flowers, with orange-red fruit when ripe.

Uses and Benefits:

- Adaptogen: Ashwagandha is renowned for its adaptogenic properties, helping the body adapt to stress and promoting overall balance.

- Energy and Stamina: It enhances vitality, endurance, and physical performance by supporting adrenal gland function and reducing fatigue.

- Mental Clarity: Ashwagandha improves cognitive function, memory, and concentration, making it beneficial for mental clarity and focus.

While generally safe for most people, pregnant women, breastfeeding mothers, and individuals with autoimmune diseases should consult healthcare providers before use.

Saw Palmetto (Serenoa repens)

Saw palmetto is a small palm tree native to the southeastern United States. It has fan-shaped leaves and produces dark berries that have been used for centuries in traditional medicine.

Uses and Benefits:

- Prostate Health: Saw palmetto is commonly used to support prostate health, reducing symptoms of benign prostatic hyperplasia (BPH) such as urinary urgency and frequency.

- Hair Loss: It may help inhibit the enzyme responsible for converting testosterone to dihydrotestosterone (DHT), which contributes to male pattern baldness.

- Anti-inflammatory: Saw palmetto has anti-inflammatory properties that may benefit conditions like chronic pelvic pain syndrome and urinary tract inflammation.

Saw palmetto may interact with hormonal medications or blood thinners. Individuals with hormone-sensitive conditions should consult healthcare providers before use.

Passionflower (Passiflora incarnata)

Passionflower is a climbing vine with intricate, showy flowers and edible fruit known as passion fruit. It is native to the southeastern United States and Central and South America.

Uses and Benefits:

- Anxiety and Insomnia: Passionflower is used to reduce symptoms of anxiety, nervousness, and insomnia by promoting relaxation and calming the mind.

- Muscle Relaxant: It has mild sedative properties that help relax muscles, making it beneficial for muscle tension, spasms, and menstrual cramps.

- Digestive Aid: Passionflower supports digestive health, alleviating symptoms of indigestion, stomach cramps, and irritable bowel syndrome (IBS).

Passionflower may cause drowsiness, so caution is advised when operating machinery or driving. It may interact with medications such as sedatives and antidepressants.

Gotu Kola (Centella asiatica)

Gotu kola is a low-growing herbaceous plant native to Asia and traditionally used in Ayurvedic and Chinese medicine. It has kidney-shaped leaves and small white or pink flowers.

Uses and Benefits:

- Cognitive Function: Gotu kola improves memory, concentration, and mental clarity by enhancing circulation to the brain and supporting nerve function.

- Skin Health: It promotes wound healing and collagen production, benefiting skin conditions like scars, stretch marks, and eczema.

- Venous Insufficiency: Gotu kola supports vascular health, reducing symptoms of varicose veins and promoting circulation in the legs.

Gotu kola is generally safe when used as directed. Pregnant women and individuals with liver disease should consult healthcare providers before use.

Rhodiola (Rhodiola rosea)

Rhodiola, also known as golden root or Arctic root, is a perennial flowering plant native to cold regions of Europe, Asia, and North America. It has succulent leaves and clusters of yellow flowers.

Uses and Benefits:

- Adaptogen: Rhodiola is valued for its adaptogenic properties, helping the body adapt to stress, fatigue, and environmental challenges.

- Energy and Endurance: It enhances physical performance, stamina, and recovery from exertion by supporting adrenal gland function.

- Mood Enhancement: Rhodiola improves mood, reduces symptoms of depression, and promotes mental clarity and focus.

Rhodiola may cause mild side effects such as dizziness or dry mouth in some individuals. Pregnant or breastfeeding women should avoid using rhodiola without medical supervision.

Bacopa (Bacopa monnieri)

Bacopa, also known as brahmi, is a creeping herb native to wetlands in India, Australia, Europe, Africa, Asia, and North and South America. It has small, succulent leaves and white or purple flowers.

Uses and Benefits:

- Cognitive Support: Bacopa improves memory, concentration, and learning ability by enhancing neurotransmitter function and promoting nerve cell communication.

- Stress Reduction: It reduces symptoms of anxiety and stress by modulating cortisol levels and promoting relaxation.

- Neuroprotective: Bacopa protects brain cells from oxidative stress and age-related cognitive decline.

Bacopa is generally well-tolerated but may cause digestive upset or nausea in some individuals. It should be used cautiously with medications that affect serotonin levels.

Holy Basil (Ocimum sanctum)

Holy basil, also known as tulsi, is a sacred herb in Hinduism and is native to the Indian subcontinent. It has aromatic green leaves and purple or white flowers.

Uses and Benefits:

- Adaptogenic: Holy basil acts as an adaptogen, helping the body cope with stress, fatigue, and anxiety while promoting balance and resilience.

- Immune Support: It enhances immune function, protecting against infections and supporting overall health and vitality.

- Anti-inflammatory: Holy basil has anti-inflammatory properties that reduce inflammation and symptoms of arthritis and respiratory conditions.

Holy basil is generally safe when used as a culinary herb or tea. Pregnant women should consult healthcare providers before using it in medicinal amounts.

Maca (Lepidium meyenii)

Maca is a cruciferous vegetable native to the high Andes mountains of Peru and Bolivia. It has a turnip-like appearance with green, yellow, or purple roots.

Uses and Benefits:

- Hormonal Balance: Maca regulates hormone levels, benefiting reproductive health, menstrual irregularities, and symptoms of menopause.

- Energy and Stamina: It enhances energy levels, endurance, and physical performance by supporting adrenal gland function.

- Libido Enhancement: Maca improves sexual function, arousal, and libido in both men and women.

Maca is generally well-tolerated but may cause digestive upset or insomnia in sensitive individuals. Individuals with thyroid conditions should use maca cautiously.

These key herbs offer a wide range of therapeutic benefits, from supporting immune health and enhancing cognitive function to promoting relaxation and aiding digestive health. Whether used individually or in combination with other herbs, they exemplify the diverse applications and holistic approach of herbal medicine in promoting overall well-being naturally. Integrating these herbs into daily routines or professional practices allows individuals to harness their medicinal properties effectively and embrace the benefits of herbal remedies.

Book 9: Growing, harvesting, and preparing each herb

A Complete Guide to Cultivating and Utilizing Herbal Remedies

Chapter 1: Cultivation and Growing Conditions

A comprehensive understanding of growing, harvesting, and preparing each herb is crucial for maximizing its medicinal potency and ensuring quality in herbal practice. Each herb requires specific conditions and techniques throughout its lifecycle, from cultivation to harvest and preparation, to preserve its beneficial properties effectively.

1) Soil and Climate Requirements

Successful cultivation begins with selecting the suitable soil and climate conditions tailored to each herb's preferences. For instance, herbs like lavender and rosemary thrive in well-drained, sandy loam soil with total sun exposure, replicating their native Mediterranean environments. On the other hand, herbs such as marshmallows and comfrey prefer moist, rich soil in partially shaded areas to mimic their natural habitat.

2) Propagation Methods

Propagation methods vary among herbs, including seeds, cuttings, division, or root propagation, chosen based on the herb's growth habits and propagation requirements. For instance, basil and cilantro are typically grown from seeds directly sown into the garden bed. At the same time, herbs like mint and lemon balm are propagated from root divisions or cuttings to maintain genetic characteristics and ensure vigorous growth.

3) Watering and Maintenance

Regular watering practices tailored to each herb's moisture needs are essential for healthy growth and optimal yield. Once established, herbs like thyme and oregano prefer drier conditions, while herbs such as parsley and chives benefit from consistent moisture to maintain lush foliage and robust growth. Proper weed control and organic pest management strategies, such as companion planting or natural predators, help maintain herb health without relying on synthetic chemicals.

Chapter 2: Harvesting Techniques

<u>Timing of Harvest</u>

Harvest timing is critical to maximize the herb's medicinal potency and flavor profile. Herbs are typically harvested when essential oils and active compounds are at their peak concentration, often just before flowering or during specific growth stages. For example, chamomile flowers are harvested in the morning after dew has evaporated to preserve their essential oils, while elderberries are harvested when fully ripe for maximum antioxidant content.

<u>Harvesting Methods</u>

Herbs are harvested using various methods depending on the plant part used and intended use. Leaves and flowers are typically harvested by hand or with small scissors to minimize damage and ensure quality. Roots like ginger and turmeric are carefully dug up, washed, and dried to preserve their medicinal properties. Berries, such as those from saw palmetto or elderberry, are harvested manually or with small tools to prevent bruising and preserve their nutrient content.

<u>Drying and Curing</u>

Proper drying and curing methods are essential to maintain the herbs' integrity and prevent spoilage. Herbs are dried in well-ventilated areas away from direct sunlight to preserve color, flavor, and medicinal properties. Hanging bundles of herbs, such as sage or thyme, upside down in a cool, dry place allows for gradual drying. Roots and seeds may be dried on screens or racks to ensure even airflow and prevent mold growth.

Chapter 3: Preparation Techniques

1) Culinary Uses

Many herbs, such as basil, cilantro, and parsley, are used fresh or dried in culinary dishes to enhance flavor and nutritional value. Fresh herbs are added near the end of cooking to retain their delicate flavors, while dried herbs are often used in soups, stews, marinades, and sauces for long-lasting flavor infusion.

2) Medicinal Applications

Herbs like echinacea, valerian, and ginkgo are prepared in various forms for medicinal use, including teas, tinctures, extracts, and capsules. Tea infusions are steeping dried or fresh herbs in hot water to extract beneficial compounds. At the same time, tinctures involve soaking herbs in alcohol or glycerin to create concentrated extracts for therapeutic use. Capsules and tablets offer convenient dosing options for standardized herbal supplements.

3) Herbal Preparations

Herbalists and practitioners often create custom herbal preparations tailored to individual health needs and preferences. Herbal oils, salves, creams, and poultices combine herbs with carrier oils or beeswax for topical applications, supporting skin health, wound healing, and muscle relaxation. Herbal syrups and elixirs blend herbs with honey or syrups for palatability and ease of consumption, which is particularly beneficial for respiratory support and immune health.

Chapter 4: Quality Assurance and Sustainability

Quality Control

Ensuring herb quality involves rigorous quality control measures at every stage, from cultivation to final product preparation. This includes testing soil health, monitoring growth conditions, and verifying harvesting techniques to maintain purity and potency. Quality standards such as organic certification or Good Agricultural Practices (GAP) further ensure herbs meet safety and efficacy standards.

Sustainability Practices

Sustainable herb cultivation practices promote biodiversity, conserve natural resources, and support local ecosystems. Crop rotation, companion planting, and organic fertilizers minimize environmental impact while enhancing soil fertility and plant resilience. Ethical wildcrafting practices for wild herbs, such as ginseng or goldenseal, prioritize species conservation and respect for native habitats.

Thorough knowledge of growing, harvesting, and preparing each herb is essential for maximizing its therapeutic benefits and ensuring quality in herbal practice. By understanding the specific cultivation needs, optimal harvesting techniques, and diverse preparation methods, herbalists and enthusiasts can cultivate, harvest, and utilize herbs effectively for culinary, medicinal, and therapeutic purposes. This holistic approach enhances herbal efficacy and promotes sustainable practices that respect natural ecosystems and support overall health and well-being.

Chapter 5: Herbal combination for synergy

Combining herbs for synergy is a practice rooted in the principles of herbal medicine. In this approach, the interaction of multiple herbs enhances their therapeutic effects, addresses specific health concerns, and optimizes overall wellness. This approach leverages the complementary actions of different herbs to achieve synergistic benefits greater than those of individual herbs alone.

Complementary Actions

Each herb possesses unique chemical constituents and therapeutic properties that can complement each other when combined thoughtfully. For example, pairing turmeric, known for its potent anti-inflammatory properties due to curcumin, with black pepper, which contains piperine, enhances curcumin absorption and bioavailability, thereby boosting its effectiveness against inflammation.

Targeted Therapeutic Effects

Herbal combinations are often formulated to target specific health concerns or conditions. For instance, a blend of ginger, peppermint, and fennel may alleviate digestive discomfort and support gastrointestinal health. Ginger aids digestion and reduces nausea, peppermint relaxes intestinal muscles and relieves gas; and fennel soothes spasms and reduces bloating, creating a comprehensive approach to digestive wellness.

Balancing Actions

Combining herbs can balance their actions to achieve a harmonious effect on the body. For example, a blend of calming herbs like chamomile, lemon balm, and passionflower may promote relaxation and reduce anxiety. Chamomile soothes the nerves and induces relaxation, lemon balm supports mood stability and eases tension, and passionflower reduces anxiety by modulating neurotransmitter activity, creating a synergistic calming effect.

Potentiating Effects

Certain herbs enhance the potency of others when combined, leading to greater efficacy. For example, combining garlic and echinacea can strengthen the immune system's response to infections. Garlic has antimicrobial properties that support immune function, while echinacea stimulates immune cell activity and enhances the body's defense mechanisms, providing a powerful synergy against pathogens.

5.1 Factors Influencing Herbal Synergy

Herbal Constituents. Understanding the primary bioactive compounds in each herb helps in selecting complementary combinations. For example, herbs rich in flavonoids (such as hawthorn and bilberry) may be combined for cardiovascular support, as flavonoids enhance blood vessel health and circulation through antioxidant and anti-inflammatory actions.

Traditional Knowledge and Empirical Evidence. Traditional herbal medicine systems, such as Ayurveda and Traditional Chinese Medicine (TCM), provide valuable insights into synergistic herb combinations based on centuries of empirical observation and clinical experience. These systems emphasize holistic approaches to health, considering the interactions between herbs and their effects on different organ systems and body functions.

Personalized Approaches. Tailoring herbal combinations to individual needs and health goals optimizes therapeutic outcomes. To design personalized formulas, herbalists and practitioners assess constitution, underlying health conditions, and medication interactions. For example, adaptogenic herbs like ashwagandha, rhodiola, and holy basil may be combined to support stress resilience and energy levels based on an individual's specific stress response and adrenal function.

5.2 Methods of Herbal Combination

Herbal Formulations

Herbalists create formulations by blending herbs in specific ratios and forms, such as teas, tinctures, capsules, or topical preparations, based on the desired therapeutic outcome. For example, a sleep blend might combine valerian, passionflower, and lemon balm in a tincture to calm the nervous system and promote restful sleep.

Sequential Therapy

Sequential therapy involves using different herbs in phases to address acute symptoms, followed by long-term support. For instance, a respiratory blend might include elderberry and mullein for immediate immune support during colds or flu, followed by licorice root and thyme for respiratory health and recovery.

Rotational Therapy

Rotational therapy alternates between different herb combinations over time to prevent tolerance and maximize effectiveness. This approach is common in chronic conditions or immune support, where the body may adapt to prolonged use of a single herb or combination.

While herbal combinations offer numerous benefits, potential herb-drug interactions, allergies, and contraindications must be considered. Consulting with a qualified herbalist or healthcare provider ensures safe and effective use, especially for individuals with existing health conditions or medications.

Using high-quality herbs from reputable sources ensures purity, potency, and therapeutic efficacy in herbal combinations. Organic certification, sustainable harvesting practices, and adherence to quality standards contribute to the overall effectiveness and safety of herbal products.

Combining herbs for synergy is a sophisticated approach to herbal medicine that enhances therapeutic outcomes by leveraging the complementary actions of different herbs. Whether targeting specific health concerns, balancing physiological functions, or potentiating therapeutic effects, herbal combinations offer versatile solutions rooted in traditional knowledge and supported by modern research. Embracing the principles of synergy allows herbalists, practitioners, and individuals to harness the full potential of nature's remedies for holistic health and well-being.

Book 10: Creating Herbal Preparations

A Practical Guide to Processing Natural Remedies

Chapter 1: Step-by-step guides for making tinctures, teas, salves, and more

Tinctures

Making a tincture is a straightforward process. You'll need dried or fresh herbs, high-proof alcohol (like vodka or brandy), glass jars with tight-fitting lids, labels, and a dark glass bottle for storage.

Preparation Steps:

Step 1: Herb Selection and Preparation: The key to a successful tincture is choosing high-quality herbs known for their medicinal properties. Clean and chop fresh herbs, or use dried herbs.

Step 2: Herb-to-Alcohol Ratio: The precise ratio, based on the herb's strength (e.g., 1:2 for fresh herbs, 1:5 for dried herbs), is crucial. Place herbs in a glass jar.

Step 3: The Magic of maceration: This step is where the transformation happens. Cover the herbs entirely with alcohol, submerging them fully. Seal the jar tightly and store it in a cool, dark place for 4-6 weeks, shaking daily. This process allows the alcohol to extract the medicinal properties from the herbs, creating a potent tincture.

Step 4: Straining: After maceration, strain the liquid through cheesecloth or a fine mesh strainer into a clean glass jar, squeezing excess liquid.

Step 5: Bottling: Pour the tincture into dark glass bottles, label with the herb name and date, and store in a cool, dark place. Tinctures typically have a shelf life of 1-3 years.

Teas

Gather dried herbs, a teapot or infuser, filtered water, and optional sweeteners like honey or lemon for herbal teas.

Preparation Steps:

Step 1: Herb Selection: Choose herbs based on desired health benefits and flavor preferences.

Step 2: Water Temperature: Boil and pour over herbs in a teapot or infuser.

Step 3: Steeping Time: Cover and steep herbs for 5-10 minutes, adjusting time based on herb strength and desired flavor.

Step 4: Straining: Remove herbs using a strainer or infuser.

Step 5: Serving: Serve hot or chilled, sweetened if desired, and store leftovers in a sealed container in the refrigerator for up to 24 hours.

Salves

To make herbal salves, gather dried herbs, carrier oils (like olive or coconut oil), beeswax, glass jars, and labels.

Preparation Steps:

Step 1: Herb Infusion: Create an herb-infused oil by placing dried herbs in a glass jar and covering them with carrier oil. Seal and put in a sunny spot for 2-4 weeks, shaking daily.

Step 2: Straining: After infusion, strain oil through cheesecloth or a fine mesh strainer into a clean glass jar, squeezing out excess oil.

Step 3: Salve Preparation: In a double boiler, gently heat infused oil and add grated beeswax (typically 1 part beeswax to 4 parts oil) until melted and combined.

Step 4: Cooling and Bottling: Pour mixture into small jars or tins, allow to cool and solidify at room temperature. Label with ingredients and date, store in a cool, dark place.

Herbal Poultices

For herbal poultices, gather fresh or dried herbs, hot water, a mortar and pestle (or blender), a clean cloth, and optional ingredients like clay or oatmeal.

Preparation Steps:

Step 1: Herb Selection: Choose herbs known for soothing or healing properties, chop or crush.

Step 2: Mixing Ingredients: Combine herbs with hot water, clay, or oatmeal to create a thick paste.

Step 3: Application: Apply paste directly to affected area, cover with clean cloth, leave on for 15-30 minutes.

Step 4: Removal and Storage: Remove the poultice, discard any leftover paste, and wash the skin. Store herbs in a cool, dry place for future use.

Herbal Infused Oils

To make herbal infused oils, gather dried herbs, carrier oils (like olive or almond oil), glass jars with lids, and labels.

Preparation Steps:

Step 1: Herb Selection: Choose dried herbs for medicinal properties and flavor.

Step 2: Herb-to-Oil Ratio: Place herbs in clean, dry glass jar, cover with carrier oil, ensuring herbs are submerged.

Step 3: Sun Infusion: Seal jar, place in sunny spot for 2-4 weeks, shaking daily to infuse oil with herbal properties.

Step 4: Straining: After infusion, strain oil through cheesecloth or fine mesh strainer into a clean glass jar, squeezing out excess oil.

Step 5: Storage: Label with herb name and date, store in cool, dark place, use within 6-12 months for best freshness. Mastering the creation of herbal preparations like tinctures, teas, salves, and poultices involves careful selection of herbs, precise preparation techniques, and attention to quality and storage practices.

Chapter 2: Dosing guidelines and safety advice

Dosage guidelines and safety tips are crucial aspects of herbal medicine to ensure the effective and safe use of herbal remedies. Understanding how to administer herbs correctly and being aware of potential interactions or side effects helps maximize therapeutic benefits while minimizing risks.

2.1 Dosage Guidelines

1) General Principles

Dosage recommendations vary widely based on the herb's potency, individual health status, age, weight, and intended use (e.g., acute or chronic conditions). Starting with lower doses and gradually increasing to assess tolerance and effectiveness is essential. Consulting with a qualified herbalist or healthcare provider can provide personalized dosage guidance tailored to specific health needs.

2) Standardized Preparations

Some herbal supplements are available in standardized forms, where the active ingredients are quantified to ensure consistent potency and dosage accuracy. Follow manufacturer instructions for dosing unless otherwise directed by a healthcare professional. Standardization helps ensure reliability and efficacy in herbal treatments.

3) Herbal Formulations

Different herbal preparations (e.g., teas, tinctures, capsules) may require specific dosage adjustments due to variations in bioavailability and absorption rates. For instance, tinctures are often concentrated and require fewer drops than teas or capsules to achieve therapeutic effects. Always follow the dosage recommendations provided for each specific preparation method.

4) Dosage Based on Herb Type

Dosage recommendations can vary widely depending on the type of herb and its intended use. For example:

Adaptogens like ashwagandha and ginseng are often taken in moderate doses over extended periods to support resilience to stress and enhance overall well-being.

Digestive Herbs such as peppermint and ginger may be used in higher doses to alleviate acute symptoms like indigestion or nausea.

Nervine Herbs like valerian and passionflower are typically used in smaller doses to promote relaxation and support sleep.

2.2 Safety Tips

Research and Education: Before using any herbal remedy, conduct thorough research or consult a knowledgeable healthcare provider to understand potential benefits, side effects, and interactions. Reliable sources of information include peer-reviewed studies, reputable herbal texts, and guidance from professional herbalists.

Start Low and Go Slow

Begin with the lowest effective dose and gradually increase if needed, observing how your body responds. This approach helps minimize the risk of adverse reactions and allows for individual tolerance and sensitivity adjustments.

Individualized Approach

When determining appropriate herbal dosages, consider individual factors such as age, weight, underlying health conditions, and medications. Children, pregnant or nursing women, and elderly individuals may require adjusted dosing regimens to ensure safety and efficacy.

Quality and Sourcing

Choose high-quality herbs from reputable sources to ensure purity, potency, and absence of contaminants. Look for organic certification or Good Manufacturing Practices (GMP) compliance when purchasing herbal products to minimize the risk of exposure to pesticides or other harmful substances.

Herb-Drug Interactions

Be aware of potential interactions between herbs and pharmaceutical medications. Certain herbs can potentiate or inhibit the effects of drugs, leading to the adverse impacts or reduced efficacy. Always disclose all medications and supplements to your healthcare provider to avoid potential interactions.

Allergies and Sensitivities

Some individuals may have allergies or sensitivities to certain herbs. When introducing new herbs, monitor for signs of allergic reactions, such as rash, itching, swelling, or difficulty breathing. Discontinue use immediately if any adverse reactions occur, and seek medical attention if necessary.

Duration of Use

Use herbs as directed and avoid prolonged or excessive use without supervision. Chronic use of certain herbs may lead to tolerance, dependency, or adverse effects on organ systems. Rotate herbs periodically or take breaks to prevent potential issues and maintain effectiveness.

Herbal Preparation Methods

Different preparation methods (e.g., teas, tinctures, and topical applications) can affect the absorption and bioavailability of herbal compounds. To achieve optimal therapeutic outcomes, follow recommended preparation guidelines and dosage instructions specific to each method.

Monitoring and Adjustments

Regularly monitor your health status and response to herbal treatments. Adjust dosages or discontinue use if symptoms persist, worsen, or new symptoms develop. Consult with a healthcare provider for guidance on adjusting herbal therapies as needed.

Storage and Shelf Life

Proper storage of herbs and herbal preparations is essential to maintain potency and safety. Store dried herbs in airtight containers in a cool, dark place away from moisture and sunlight. Check expiration dates on herbal products and discard any expired or deteriorated items.

Dosage guidelines and safety tips are fundamental aspects of responsible herbal medicine practice. By understanding appropriate dosing principles, considering individual health factors, and adhering to safety precautions, individuals can effectively harness the therapeutic benefits of herbs while minimizing potential risks. Consulting with qualified herbalists or healthcare providers ensures personalized guidance and enhances the safe and effective use of herbal remedies for promoting overall health and well-being.

Chapter 3: Recipes for specific ailments

Digestive Health

Peppermint and Ginger Tea:

Ingredients:

- 1 teaspoon dried peppermint leaves
- 1 teaspoon dried ginger root
- 1 cup boiling water

Instructions:

- Place dried peppermint leaves and dried ginger root in a teapot or mug.
- Pour boiling water over the herbs.
- Cover and steep for 10 minutes.
- Strain and drink 1-2 cups daily to relieve indigestion, bloating, and nausea.

Sleep and Relaxation

Chamomile Lavender Sleep Tincture:

Ingredients:

- 1 part dried chamomile flowers
- 1 part dried lavender flowers
- High-proof alcohol (enough to cover the herbs)

Instructions:

- Fill a glass jar halfway with dried chamomile flowers and dried lavender flowers.
- Cover the herbs with high-proof alcohol, ensuring they are fully submerged.
- Seal the jar tightly and store in a cool, dark place for 4-6 weeks, shaking daily.
- Strain the tincture through cheesecloth or a fine mesh strainer into a clean glass jar.
- Take 1-2 droppers before bedtime to promote relaxation and improve sleep quality.

Immune Support

Elderberry Syrup:

Ingredients:

- 1 cup dried elderberries
- 3 cups water
- 1 cup honey

Instructions:

- In a saucepan, combine dried elderberries and water.
- Bring to a boil, then reduce heat and simmer for 30 minutes.
- Mash the elderberries with a spoon or potato masher.
- Strain the mixture through a fine mesh strainer or cheesecloth.
- Stir in honey while the liquid is still warm.
- Store in a glass jar in the refrigerator and take 1 tablespoon daily during cold and flu season to boost immune function.

Respiratory Health

Thyme and Eucalyptus Steam Inhalation:

Ingredients:

- Handful of fresh thyme leaves or 2 tablespoons dried thyme

- 1-2 drops eucalyptus essential oil

- Boiling water

Instructions:

- Place fresh thyme leaves or dried thyme in a heatproof bowl.
- Add 1-2 drops of eucalyptus essential oil.
- Pour boiling water over the herbs and oil.
- Lean over the bowl with a towel draped over your head to trap steam.
- Inhale the steam for 5-10 minutes to clear congestion and support respiratory health.

Skin Irritations

Calendula Salve:

Ingredients:

- 1 cup dried calendula flowers

- 1 cup carrier oil (e.g., olive or almond oil)

- 1/4 cup beeswax

Instructions:

- In a clean, dry glass jar, combine dried calendula flowers and carrier oil.
- Seal the jar tightly and place in a sunny spot for 2-4 weeks, shaking daily to infuse the oil.

- Strain the oil through cheesecloth or a fine mesh strainer into a clean glass jar.
- In a double boiler, gently heat the infused oil and add beeswax.
- Stir until the beeswax is completely melted and combined with the oil.
- Pour the mixture into small jars or tins and allow to cool and solidify at room temperature.
- Apply the salve to cuts, burns, or rashes to soothe inflammation and promote healing.

Considerations

- **Dosage and Frequency**: Follow the recommended dosages and usage instructions for each recipe to ensure safety and effectiveness.

- **Individual Sensitivities**: Monitor for any allergic reactions or sensitivities to ingredients used in the recipes. Discontinue use if adverse reactions occur and consult with a healthcare provider.

- **Quality of Ingredients**: Use high-quality, organic herbs and natural ingredients to maximize therapeutic benefits and minimize exposure to contaminants.

Stress and Anxiety Relief

Lemon Balm and Passionflower Tea:

Ingredients:

- 1 teaspoon dried lemon balm leaves

- 1 teaspoon dried passionflower

- 1 cup boiling water

Instructions:

- Place dried lemon balm leaves and dried passionflower in a teapot or mug.
- Pour boiling water over the herbs.
- Cover and steep for 10-15 minutes.

- Strain and drink 1-2 cups daily to promote relaxation and alleviate stress and anxiety.

Joint Pain and Inflammation

Turmeric Golden Milk:

Ingredients:

- 1 teaspoon ground turmeric
- 1/2 teaspoon ground cinnamon
- Pinch of ground black pepper (increases turmeric absorption)
- 1 cup milk (dairy or non-dairy)
- 1 teaspoon honey (optional)

Instructions:

- In a small saucepan, whisk together turmeric, cinnamon, black pepper, and milk.
- Heat over medium-low heat until hot but not boiling, stirring occasionally.
- Remove from heat and stir in honey if desired.
- Drink warm daily to reduce joint pain and inflammation.

Menstrual Cramps

Cramp Bark and Chamomile Tea:

Ingredients:

- 1 teaspoon dried cramp bark
- 1 teaspoon dried chamomile flowers
- 1 cup boiling water

Instructions:

- Place dried cramp bark and chamomile flowers in a teapot or mug.

- Pour boiling water over the herbs.
- Cover and steep for 10-15 minutes.
- Strain and drink 1-2 cups daily during menstruation to relieve menstrual cramps and discomfort.

Headache Relief

Feverfew and Peppermint Herbal Infusion:

Ingredients:

- 1 teaspoon dried feverfew leaves
- 1 teaspoon dried peppermint leaves
- 1 cup boiling water

Instructions:

- Place dried feverfew leaves and peppermint leaves in a teapot or mug.
- Pour boiling water over the herbs.
- Cover and steep for 10-15 minutes.
- Strain and drink 1-2 cups daily as needed to alleviate headaches and migraines.

Allergy Relief

Nettle Leaf Infusion:

Ingredients:

- 1 tablespoon dried nettle leaves
- 1 cup boiling water

Instructions:

- Place dried nettle leaves in a teapot or mug.
- Pour boiling water over the herbs.
- Cover and steep for 10-15 minutes.
- Strain and drink 1-2 cups daily during allergy season to reduce allergy symptoms such as sneezing and congestion.

Book 11: Remedies for Common Ailments

Simple Solutions from Nature's Pharmacy

Chapter 1: Herbal solutions for everyday health problems

Colds and Respiratory Issues

Elderberry Syrup:

Ingredients:

- 1 cup dried elderberries
- 3 cups water
- 1 cup honey

Instructions:

- Combine elderberries and water in a saucepan.
- Bring to a boil, then reduce heat and simmer for 30 minutes.
- Mash the elderberries with a spoon or potato masher.
- Strain the mixture through a fine mesh strainer or cheesecloth.
- Stir in honey while the liquid is still warm.
- Store in a glass jar in the refrigerator.
- Take 1 tablespoon daily during cold and flu season.

Echinacea Tea:

Ingredients:

- 1 teaspoon dried echinacea root
- 1 cup boiling water

Instructions:

- Place dried echinacea root in a teapot or mug.
- Pour boiling water over the herb.
- Cover and steep for 10 minutes.
- Strain and drink 1-2 cups daily at the first sign of a cold.

Peppermint and Eucalyptus Steam Inhalation:

Ingredients:

- Handful of fresh peppermint leaves or 2 tablespoons dried peppermint
- 1-2 drops eucalyptus essential oil
- Boiling water

Instructions:

- Place peppermint and eucalyptus oil in a heatproof bowl.
- Pour boiling water over the herbs and oil.
- Lean over the bowl with a towel draped over your head to trap steam.
- Inhale the steam for 5-10 minutes to clear nasal congestion.

Digestive Problems

Ginger Tea:

Ingredients:

- 1 teaspoon grated fresh ginger

- 1 cup boiling water

Instructions:

- Place grated ginger in a teapot or mug.
- Pour boiling water over the ginger.
- Cover and steep for 10 minutes.
- Strain and drink before meals to aid digestion.

Peppermint Tea:

Ingredients:

- 1 teaspoon dried peppermint leaves
- 1 cup boiling water

Instructions:

- Place peppermint leaves in a teapot or mug.
- Pour boiling water over the leaves.
- Cover and steep for 10 minutes.
- Strain and drink after meals to relieve indigestion.

Fennel Seed Tea:

Ingredients:

- 1 teaspoon crushed fennel seeds
- 1 cup boiling water

Instructions:

- Place crushed fennel seeds in a teapot or mug.
- Pour boiling water over the seeds.
- Cover and steep for 10 minutes.
- Strain and drink to ease bloating and improve digestion.

Skin Conditions

Calendula Salve:

Ingredients:

- 1 cup dried calendula flowers
- 1 cup carrier oil (e.g., olive or almond oil)
- 1/4 cup beeswax

Instructions:

- Combine dried calendula flowers and carrier oil in a glass jar.
- Seal the jar and place it in a sunny spot for 2-4 weeks, shaking daily.
- Strain the oil through cheesecloth or a fine mesh strainer.
- Heat the infused oil with beeswax in a double boiler until melted.
- Pour the mixture into small jars or tins and allow to cool.
- Apply to cuts, burns, or rashes to soothe and heal the skin.

Aloe Vera Gel:

Ingredients:

- Fresh aloe vera leaf

Instructions:

- Cut an aloe vera leaf and scoop out the gel.
- Apply the gel directly to sunburn, minor burns, or dry skin.
- Store any unused gel in the refrigerator.

Tea Tree Oil Spot Treatment:

Ingredients:

- Tea tree essential oil
- Carrier oil (e.g., coconut or jojoba oil)

Instructions:

- Dilute tea tree oil with a carrier oil (1-2 drops of tea tree oil per teaspoon of carrier oil).
- Apply the mixture to acne spots with a cotton swab.
- Use daily until the acne clears.

Everyday Health Maintenance

Nettle Leaf Tea:

Ingredients:

- 1 tablespoon dried nettle leaves
- 1 cup boiling water

Instructions:

- Place dried nettle leaves in a teapot or mug.
- Pour boiling water over the leaves.
- Cover and steep for 10 minutes.
- Strain and drink daily to boost overall health and reduce inflammation.

Ashwagandha Tincture:

Ingredients:

- 1 part dried ashwagandha root

- High-proof alcohol (enough to cover the herbs)

Instructions:

- Fill a jar halfway with dried ashwagandha root.
- Cover the root with high-proof alcohol, ensuring it is fully submerged.
- Seal the jar and store it in a cool, dark place for 4-6 weeks, shaking daily.
- Strain the tincture through cheesecloth or a fine mesh strainer.
- Take 1-2 droppers daily to reduce stress and boost energy levels.

Turmeric Golden Milk:

Ingredients:

- 1 teaspoon ground turmeric
- 1/2 teaspoon ground cinnamon
- Pinch of black pepper
- 1 cup milk (dairy or non-dairy)
- 1 teaspoon honey (optional)

Instructions:

- In a small saucepan, whisk together ground turmeric, ground cinnamon, black pepper, and milk.
- Heat over medium-low heat until hot but not boiling.
- Stir in honey if desired.
- Drink daily to reduce inflammation and support overall health.

Insomnia and Sleep Disorders

Valerian Root Tea:

Ingredients:

- 1 teaspoon dried valerian root
- 1 cup boiling water

Instructions:

- Place dried valerian root in a teapot or mug.
- Pour boiling water over the herb.
- Cover and steep for 10-15 minutes.
- Strain and drink 30 minutes before bedtime to promote restful sleep.

Lavender Chamomile Sleep Sachet:

Ingredients:

- 1/2 cup dried lavender flowers
- 1/2 cup dried chamomile flowers
- Small cloth bag or sachet

Instructions:

- Mix dried lavender flowers and chamomile flowers together.
- Fill the small cloth bag or sachet with the mixture.
- Place the sachet under your pillow to help induce relaxation and sleep.

Boosting Energy and Combating Fatigue

Ginseng Tonic:

Ingredients:

- 1 teaspoon dried ginseng root
- 1 cup boiling water
- Honey (optional)

Instructions:

- Place dried ginseng root in a teapot or mug.
- Pour boiling water over the herb.
- Cover and steep for 10-15 minutes.
- Strain and drink in the morning to boost energy and combat fatigue.
- Add honey if desired for taste.

Rosemary and Peppermint Bath:

Ingredients:

- 1/2 cup dried rosemary
- 1/2 cup dried peppermint
- Muslin bag or cheesecloth

Instructions:

- Place dried rosemary and peppermint in a muslin bag or wrap in cheesecloth.
- Hang the bag under the hot water tap while filling the bathtub.
- Soak in the rosemary and peppermint bath for 20-30 minutes to invigorate and refresh your body.

Immune System Support

Astragalus Root Soup:

Ingredients:

- 2 tablespoons dried astragalus root
- 8 cups water
- 2 carrots, chopped
- 2 celery stalks, chopped
- 1 onion, chopped
- Salt and pepper to taste

Instructions:

- Combine dried astragalus root and water in a large pot.
- Bring to a boil, then reduce heat and simmer for 20 minutes.
- Add chopped carrots, celery, and onion.
- Simmer for another 30 minutes until vegetables are tender.
- Season with salt and pepper to taste.
- Strain out the astragalus root before serving.
- Drink the soup regularly to boost the immune system.

Reishi Mushroom Tea:

Ingredients:

- 1 tablespoon dried reishi mushroom slices
- 3 cups water

Instructions:

- Combine dried reishi mushroom slices and water in a saucepan.

- Bring to a boil, then reduce heat and simmer for 30 minutes.
- Strain the tea and drink 1 cup daily to enhance immune function.

Pain Relief

White Willow Bark Tea:

Ingredients:

- 1 teaspoon dried white willow bark
- 1 cup boiling water

Instructions:

- Place dried white willow bark in a teapot or mug.
- Pour boiling water over the herb.
- Cover and steep for 10-15 minutes.
- Strain and drink 1-2 cups daily to relieve pain and reduce inflammation.

Arnica Salve:

Ingredients:

- 1 cup dried arnica flowers
- 1 cup carrier oil (e.g., olive or coconut oil)
- 1/4 cup beeswax

Instructions:

- Infuse dried arnica flowers in carrier oil for 2-4 weeks, shaking daily.
- Strain the oil through cheesecloth or a fine mesh strainer.
- Heat the infused oil with beeswax in a double boiler until melted.
- Pour the mixture into small jars or tins and allow to cool.

- Apply to bruises, sprains, and sore muscles to reduce pain and inflammation.

Cognitive Function and Memory

Ginkgo Biloba Tea:

Ingredients:

- 1 teaspoon dried ginkgo biloba leaves
- 1 cup boiling water

Instructions:

- Place dried ginkgo biloba leaves in a teapot or mug.
- Pour boiling water over the herb.
- Cover and steep for 10-15 minutes.
- Strain and drink 1-2 cups daily to enhance cognitive function and memory.

Rosemary and Sage Infused Oil:

Ingredients:

- 1/2 cup dried rosemary
- 1/2 cup dried sage
- 1 cup carrier oil (e.g., olive or almond oil)

Instructions:

- Combine dried rosemary and sage in a glass jar.
- Cover the herbs with carrier oil.
- Seal the jar and place it in a sunny spot for 2-4 weeks, shaking daily.
- Strain the oil through cheesecloth or a fine mesh strainer.
- Massage a small amount of the infused oil into your temples and scalp to stimulate brain function and improve memory.

Chapter 2: Case studies and testimonials

Herbal remedies have a long history of use across various cultures and traditions. Both historical anecdotes and modern testimonials often support their efficacy. Here, we present several case studies and testimonials from individuals who have experienced the benefits of herbal remedies firsthand. These stories highlight the potential of herbal treatments to improve health and well-being.

Case Study 1: Overcoming Chronic Indigestion with Ginger Tea

Sarah, a 34-year-old marketing executive, had been suffering from chronic indigestion and bloating for several years. She tried numerous over-the-counter medications, but the relief was always temporary.

Upon a friend's recommendation, Sarah decided to try ginger tea. She prepared the tea by steeping one teaspoon of grated fresh ginger in a cup of boiling water for 10 minutes and drinking it before meals. It's important to note that the tea should not be too hot when consumed to avoid any potential damage to the digestive system.

Within a week, Sarah noticed significant improvements in her digestion. The bloating and discomfort she typically felt after meals were significantly reduced. After a month of regular ginger tea consumption, her chronic indigestion had almost wholly disappeared. She now incorporates ginger tea into her daily routine and reports feeling much better overall. The relief provided by the ginger tea lasted for several hours after each meal, indicating its long-lasting effectiveness.

"I was initially skeptical, but ginger tea has made a difference. I no longer dread meals, and my digestive system feels more balanced and comfortable. It's a simple and effective remedy that I highly recommend."

Case Study 2: Managing Stress with Ashwagandha Tincture

John, a 45-year-old financial analyst, struggled with high levels of stress due to his demanding job. His stress led to insomnia and a constant feeling of fatigue.

John started taking ashwagandha tincture as an adaptogenic herb known to help the body manage stress. He took one dropperful of tincture daily, diluted in a small amount of water.

After two weeks, John began to notice a reduction in his stress levels. He felt more relaxed and fell asleep more easily at night. Over the next two months, his overall well-being improved significantly, and he felt more energized during the day. This improvement in his overall well-being gave him a new sense of hope and optimism.

"Ashwagandha tincture has been a game-changer for me. It's incredible how much it has helped me manage my stress and improve my sleep. I feel more balanced and less overwhelmed by daily challenges."

Case Study 3: Treating Eczema with Calendula Salve

Emily, a 29-year-old teacher, had been battling eczema for most of her life. The itching and redness caused by the condition were persistent and uncomfortable.

Emily decided to try a natural approach with calendula salve. She applied the salve to the affected areas twice daily.

Within a few days, Emily noticed a reduction in redness and itching. After consistent use for three weeks, her eczema patches began to heal, and her skin felt more moisturized and less irritated.

"I've tried so many treatments for my eczema, but nothing worked as well as calendula salve. It's soothing, natural, and effective. My skin has never felt better, and its relief is amazing."

Case Study 4: Enhancing Immunity with Elderberry Syrup

Mike, a 52-year-old carpenter, was prone to frequent colds and respiratory infections, especially during winter.

Mike started taking elderberry syrup daily during the cold and flu season. He took one tablespoon each morning as a preventive measure.

Throughout the winter, Mike experienced fewer colds than usual. When he did catch a cold, the symptoms were milder and the duration was shorter. He credited elderberry syrup for boosting his immune system.

"Elderberry syrup has become a staple in our household. Since taking it, I've fended off colds much more effectively. It's a natural remedy that truly works."

Case Study 5: Relieving Pain with White Willow Bark Tea

Linda, a 60-year-old retiree, suffered from chronic joint pain due to arthritis. Traditional pain medications provided relief but came with unwanted side effects.

Linda began drinking white willow bark tea twice a day. She prepared the tea by steeping one teaspoon of dried white willow bark in a cup of boiling water for 10-15 minutes.

After a week, Linda noticed a reduction in her pain levels. Over the next month, the tea helped manage her arthritis symptoms more effectively than some of the medications she had been taking.

"White willow bark tea has been a fantastic natural alternative for managing my arthritis pain. It's gentle on my stomach and provides consistent relief. I'm so grateful for this herbal remedy."

Case Study 6: Reducing Anxiety with Lavender Essential Oil

Rebecca, a 38-year-old software engineer, experienced high levels of anxiety, particularly during work deadlines. This anxiety often manifested as physical symptoms, such as a racing heart and difficulty concentrating.

Rebecca began using lavender essential oil for aromatherapy. She added a few drops to her diffuser and inhaled the scent for 30 minutes each evening.

After a week, Rebecca noticed a marked reduction in her anxiety levels. The calming effect of lavender helped her feel more relaxed and better manage stress. Her physical symptoms of anxiety also diminished.

"Lavender essential oil has been incredibly soothing. It helps me unwind after a stressful day and significantly reduces my anxiety. I highly recommend it to anyone looking for a natural way to manage stress."

Case Study 7: Improving Digestive Health with Peppermint Tea

Thomas, a 50-year-old chef, struggled with frequent episodes of indigestion and gas, especially after heavy meals. This discomfort affected his daily activities and overall well-being.

Thomas started drinking peppermint tea after meals. He prepared the tea by steeping one teaspoon of dried peppermint leaves in a cup of boiling water for 10 minutes.

Within a few days, Thomas experienced a noticeable improvement in his digestion. The tea helped reduce gas and discomfort, making it easier for him to enjoy his meals and perform his duties as a chef. The relief from discomfort was a welcome change for Thomas, making his days more bearable.

"Peppermint tea has been a lifesaver for my digestion. It's simple to make and effective at easing discomfort after meals. I feel much better and more energized throughout the day."

Case Study 8: Alleviating Menstrual Cramps with Chamomile Tea

Jessica, a 26-year-old student, suffered from severe menstrual cramps that often disrupted her studies and daily life. Over-the-counter pain relievers provided limited relief.

Jessica began drinking chamomile tea during her menstrual cycle. She prepared the tea by steeping two teaspoons of dried chamomile flowers in a cup of boiling water for 15 minutes.

Jessica found that chamomile tea significantly reduced her menstrual cramps. The soothing effect of the tea also helped improve her mood and overall comfort during her period.

"Chamomile tea has been wonderful for my menstrual cramps. It's not only effective but also calming, which helps me get through the day more comfortably. I no longer rely on painkillers as much as I used to."

Case Study 9: Enhancing Skin Health with Aloe Vera Gel

Megan, a 42-year-old office manager, had persistent issues with dry skin and occasional sunburns, which were difficult to manage with regular moisturizers.

Megan started using fresh aloe vera gel directly on her skin. She cut an aloe vera leaf, scooped out the gel, and applied it to the affected areas.

Megan noticed a significant improvement in her skin's hydration and overall health. The aloe vera gel helped soothe her sunburns and kept her skin moisturized and smooth.

"Aloe vera gel has made a huge difference for my skin. It's incredibly hydrating and soothing, especially after sun exposure. I use it daily, and my skin has never felt better."

Case Study 10: Easing Muscle Soreness with Arnica Salve

Mark, a 35-year-old fitness trainer, experienced frequent muscle soreness and minor injuries due to his intense workout regimen. Traditional pain relief methods were not always effective or convenient.

Mark began using arnica salve on his sore muscles and minor injuries. He applied the salve twice daily to the affected areas.

Within days, Mark felt a significant reduction in muscle soreness and faster recovery from minor injuries. The arnica salve provided effective pain relief and helped him maintain his fitness routine.

"Arnica salve has been fantastic for my muscle soreness. It's easy to apply and works quickly to reduce pain and inflammation. It's a must-have for anyone who exercises regularly."

Case Study 11: Combating Cold Symptoms with Echinacea Tea

Sophia, a 29-year-old teacher, frequently caught colds due to her constant exposure to germs in the classroom. These colds often led to missed work and general discomfort.

Sophia started drinking echinacea tea at the first sign of a cold. She prepared the tea by steeping one teaspoon of dried echinacea root in a cup of boiling water for 10 minutes.

Sophia found that echinacea tea helped shorten the duration and severity of her colds. She missed fewer work days and felt better equipped to manage her symptoms.

"Echinacea tea has been a great addition to my routine. It helps me bounce back quickly when I feel a cold coming on. I feel healthier and more resilient against infections."

These case studies and testimonials provide compelling evidence of the effectiveness of herbal remedies in addressing various health issues. The experiences of these individuals demonstrate the potential benefits of incorporating herbal treatments into daily routines. While individual results may vary, these stories highlight the positive impact that natural remedies can have on health and well-being. Always consult a healthcare provider before starting any new treatment to ensure it is appropriate for your health needs.

Book 12: Detox and Cleanse with Barbara O'Neill's Methods

Revitalize Your Health with Natural Detox Strategies and Holistic Wellness Practices

Chapter 1: Understanding Detoxification

1.1 What is Detoxification?

Detoxification, in the context of natural healing and wellness, refers to eliminating toxins and waste products from the body. It is a fundamental principle in Barbara O'Neill's approach to health, emphasizing the body's innate ability to cleanse and heal itself through natural methods. Detoxification is not just a physical process but also encompasses mental, emotional, and spiritual aspects, aiming to restore balance and promote overall well-being.

Physical Detoxification:

Elimination of Toxins: The body accumulates toxins from various sources, including environmental pollutants, processed foods, medications, and metabolic by-products. Detoxification processes such as liver metabolism, kidney filtration, and intestinal elimination are essential for removing these toxins from the bloodstream and organs.

Supporting Organs: Detoxification supports the organs involved in toxin elimination, primarily the liver, kidneys, lungs, skin, and digestive system. These organs work synergistically to neutralize and eliminate toxins through sweat, urine, feces, and exhalation.

Methods of Detoxification:

Nutritional Support: A diet rich in antioxidants, vitamins, minerals, and fiber supports detoxification by providing essential nutrients for metabolic processes and enhancing the body's natural detox pathways.

Hydration: Adequate hydration with water and herbal teas promotes kidney function and helps flush toxins from the body. Hydration is essential for maintaining optimal detoxification processes.

Emotional and Mental Detoxification:

Stress Management: Chronic stress can impair detoxification pathways and contribute to toxin accumulation. Practices such as mindfulness, meditation, and deep breathing support mental and emotional detoxification by reducing stress hormone levels.

Healthy Relationships: Cultivating supportive relationships and addressing emotional traumas are integral to mental detoxification. Emotional well-being influences overall health and detoxification capacity.

Spiritual Detoxification:

Mind-Body Connection: Practices that enhance the mind-body connection, such as yoga, tai chi, and qigong, facilitate spiritual detoxification by promoting energy flow, emotional release, and spiritual alignment.

Nature Connection: Spending time in nature and connecting with the natural environment promotes spiritual detoxification by fostering a sense of grounding, peace, and harmony with the Earth.

Benefits of Detoxification:

Improved Energy Levels: By reducing the burden of toxins on the body, detoxification enhances energy production and vitality.

Enhanced Immune Function: Supporting detoxification pathways strengthens the immune system's ability to defend against infections and diseases.

1.2 The Body's Natural Detox Systems

The human body possesses sophisticated natural detoxification systems designed to eliminate toxins and maintain optimal health. Understanding these systems is fundamental to Barbara O'Neill's approach to natural healing, emphasizing the importance of supporting and enhancing these innate processes.

Liver Detoxification:

Metabolic Cleansing: The liver is the primary organ responsible for detoxification. It metabolizes toxins into less harmful substances that can be excreted through bile or urine. This phase involves enzymatic reactions that break down toxins into water-soluble compounds for easier elimination.

Nutrient Support: Essential nutrients such as vitamins B, C, E and minerals like zinc and selenium support liver detoxification pathways. These nutrients act as cofactors for enzymes involved in detoxification processes.

Kidney Filtration:

Blood Filtration: The kidneys filter waste products, excess minerals, and toxins from the bloodstream, regulating water and electrolyte balance. They excrete toxins through urine, ensuring the body maintains proper fluid and electrolyte levels.

Hydration Importance: Adequate hydration supports kidney function by facilitating urine production and flushing out toxins. Water and herbal teas are essential for maintaining optimal kidney filtration and detoxification.

Intestinal Elimination:

Digestive Clearance: The gastrointestinal tract plays a crucial role in detoxification by eliminating waste products and toxins through bowel movements. Fiber-rich foods support regular bowel movements, preventing the reabsorption of toxins into the bloodstream.

Microbiome Balance: A healthy gut microbiome supports detoxification by metabolizing toxins, producing vitamins, and enhancing nutrient absorption. Probiotics and prebiotics promote a balanced microbiome, aiding in intestinal detoxification.

Lymphatic System:

Toxin Transport: The lymphatic system transports cellular waste, toxins, and pathogens through lymphatic vessels and nodes. Lymphatic drainage techniques, exercise, and hydration support lymphatic circulation and detoxification.

Immune Support: The lymphatic system plays a vital role in immune function, helping to defend against infections and supporting overall immune health through detoxification.

Skin Detoxification:

Sweat Secretion: The skin eliminates toxins through sweat glands, regulating body temperature and removing metabolic waste products. Regular exercise, saunas, and dry brushing support skin detoxification by promoting sweating and toxin excretion.

Barrier Function: Maintaining skin health and integrity is crucial for effective detoxification. Proper hygiene, moisturizing, and avoiding harsh chemicals support the skin's barrier function and detoxification capabilities.

Respiratory System:

Gas Exchange: The respiratory system removes carbon dioxide and volatile toxins through breathing. Deep breathing exercises, fresh air exposure, and air purification enhance respiratory detoxification and support lung health.

Air Quality: Avoiding environmental pollutants and secondhand smoke protects respiratory health and supports natural detoxification processes through improved air quality.

The body's natural detoxification systems work synergistically to eliminate toxins and maintain health. Barbara O'Neill's holistic approach emphasizes supporting liver function, kidney filtration, intestinal health, lymphatic circulation, skin detoxification, and respiratory detoxification through nutrition, hydration, exercise, and mindful practices. Understanding and enhancing these natural detox systems are key to promoting longevity, vitality, and overall well-being in natural healing practices.

1.3 Benefits of Regular Detox Practices

Regular detox practices, such as fasting, dietary changes, and herbal supplements, offer many benefits that support overall health and well-being, aligning with Barbara O'Neill's holistic approach to natural healing. These practices aim to enhance the body's natural detoxification processes and promote the optimal functioning of organs and systems for eliminating toxins.

1. Enhanced Energy Levels: Regular detoxification helps reduce the burden of toxins on the body, allowing organs like the liver and kidneys to function more efficiently. This efficiency translates into increased energy production, promoting vitality and reducing feelings of fatigue. [Reference to a study on the effects of detoxification on energy levels].

2. Improved Digestive Health: Detox practices such as dietary changes and herbal supplements can support gastrointestinal health by promoting regular bowel movements, reducing bloating, and improving nutrient absorption. Removing toxins from the intestines supports a healthy microbiome balance, which is crucial for overall digestive function.

3. Strengthened Immune System: Supporting detoxification pathways enhances immune function by reducing the load of toxins that can compromise immune response. A healthy immune system helps defend against infections and supports overall resilience to illness.

4. Clearer Skin and Radiant Complexion: Detoxifying the body can lead to clearer skin and a more radiant complexion by eliminating toxins contributing to skin issues like acne, eczema, and inflammation. Skin detoxification practices such as sweating through exercise or saunas can also improve skin appearance.

5. Weight Management Support: Detox practices often include dietary adjustments and increased physical activity, which can contribute to weight loss and weight management goals. Detoxification may support metabolic processes and promote a healthy weight by eliminating toxins and reducing inflammation.

6. Mental Clarity and Emotional Balance: Toxins can affect cognitive function and mood stability. Detox practices that support liver health and reduce toxin exposure play a crucial role in promoting a sense of balance, contributing to improved mental clarity, enhanced focus, and emotional balance.

7. Enhanced Respiratory Function: Detoxification practices that support lung health, such as deep breathing exercises and avoiding environmental pollutants, can enhance respiratory function. Clearing toxins from the respiratory system supports efficient oxygen exchange and overall lung health.

8. Hormonal Balance: Certain toxins can disrupt hormone balance in the body. Detox practices that support liver function and reduce exposure to endocrine-disrupting chemicals may help maintain hormonal balance and support reproductive health.

9. Overall Vitality and Longevity: Regular detox practices contribute to overall vitality and longevity by reducing the toxic burden on organs and systems. Supporting the body's natural detoxification processes not only helps maintain optimal health but also leaves you feeling refreshed and revitalized, ready to take on life's challenges.

Chapter 2: Preparing for a Detox

2.1 Assessing Your Current Health

Assessing your current health is a crucial step in Barbara O'Neill's holistic approach to natural healing, providing a foundation for understanding your body's needs and implementing effective wellness practices. This assessment involves evaluating various aspects of physical, mental, and emotional well-being to identify areas for improvement and develop personalized health goals.

1. Physical Health Assessment: Begin by evaluating your physical health through a comprehensive review of your body's systems and functions. Consider factors such as:

- Nutritional Status: Assess your diet for balance, adequacy of essential nutrients, and potential deficiencies. Consider consulting with a nutritionist or dietitian for a detailed dietary analysis.

- Physical Activity: Evaluate your exercise routine and overall physical fitness level. Assess whether you are meeting recommended guidelines for aerobic exercise, strength training, and flexibility.

- Medical History: Review your medical history, including chronic conditions, past surgeries, and current medications. Identify any health concerns or symptoms that may require attention.

- Vital Signs: Monitor your vital signs, including blood pressure, heart rate, and cholesterol levels. Regular health screenings can provide valuable insights into your cardiovascular health and metabolic function.

- Body Composition: Assess your body composition, including body mass index (BMI), percentage of body fat, and muscle mass. Understanding your body composition helps set realistic weight management goals.

2. Mental and Emotional Well-being: Evaluate your mental and emotional well-being to assess stress levels, emotional resilience, and overall psychological health:

- Stress Management: Identify sources of stress in your life and assess your coping mechanisms. Practice stress-reduction techniques such as mindfulness meditation, deep breathing exercises, or journaling.

- Sleep Patterns: Evaluate your sleep quality and duration. Poor sleep can impact mental clarity, mood stability, and overall well-being. Establish a bedtime routine and create a sleep-friendly environment.

- Emotional Balance: Assess your emotional state and identify any symptoms of anxiety, depression, or mood disorders. Seek support from a mental health professional if needed to address emotional challenges effectively.

3. Lifestyle Habits and Environmental Factors: Evaluate your lifestyle habits and environmental factors that may impact your health:

- Smoking and Alcohol Consumption: Assess your habits regarding smoking and alcohol consumption. Consider cessation programs or strategies to reduce intake if necessary.

- Environmental Exposures: Identify potential environmental toxins or pollutants in your home and workplace. Take steps to minimize exposure and enhance indoor air quality.

- Hydration and Nutrition: Evaluate your daily intake of water and nutrient-rich foods. Ensure adequate hydration and consume a balanced diet rich in fruits, vegetables, whole grains, and lean proteins.

4. Social and Support Networks: Assess your social connections and support networks, which play a vital role in overall well-being:

- Social Relationships: Evaluate the quality of your relationships with family, friends, and community members. Cultivate supportive relationships that contribute positively to your emotional health.

- Support Systems: Identify sources of support during challenging times, such as family members, friends, or support groups. Maintain open communication and seek assistance when needed.

5. Holistic Health Perspective: Consider a holistic health perspective that integrates physical, mental, emotional, and spiritual dimensions of well-being:

- Mind-Body Connection: Evaluate practices that promote mind-body harmony, such as yoga, tai chi, or meditation. These practices enhance overall resilience and well-being.

- Spiritual Well-being: Assess your sense of purpose, values, and spiritual beliefs. Engage in activities that nurture your spiritual health and promote a sense of meaning in life.

2.2 Setting Realistic Goals for Detox

Setting realistic goals for detox is essential in Barbara O'Neill's approach to natural healing, emphasizing gradual and sustainable changes to support the body's detoxification processes effectively. Whether you're embarking on a short-term detox program or integrating detox practices into your daily life, establishing achievable goals ensures you stay motivated and experience meaningful health improvements.

1. Identify Your Motivation: Begin by identifying your reasons for pursuing detoxification. Whether it's to improve energy levels, support weight management, enhance skin health, or promote overall well-being, understanding your motivations provides a foundation for setting meaningful goals.

2. Start with Small Steps: Set achievable goals that align with your current lifestyle and health status. Begin with small changes, such as increasing water intake, incorporating more fruits and vegetables into your diet, or reducing processed foods and sugar. Gradually build upon these changes to create sustainable habits.

3. Define Specific Objectives: Outline specific detox objectives based on your personal health assessment. For example, you may aim to eliminate caffeine or alcohol for a specified period, increase daily physical activity, or implement regular relaxation practices to reduce stress levels.

4. Consider Timeframes and Milestones: Establish realistic timeframes for achieving your detox goals. Break down larger objectives into smaller milestones to track progress and celebrate achievements along the way. For instance, set weekly or monthly targets for reducing intake of refined sugars or completing a certain number of exercise sessions.

5. Focus on Balanced Nutrition: Prioritize nutrition goals that support detoxification, such as consuming a variety of nutrient-dense foods, incorporating herbal teas or detoxifying herbs, and emphasizing whole foods over processed options. Aim for a balanced diet that includes adequate fiber, vitamins, and minerals to support liver and kidney function.

6. Incorporate Detox Practices: Integrate detox practices into your daily routine, such as dry brushing to stimulate lymphatic circulation, practicing deep breathing exercises for respiratory detoxification, or scheduling regular sauna sessions to promote sweat-based detoxification. Consistency is key to maximizing the benefits of detox practices.

7. Monitor and Adjust as Needed: Regularly assess your progress towards achieving detox goals and make adjustments as needed. Pay attention to how your body responds to detox practices and modify your approach based on feedback from your health assessment and personal experiences.

8. Seek Professional Guidance if Necessary: Consult with a healthcare provider, nutritionist, or holistic practitioner for personalized guidance and support in setting detox goals. They can provide expert advice, recommend appropriate detox protocols, and address any health concerns or specific dietary needs.

2.3 Creating a Supportive Environment

Creating a supportive environment is crucial in Barbara O'Neill's approach to natural healing and detoxification, as it enhances the effectiveness of detox practices and promotes overall well-being. A supportive environment encompasses physical, social, and emotional aspects that foster a healthy lifestyle and encourage positive health outcomes.

1. Physical Environment: Ensure your physical surroundings support detox goals by creating a clean, toxin-free space at home and work. Consider the following:

- Air Quality: Improve indoor air quality by ventilating spaces, using air purifiers, and reducing exposure to pollutants such as cigarette smoke and household chemicals.

- Toxin-Free Living: Choose natural cleaning products, cosmetics, and personal care items free from harmful chemicals like parabens, phthalates, and synthetic fragrances.

- Organic Foods: Opt for organic produce and minimize exposure to pesticides and additives in your diet.

2. Nutrient-Rich Diet: Support detoxification by stocking your kitchen with nutrient-dense foods that promote liver health and overall wellness:

- Whole Foods: Emphasize fresh fruits, vegetables, whole grains, lean proteins, and healthy fats to provide essential vitamins, minerals, and antioxidants.

- Hydration: Keep filtered water and herbal teas readily available to support kidney function and flush out toxins from the body.

3. Social Support: Surround yourself with supportive relationships and communities that encourage healthy habits and positive lifestyle choices:

- Family and Friends: Engage in activities that promote well-being, such as outdoor walks, cooking nutritious meals together, or practicing relaxation techniques.

- Support Groups: Join local or online support groups focused on detoxification, nutrition, or holistic health to share experiences and receive encouragement.

4. Emotional Well-being: Prioritize mental and emotional health practices that reduce stress and promote relaxation:

- Stress Management: Practice mindfulness, meditation, yoga, or deep breathing exercises to reduce cortisol levels and support adrenal health.

- Work-Life Balance: Establish boundaries between work and personal life to prevent burnout and prioritize self-care activities.

5. Physical Activity: Incorporate regular exercise into your routine to support lymphatic circulation, cardiovascular health, and overall detoxification:

- Movement: Choose activities you enjoy, such as walking, jogging, swimming, or yoga, to promote sweat-based detoxification and enhance mood.

6. Holistic Practices: Integrate holistic practices that promote mind-body harmony and support detoxification:

- Massage Therapy: Schedule regular massages to stimulate lymphatic drainage and promote relaxation.

- Acupuncture or Acupressure: Consider alternative therapies that support energy flow and overall well-being.

7. Education and Awareness: Stay informed about detoxification techniques, nutritional strategies, and holistic health practices to make informed decisions:

- Continued Learning: Attend workshops, read books, or listen to podcasts related to natural healing and detoxification.

- Personal Growth: Reflect on your health journey, celebrate achievements, and set new goals to maintain motivation and progress.

Chapter 3: Dietary Detoxification

3.1 Detox Diet Principles

Detox diets are centered around principles that support the body's natural detoxification processes and promote overall health and vitality. Barbara O'Neill emphasizes these principles to guide individuals in adopting a detox diet that enhances well-being through nutrient-dense foods, hydration, and mindful eating practices.

1. Whole, Plant-Based Foods: Emphasize a diet rich in whole, plant-based foods such as fruits, vegetables, legumes, nuts, seeds, and whole grains. These foods are high in fiber, vitamins, minerals, and antioxidants, supporting liver function and promoting overall health.

2. Hydration: Drink plenty of water throughout the day. Water supports kidney function and helps flush out toxins from the body. Herbal teas and infused water also benefit hydration and add variety to your beverage choices.

3. Organic and Chemical-Free: Choose organic produce whenever possible to minimize exposure to pesticides, herbicides, and synthetic fertilizers. Opt for chemical-free cleaning products, cosmetics, and personal care items to reduce toxin intake through environmental sources.

4. Nutrient Density: Focus on nutrient-dense foods that provide essential vitamins (like vitamin C and B vitamins) and minerals (such as magnesium and zinc) that support detoxification pathways. Incorporate a variety of colorful fruits and vegetables to maximize antioxidant intake and promote cellular health.

5. Lean Proteins: Include lean protein sources such as legumes, tofu, tempeh, and lean cuts of poultry or fish. Protein is essential for tissue repair and supports liver function in processing toxins. Choose organic and sustainably sourced options when possible.

6. Limit Processed Foods and Sugars: Minimize consumption of processed foods, refined sugars, and artificial additives that contribute to inflammation and burden the liver. Opt for natural sweeteners like honey or maple syrup in moderation, and choose whole grains over refined grains.

7. Detoxifying Herbs and Spices: Incorporate detoxifying herbs and spices into your meals, such as turmeric, ginger, garlic, cilantro, and parsley. These culinary ingredients support liver detoxification pathways and add flavor and nutritional benefits to dishes.

8. Balanced Macronutrients: Maintain a balanced ratio of macronutrients (carbohydrates, proteins, and fats) to support overall health and energy levels. Include healthy fats from sources like avocado, nuts, seeds, and olive oil to promote satiety and support cellular function.

9. Mindful Eating Practices: Practice mindful eating by paying attention to hunger and fullness cues, chewing food thoroughly, and savoring the flavors and textures of your meals. Mindful eating promotes digestion, nutrient absorption, and overall enjoyment of food.

10. Consider Individual Needs: Tailor your detox diet to meet your individual health needs, preferences, and goals. Consult with a healthcare provider or nutritionist for personalized guidance, especially if you have specific dietary restrictions, medical conditions, or nutritional concerns.

3.2 Importance of Whole Foods and Hydration

In Barbara O'Neill's approach to natural healing and detoxification, the importance of whole foods and hydration cannot be overstated. These foundational principles support the body's detoxification processes and promote overall health and vitality.

1. Nutrient Density and Support for Detoxification: Whole foods, such as fruits, vegetables, whole grains, nuts, seeds, and legumes, are rich in essential nutrients like vitamins, minerals, antioxidants, and dietary fiber. These nutrients play a crucial role in supporting liver function, which is central to detoxification. Antioxidants, for example, help neutralize free radicals and reduce oxidative stress on cells, while fiber supports digestive health and promotes regular bowel movements, aiding in the elimination of toxins from the body.

2. Hydration and Kidney Function: Proper hydration is essential for kidney function and plays a vital role in detoxification. Water helps flush out toxins through urine, maintaining kidney health and supporting the body's natural filtration system. Additionally, staying well-hydrated ensures optimal cellular function, promotes healthy skin, and helps regulate body temperature. Herbal teas and infused water can also contribute to hydration while providing additional health benefits through their antioxidant and phytonutrient content.

3. Reduction of Toxin Load: Whole foods are typically free from additives, preservatives, and artificial ingredients commonly found in processed foods. Individuals choose whole foods to reduce their exposure to toxins and chemicals that can burden the liver and other detoxification organs. Organic produce further minimizes exposure to pesticides and synthetic fertilizers, supporting overall health and reducing environmental impact.

4. Sustainable Energy and Vitality: The balanced nutrients found in whole foods provide sustained energy levels and support overall vitality. Unlike refined sugars and processed foods, which can lead to energy crashes and spikes in blood sugar levels, whole foods provide a steady energy source and promote stable mood and concentration throughout the day. Healthy fats from sources like avocado, nuts, and olive oil contribute to satiety and support brain health.

5. Mindful Eating and Digestive Health: Practicing mindful eating, such as chewing food thoroughly and savoring each bite, enhances digestion and nutrient absorption. This cautious approach to eating supports gastrointestinal health and ensures that the body efficiently utilizes the nutrients from whole foods. A well-functioning digestive system is essential for detoxification, as it helps eliminate waste and toxins from the body effectively.

Incorporating whole foods and maintaining adequate hydration are fundamental aspects of Barbara O'Neill's holistic approach to natural healing and detoxification. By prioritizing nutrient-dense foods and mindful eating practices, individuals support their body's detoxification processes, promote overall health, and sustain long-term vitality. These foundational principles contribute to physical well-being and enhance mental clarity, emotional balance, and overall quality of life.

3.3 Foods to Include and Avoid

By choosing nutrient-dense options and steering clear of substances that burden the body, individuals cannot only optimize their health and vitality but also feel inspired and motivated by the benefits of their dietary choices.

1. Foods to Include:

a. Fresh Fruits and Vegetables: Incorporate a variety of colorful fruits and vegetables rich in vitamins, minerals, antioxidants, and fiber. Examples include leafy greens like spinach and kale, berries, citrus fruits, cruciferous vegetables such as broccoli and Brussels sprouts, and vibrant peppers.

b. Whole Grains: Opt for whole grains like quinoa, brown rice, oats, and whole wheat, which provide complex carbohydrates for sustained energy and fiber to support digestive health.

c. Lean Proteins: Choose lean protein sources such as poultry, fish, tofu, tempeh, legumes (beans and lentils), and nuts/seeds. Protein supports muscle repair, immune function, and overall cellular health.

d. Healthy Fats: Incorporate sources of healthy fats such as avocados, nuts, seeds, olive oil, and fatty fish (like salmon and sardines). These fats provide essential fatty acids that support brain function, cardiovascular health, and cellular integrity.

e. Herbal Teas: Include herbal teas such as chamomile, ginger, peppermint, and dandelion root, which offer hydration and may provide additional health benefits, including digestive support and antioxidant properties.

2. Foods to Avoid:

It's crucial to minimize the consumption of processed foods, which are often high in refined sugars, artificial additives, and trans fats. Being aware of the negative effects of these substances can help individuals make more cautious and informed dietary choices.

b. Sugary Beverages: Limit or avoid sugary drinks such as sodas, energy drinks, and sweetened beverages, leading to blood sugar spikes, weight gain, and increased risk of chronic diseases.

c. Excessive Alcohol: Reduce alcohol consumption, as it can impair liver function and contribute to oxidative stress. If consumed, opt for moderation and consider alcohol-free periods to support detoxification.

d. High-Sodium Foods: Cut back on foods high in sodium, such as processed meats, canned soups, and salty snacks. High sodium intake can lead to water retention, elevated blood pressure, and kidney strain.

By choosing organic produce whenever possible, individuals can take control of their health and reduce their exposure to pesticides and synthetic chemicals that may interfere with detoxification pathways and overall health.

3.4 Juice Fasting and Smoothie Cleanses

These practices involve consuming nutrient-rich juices or blended smoothies made from fresh fruits, vegetables, and herbs for a specified period, providing concentrated vitamins, minerals, antioxidants, and phytonutrients while allowing the digestive system to rest.

1. Juice Fasting: Juice fasting typically involves consuming freshly squeezed juices from fruits, vegetables, and herbs for a limited duration, ranging from a few days to several weeks. This practice provides essential nutrients in an easily digestible form, supporting detoxification pathways without the need for solid foods. Juice fasting is believed to allow the digestive system to rest, redirecting energy towards cellular repair and elimination of toxins.

2. Benefits of Juice Fasting:

- **Nutrient Absorption:** Juices deliver a concentrated dose of vitamins, minerals, and antioxidants directly into the bloodstream, promoting cellular repair and supporting immune function.

- **Hydration:** Juices are hydrating and help flush toxins from the body, supporting kidney function and maintaining electrolyte balance.

- **Weight Management:** Juice fasting may aid in weight loss by reducing calorie intake while providing essential nutrients, promoting detoxification, and supporting metabolism.

- **Digestive Rest:** By eliminating solid foods, juice fasting allows the digestive system to rest and may alleviate digestive discomfort or bloating.

3. Smoothie Cleanses: Smoothie cleanses involve consuming blended mixtures of fruits, vegetables, nuts, seeds, and superfoods like spirulina or chia seeds. These nutrient-dense beverages provide fiber and protein, promoting satiety and supporting detoxification while maintaining energy levels throughout the cleanse.

4. Benefits of Smoothie Cleanses:

- **Fiber Content:** Smoothies retain fiber from whole fruits and vegetables, promoting digestive health, regulating blood sugar levels, and supporting bowel regularity.

- **Sustained Energy:** Blended smoothies provide a steady release of nutrients and energy, reducing cravings and supporting overall vitality during the cleanse.

- **Customization:** Smoothie recipes can be customized with ingredients like leafy greens, ginger, turmeric, and probiotic-rich foods to enhance detoxification, support immune function, and promote gut health.

5. Considerations and Precautions:

- **Nutrient Balance:** While juice fasting and smoothie cleanses offer concentrated nutrients, they may lack sufficient protein, fats, and some essential nutrients found in whole foods. Consider incorporating small amounts of protein-rich foods like nuts, seeds, or plant-based proteins to maintain nutrient balance.

- **Duration:** Consult with a healthcare professional before embarking on an extended juice fast or cleanse, especially if you have underlying health conditions or are pregnant or nursing.

- **Hydration:** Drink plenty of water alongside juices and smoothies to support hydration and aid in detoxification.

When practiced mindfully and with consideration for individual health needs, these methods can contribute to overall well-being, enhance detoxification processes, and support sustainable health practices.

Chapter 4: Herbal Detox Remedies

4.1 Key Herbs for Detoxification

1. Dandelion Root: Known for its liver-cleansing properties, dandelion root stimulates bile production and enhances liver function, supporting the breakdown and elimination of toxins from the body. It can be consumed as a tea or supplement to promote detoxification and digestive health.

2. Milk Thistle: Milk thistle contains a compound called silymarin, which protects liver cells from damage and supports regeneration. It is commonly used to promote liver detoxification and may help alleviate symptoms of liver conditions such as fatty liver disease and hepatitis.

3. Turmeric: Renowned for its anti-inflammatory and antioxidant properties, turmeric contains curcumin, which supports liver detoxification pathways and helps reduce inflammation throughout the body. It can be used fresh or in powdered form in cooking or as a supplement.

4. Ginger: Ginger aids digestion, reduces inflammation, and supports detoxification by stimulating circulation and promoting sweating, which helps eliminate toxins through the skin. It can be consumed fresh, as a tea, or added to meals for its spicy and aromatic flavor.

5. Cilantro: Cilantro (coriander) helps remove heavy metals from the body, acting as a natural chelator to bind to toxic metals and facilitate their elimination through urine and feces. It is often used fresh in salads, soups, or smoothies for its detoxifying benefits.

6. Parsley: Rich in vitamins A, C, and K, as well as folate and iron, parsley supports kidney function and helps eliminate toxins through urine. It can be added to dishes as a garnish or incorporated into juices and smoothies for its cleansing properties.

7. Burdock Root: Burdock root is valued for its blood-purifying properties and supports liver detoxification. It contains antioxidants and prebiotic fibers that promote digestive health and elimination of waste products from the body. Burdock root can be consumed as a tea, in soups, or as a supplement.

8. Peppermint: Peppermint aids digestion, relieves bloating, and supports detoxification by calming the digestive tract and promoting bile flow. It can be consumed as a tea or added to dishes for its refreshing taste and digestive benefits.

9. Fenugreek: Fenugreek seeds are rich in fiber and antioxidants, supporting digestive health and detoxification by promoting bowel regularity and removing waste products from the body. Fenugreek can be used as a spice in cooking or taken as a supplement.

10. Garlic: Garlic contains sulfur compounds that support liver detoxification pathways and enhance immune function. It has antimicrobial properties and may help eliminate toxins and harmful bacteria from the body. Garlic can be used fresh in cooking or as a supplement.

Incorporating these key herbs into daily routines can support the body's natural detoxification processes, enhance liver function, and promote overall health and vitality. Barbara O'Neill's approach emphasizes the therapeutic benefits of these herbs in supporting detoxification, reducing inflammation, and promoting optimal wellness through natural healing practices.

4.2 How to Prepare and Use Herbal Detox Teas

Herbal detox teas are instrumental in supporting the body's natural cleansing processes and promoting overall health. Crafted from a blend of herbs renowned for their detoxification properties, these teas offer a convenient and enjoyable way to integrate natural healing into daily routines.

1. Selecting Herbs: Choose high-quality organic herbs known for their detoxifying benefits. Common choices include dandelion root, burdock root, milk thistle, ginger, turmeric, cilantro, parsley, peppermint, fenugreek, and garlic. Each herb contributes unique properties that support liver function, aid digestion, and promote toxin elimination.

2. Preparation Methods:

- **Infusion Method:** Use this method for delicate herbs like peppermint, parsley, and cilantro. Bring water to a boil and pour over fresh or dried herbs in a heat-safe container. Cover and steep for 5-10 minutes, then strain and enjoy.

- **Decoction Method:** Suitable for tougher roots and seeds such as dandelion root, burdock root, and fenugreek. Simmer herbs in water over low heat for 15-20 minutes to extract their medicinal properties. Strain and drink warm or cold.

3. Blending Teas: Experiment with different combinations of herbs to create custom blends tailored to specific detoxification goals. For example, combine dandelion root, burdock root, and milk thistle for a liver-supporting blend, or mix ginger, turmeric, and garlic for an anti-inflammatory and immune-boosting blend.

4. Incorporating Teas into Daily Routine:

- **Morning Ritual:** Start the day with a cup of herbal detox tea to kickstart metabolism, support digestion, and hydrate the body after sleep.

- **Between Meals:** Sip on herbal teas between meals to curb cravings, stay hydrated, and support detoxification throughout the day.

- **Evening Relaxation:** Wind down in the evening with a soothing herbal tea blend to promote relaxation, aid digestion, and prepare the body for restorative sleep.

5. Enhancing Tea Benefits:

- **Lemon:** Add a squeeze of fresh lemon juice to herbal teas to enhance detoxification benefits and boost vitamin C content.

- **Honey or Stevia:** Sweeten herbal teas naturally with raw honey or stevia for added flavor without compromising health benefits.

- **Cold Brew:** Prepare herbal teas using the cold brew method for a refreshing alternative during warmer months, preserving delicate flavors and nutrients.

6. Consistency and Moderation: To experience the full benefits of herbal detox teas, consume them consistently as part of a balanced diet and healthy lifestyle. However, avoid excessive consumption, particularly if you have underlying health conditions or are pregnant or nursing. Consult with a healthcare provider before starting any new herbal regimen.

Herbal detox teas provide a natural and effective way to support detoxification, enhance liver function, and promote overall well-being. By selecting quality herbs, experimenting with blends, and integrating teas into daily routines, individuals can harness the therapeutic benefits to optimize health and vitality.

4.3 Making Herbal Detox Tinctures and Tonics

Creating herbal detox tinctures and tonics is a powerful method to harness the cleansing properties of herbs recommended for detoxification. These preparations offer concentrated forms of medicinal plants that can support liver function, aid digestion, and promote overall wellness.

1. Choosing Herbs: Select herbs known for their detoxifying benefits, such as dandelion root, milk thistle, burdock root, turmeric, ginger, and cilantro. Each herb brings unique properties that enhance detoxification pathways and support the body's natural cleansing processes.

2. Preparation Methods:

- **Tinctures:** Tinctures are concentrated herbal extracts made by steeping herbs in alcohol or glycerin to extract their active compounds. To prepare a tincture, chop fresh or dried herbs finely and place them in a glass jar. Cover with alcohol (like vodka or rum) or glycerin, ensuring the herbs are fully submerged. Seal the jar and let it sit for 4-6 weeks in a cool, dark place, shaking it daily. After steeping, strain the liquid through cheesecloth or a fine mesh sieve into dark glass dropper bottles for storage.

- **Tonics:** Herbal tonics are liquid preparations made by simmering herbs in water to extract their medicinal properties. Start by combining water and herbs in a saucepan, bring to a boil, then reduce heat and simmer for 15-20 minutes. Let it cool, strain the liquid, and store in glass bottles in the refrigerator for up to a week. Tonics can be consumed daily to support detoxification, digestion, and overall health.

3. Custom Blends:

Experiment with different combinations of herbs to create custom tincture and tonic blends tailored to specific health goals. For example, combine dandelion root, burdock root, and milk thistle for a liver-supporting tincture, or mix ginger, turmeric, and cilantro for an anti-inflammatory and digestive tonic.

4. Usage and Dosage:

- **Tinctures:** Take tinctures by diluting a few drops in water or juice, up to three times a day, depending on the herb and individual needs. Start with a lower dosage and gradually increase as tolerated.

- **Tonics:** Drink herbal tonics as is or diluted with water throughout the day. They can be taken on an empty stomach or with meals to aid digestion and support detoxification.

5. Safety Considerations:

- Research individual herbs and their potential interactions with medications or existing health conditions before preparing tinctures and tonics.

- Pregnant or nursing women, as well as individuals with chronic health conditions, should consult a healthcare professional before incorporating herbal preparations into their regimen.

By crafting herbal detox tinctures and tonics using quality ingredients and following proper preparation methods, individuals can enhance their detoxification efforts naturally. These concentrated herbal preparations offer a convenient and effective way to support liver health, aid digestion, and promote overall wellness as recommended by natural health practices.

Book 13: Colon Cleansing Techniques

Effective Methods for Detoxifying and Revitalizing Your Digestive Health

Chapter 1: Importance of Colon Health in Detoxification

Colon health plays a crucial role in the body's detoxification processes, influencing overall wellness and vitality. Barbara O'Neill emphasizes the significance of maintaining a healthy colon to support effective toxin elimination and promote optimal digestive function.

Elimination of Toxins: The colon, also known as the large intestine, is responsible for the final stages of digestion and eliminating waste products from the body. A healthy colon ensures the efficient removal of toxins, metabolic waste, and harmful substances that can accumulate in the digestive system.

Absorption of Nutrients: A clean and healthy colon facilitates the absorption of nutrients from food and supplements. When the colon is clogged with toxins and impacted waste, nutrient absorption can be impaired, leading to deficiencies and compromised overall health.

Balancing Gut Microbiota: The colon is home to a diverse community of beneficial bacteria that play a crucial role in digestion, immune function, and detoxification. Maintaining a healthy balance of gut microbiota supports optimal colon function and overall well-being.

Prevention of Toxin Reabsorption: A sluggish or congested colon may lead to reabsorbing toxins and waste products back into the bloodstream, compromising detoxification efforts. This can burden the liver and other organs involved in detoxification, potentially leading to systemic inflammation and health issues.

Promoting Regular Bowel Movements: Regular bowel movements are essential for maintaining colon health and supporting detoxification. Adequate fiber intake, hydration, and a balanced diet rich in whole foods help promote bowel regularity and prevent constipation, which can contribute to toxin buildup.

Natural Detoxification Support: Barbara O'Neill recommends natural methods to support colon health and enhance detoxification efforts. These include dietary fiber from fruits, vegetables, and whole grains, hydration with water and herbal teas, and regular physical activity to promote bowel motility.

Colon Cleansing Practices: Periodic colon cleansing practices, such as herbal teas, probiotics, and enemas, can help remove impacted waste and toxins from the colon. These practices should be undertaken cautiously and under the guidance of a qualified healthcare practitioner to ensure safety and effectiveness.

Maintaining colon health is essential for effective detoxification and overall wellness. By adopting a fiber-rich diet, staying hydrated, promoting regular bowel movements, and considering natural colon cleansing practices, individuals can support their body's natural detoxification processes and enhance overall health, as Barbara O'Neill's holistic approach recommends.

Chapter 2: Natural Colon Cleansing Methods

Natural methods for cleansing the colon emphasize gentle yet effective approaches to remove accumulated toxins and support overall health. These methods promote digestive function and regularity, enhancing well-being through natural practices:

*Dietary Fiber:*Incorporate high-fiber foods such as fruits, vegetables, whole grains, and legumes into your daily diet. Fiber acts as a natural bulking agent, promoting regular bowel movements and aiding in removing waste and toxins from the colon.

*Hydration:*Drink an ample amount of water throughout the day to support colon health and detoxification. Water softens stool, facilitates waste elimination, and helps prevent constipation, promoting regularity and cleansing.

*Herbal Teas:*Utilize herbal teas containing detoxifying herbs like senna, cascara sagrada, and licorice root to stimulate bowel movements and aid in colon cleansing. Use these teas intermittently and under guidance to maintain bowel health effectively.

*Probiotics:*Consume probiotic-rich foods such as yogurt, kefir, sauerkraut, and kimchi to maintain a healthy balance of gut bacteria. Probiotics support digestion, enhance immune function, and contribute to regular bowel movements, thereby supporting colon health naturally.

Physical Activity: Engage in regular physical exercise such as walking, jogging, yoga, or cycling to stimulate bowel motility and enhance digestion. Physical activity promotes efficient waste elimination and supports overall colon health and detoxification.

Enemas and Colon Hydrotherapy: These practices involve using water or a gentle solution to flush the colon and remove impacted waste and toxins. While beneficial for some, these methods should be approached cautiously and preferably under professional guidance to avoid potential complications.

Whole Foods Diet: Emphasize a diet rich in whole foods while minimizing processed foods, refined sugars, and unhealthy fats. Whole foods provide essential nutrients and antioxidants that support digestive health and aid in the natural elimination of toxins from the body.

Stress Management: Practice stress-reducing techniques such as meditation, deep breathing, yoga, or mindfulness to support colon health. Chronic stress can adversely affect digestive function, so managing stress effectively promotes relaxation and reduces digestive disturbances.

These practices provide holistic benefits for overall well-being without the need for harsh or invasive treatments.

Chapter 3: Fiber-Rich Foods, Herbal Laxatives, and Enemas

Effective colon cleansing methods include incorporating fiber-rich foods, herbal laxatives, and occasional enemas to support digestive health and detoxification.

1. Fiber-Rich Foods: Dietary fiber plays a crucial role in maintaining regular bowel movements and promoting colon health. It acts as a natural bulking agent, helping to move waste through the digestive tract and preventing constipation. Foods such as fruits (apples, berries), vegetables (broccoli, spinach), whole grains (oats, quinoa), and legumes (beans, lentils) are excellent sources of fiber. Including these foods in your diet can support natural colon cleansing and enhance overall digestive function.

2. Herbal Laxatives: Certain herbs are known for their laxative properties and can be used to stimulate bowel movements and support colon cleansing. Examples include senna, cascara sagrada, rhubarb root, and aloe vera. These herbs work by increasing bowel motility and promoting the elimination of waste from the colon. Herbal laxatives should be used judiciously and under the guidance of a healthcare professional to avoid dependency and ensure safe usage.

3. Enemas: An enema involves flushing liquid (usually water or a saline solution) into the rectum to cleanse the colon. It can help remove impacted feces, toxins, and waste buildup from the lower part of the colon. Enemas are sometimes used for therapeutic purposes, such as preparing for medical procedures or to relieve severe constipation. However, they should be administered with caution and preferably under the supervision of a qualified healthcare provider to avoid potential risks and complications.

Combining fiber-rich foods with herbal laxatives and occasional enemas can provide a comprehensive approach to colon cleansing. Fiber supports regularity and digestive health, while herbal laxatives can offer additional support for bowel movement stimulation. Enemas, when used sparingly and appropriately, can help in cases of severe constipation or as part of a detoxification regimen. It's essential to maintain hydration and listen to your body's cues when incorporating these methods into your routine.

By incorporating fiber-rich foods, herbal laxatives, and occasional enemas into your approach to colon health, you can support natural colon cleansing and promote overall digestive wellness. These methods provide gentle yet effective ways to enhance detoxification and maintain regular bowel movements, contributing to your overall health and well-being. Always consult with a healthcare professional before starting any new regimen, especially if you have underlying health conditions or concerns.

Chapter 4: Step-by-Step Guide to Safe Colon Cleansing

Safe colon cleansing involves adopting gentle yet effective practices to support digestive health and enhance detoxification. Here's a step-by-step guide to help you navigate the process:

1. Assess Your Health:

Before embarking on a colon cleansing regimen, it's crucial to assess your current health status. Take into account any existing medical conditions or medications you are taking. For a comprehensive understanding, consult with a healthcare professional, especially if you have gastrointestinal issues or concerns. This professional guidance will ensure you are on the right track and make you feel secure in your journey towards digestive health.

2. Increase Fiber Intake:

Start your journey by incorporating fiber-rich foods into your daily diet. Fruits, vegetables, whole grains, and legumes are not just excellent sources of dietary fiber, but they also support regular bowel movements and help cleanse the colon naturally. Aim for at least 25-30 grams of fiber per day from food sources, and you'll soon start feeling the benefits, which will keep you motivated on your path to digestive health.

3. Hydrate Adequately:

Water is a powerful ally in your quest for digestive health. Drinking plenty of water throughout the day not only maintains hydration but also supports bowel function. It helps soften stool and facilitates waste movement through the digestive system, aiding in natural colon cleansing. Understanding this role of water will empower you to take control of your digestive health.

4. Include Herbal Laxatives Sparingly:

To stimulate bowel movements, consider incorporating herbal laxatives like senna, cascara sagrada, or rhubarb root. Use these herbs sparingly and under the guidance of a healthcare professional to avoid dependency and ensure safe usage.

5. Try Enemas or Colon Hydrotherapy:

Consider using enemas or colon hydrotherapy (colonics) to further cleanse the colon. These procedures involve flushing the colon with water or a gentle solution to remove impacted waste and toxins. Ensure trained professionals administer these procedures in a safe and sanitary environment.

6. Maintain a Balanced Diet:

Continue prioritizing a balanced diet rich in whole foods while minimizing processed foods, refined sugars, and unhealthy fats. Whole foods provide essential nutrients and antioxidants that support digestive health and aid in eliminating toxins from the body.

7. Practice Regular Physical Activity:

Regular physical exercise promotes bowel motility and enhances overall digestive function. Activities such as walking, jogging, yoga, or cycling stimulate the muscles of the digestive tract and support natural colon cleansing.

8. Manage Stress:

Stress can impact digestive health and bowel function. To promote relaxation and reduce digestive disturbances, incorporate stress-reducing practices such as meditation, deep breathing, or mindfulness.

9. Listen to Your Body:

Pay attention to your body's signals and adjust your colon cleansing regimen accordingly. If you experience discomfort, irregular bowel movements, or other adverse symptoms, discontinue the practice and consult a healthcare provider.

10. Monitor Results:

Monitor how your body responds to colon cleansing practices. Evaluate improvements in digestion, bowel regularity, and overall well-being. Adjust your approach based on feedback from your body and continue to prioritize long-term digestive health.

Chapter 5: Liver and Kidney Detox

5.1 Understanding the Liver's Role in Detoxification

The liver is a vital organ responsible for detoxifying the body by processing and filtering toxins from the bloodstream. Barbara O'Neill emphasizes the liver's crucial role in maintaining overall health through effective detoxification processes.

1. **Metabolic Processing:** The liver plays a central role in metabolizing various substances, including medications, hormones, and nutrients. It transforms these substances into forms that the body can either utilize or eliminate.

2. **Detoxification Pathways:** The liver detoxifies harmful compounds through two primary pathways: Phase I and Phase II detoxification. In Phase I, enzymes modify toxins to make them more water-soluble. In Phase II, conjugation reactions further process these substances for excretion.

3. **Bile Production:** The liver produces bile, a digestive fluid that aids in the breakdown and absorption of fats and fat-soluble vitamins. Bile also serves as a vehicle for excreting waste products, including toxins and excess cholesterol, into the intestines.

4. **Antioxidant Production:** The liver synthesizes antioxidants such as glutathione, which neutralize free radicals and protect cells from oxidative damage. These antioxidants are crucial for supporting the liver's detoxification functions and overall cellular health.

5. **Nutrient Storage:** The liver stores essential nutrients such as vitamins (A, D, E, K) and minerals (iron, copper). These nutrients are released as needed to support various metabolic processes and detoxification pathways.

6. **Supporting Detoxification:** Barbara O'Neill recommends supporting liver function through a balanced diet rich in antioxidants, fiber, and essential nutrients. This includes consuming plenty of fruits, vegetables, whole grains, and lean proteins while minimizing processed foods and alcohol consumption.

7. **Healthy Lifestyle Practices:** Maintaining a healthy weight, engaging in regular exercise, managing stress effectively, and avoiding exposure to environmental toxins further supports liver health and enhances its detoxification capabilities.

Understanding the liver's role in detoxification underscores the importance of maintaining its optimal function for overall health and well-being. By adopting a holistic approach that supports liver health through nutrition, lifestyle, and natural detoxification practices, individuals can promote long-term vitality and resilience as recommended by Barbara O'Neill.

5.2 Natural Remedies for Liver Health

Barbara O'Neill advocates for natural remedies that support liver health, emphasizing holistic approaches to maintain this crucial organ's function and enhance overall well-being.

1. **Milk Thistle:** Known for its antioxidant and anti-inflammatory properties, milk thistle (Silybum marianum) supports liver health by promoting regeneration of liver cells and protecting against toxins and free radicals.

2. **Dandelion Root:** Dandelion root (Taraxacum officinale) stimulates bile production and liver detoxification, aiding in the elimination of toxins from the body. It also supports digestion and may help reduce inflammation.

3. **Turmeric:** Curcumin, the active compound in turmeric (Curcuma longa), has potent antioxidant and anti-inflammatory effects. It supports liver function by enhancing bile production, promoting detoxification pathways, and protecting liver cells from damage.

4. **Artichoke:** Artichoke leaf extract stimulates bile flow and liver detoxification processes, aiding in the elimination of toxins and promoting overall digestive health.

5. **Schisandra:** Schisandra (Schisandra chinensis) berries contain compounds that support liver function by enhancing detoxification processes and protecting liver cells from damage caused by toxins and stress.

6. **Green Tea:** Rich in antioxidants such as catechins, green tea (Camellia sinensis) supports liver health by reducing oxidative stress, enhancing liver function, and promoting detoxification pathways.

7. **Licorice Root:** Licorice root (Glycyrrhiza glabra) has anti-inflammatory and antioxidant properties that support liver health. It may help protect liver cells from damage and support detoxification processes.

8. **Healthy Diet:** Consuming a balanced diet rich in fruits, vegetables, whole grains, lean proteins, and healthy fats provides essential nutrients and antioxidants that support liver health and overall well-being.

9. **Hydration:** Adequate hydration supports liver function by facilitating the elimination of toxins and waste products from the body. Drinking enough water throughout the day helps maintain optimal liver health.

10. **Lifestyle Factors:** Maintaining a healthy weight, engaging in regular physical activity, managing stress effectively, and avoiding excessive alcohol consumption and exposure to environmental toxins are crucial for supporting liver health.

5.3 Supporting Kidney Function During Detox

During detoxification, it's essential to support kidney function as the kidneys play a crucial role in filtering toxins and waste products from the bloodstream. Barbara O'Neill emphasizes holistic approaches to support kidney health during detox.

Hydration: Adequate hydration is vital for kidney function and overall detoxification. Drinking plenty of water helps flush out toxins and waste products through urine, supporting kidney function and maintaining optimal hydration levels.

Herbal Teas: Certain herbal teas such as dandelion root, nettle leaf, and parsley can support kidney health by promoting urine production and aiding in the elimination of toxins. These teas have diuretic properties that help flush out excess fluids and waste from the kidneys.

Cranberry Juice: Cranberry juice is known for its ability to support urinary tract health and may help prevent urinary tract infections (UTIs). It contains antioxidants that can help protect the kidneys from oxidative stress and promote overall urinary health.

Limit Sodium Intake: Excessive sodium consumption can put strain on the kidneys by increasing fluid retention and blood pressure. Barbara O'Neill recommends limiting sodium intake to support kidney function during detoxification.

Potassium-Rich Foods: Consuming foods rich in potassium, such as bananas, avocados, spinach, and sweet potatoes, can help maintain electrolyte balance and support kidney health. Potassium helps regulate fluid balance and blood pressure, crucial for kidney function.

Avoid Alcohol and Caffeine: Limiting alcohol and caffeine intake during detox can help reduce the burden on the kidneys. Both substances can dehydrate the body and affect kidney function, hindering their ability to effectively filter toxins from the bloodstream.

Maintain a Balanced Diet: Eating a balanced diet that includes plenty of fruits, vegetables, whole grains, and lean proteins supports overall kidney health. These foods provide essential nutrients and antioxidants that support kidney function and overall well-being.

Monitor Electrolyte Levels: During detoxification, it's essential to monitor electrolyte levels to ensure they remain balanced. Electrolytes such as sodium, potassium, and magnesium play critical roles in kidney function and overall health.

Consult with a Healthcare Professional: Before starting any detoxification, regimen or making significant dietary changes, it's important to consult with a healthcare professional, especially if you have pre-existing kidney conditions or concerns.

By incorporating these practices into your detoxification regimen, you can support kidney function, promote overall detoxification, and enhance your body's natural ability to eliminate toxins as advocated by Barbara O'Neill. Taking a holistic approach to kidney health ensures that detoxification supports overall well-being without compromising vital organ function.

Chapter 6: Skin and Lymphatic System Detox

6.1 Skin as an Organ of Elimination

The skin serves a critical role as an organ of elimination in the body's detoxification processes. Understanding how the skin functions in eliminating toxins can enhance overall health and well-being.

Sweat Production: Sweat glands release sweat, a fluid that contains water, electrolytes, and small amounts of waste products like urea and lactic acid. Sweating helps regulate body temperature and eliminates toxins from the body.

Pores and Sebum Production: Pores on the skin's surface release sebum, an oily substance that moisturizes and protects the skin. Sebum also eliminates waste products and maintains the skin's barrier function against harmful substances.

Detoxification through Skin Care: Proper skincare practices support the skin's detoxification function. Regular cleansing removes dirt, oil, and pollutants from the skin's surface, allowing pores to function effectively. Natural skincare products without harsh chemicals can further aid the skin's natural detoxification process.

Dry Brushing: Dry brushing is a technique that stimulates circulation and lymphatic drainage, facilitating the removal of toxins through the skin. By gently exfoliating the skin's surface with a dry brush, dry brushing promotes detoxification and enhances overall skin health.

Hydration: Adequate hydration is crucial for maintaining healthy skin and supporting its detoxification function. Drinking sufficient water helps keep the skin hydrated, promotes sweat production, and aids in flushing out toxins through the skin.

Sauna Therapy: Saunas promote detoxification through the skin by increasing sweat production and enhancing circulation. The heat and humidity in saunas open pores, releasing toxins through sweat, thereby supporting overall detoxification processes.

Healthy Lifestyle Practices: Adopting healthy lifestyle habits such as regular exercise, a balanced diet rich in antioxidants and nutrients, and effective stress management supports skin health and its role in detoxification. These practices contribute to maintaining radiant and healthy skin.

Understanding the skin's function as an organ of elimination highlights its importance in detoxification and overall health. By implementing proper skincare routines, staying hydrated, and embracing a healthy lifestyle, individuals can optimize skin health and effectively support its natural detoxification processes.

6.2 Dry Brushing and Its Benefits

Dry brushing is a practice that offers numerous benefits for skin health and overall well-being. This technique involves gently brushing the skin with a dry, natural-bristled brush in specific motions, typically before showering. Barbara O'Neill advocates dry brushing for its potential detoxification benefits and skin-enhancing properties.

1. Exfoliation: Dry brushing effectively exfoliates the skin by removing dead skin cells from the surface. This process helps unclog pores, allowing the skin to breathe and function more efficiently in eliminating toxins.

2. Stimulation of Circulation: The brushing motion stimulates blood circulation and lymphatic drainage. Improved circulation helps deliver oxygen and nutrients to the skin while aiding in the removal of metabolic waste products and toxins.

3. Lymphatic System Support: Dry brushing supports the lymphatic system, which plays a vital role in immune function and detoxification. By stimulating lymphatic flow, dry brushing encourages the removal of cellular waste and toxins from the body.

4. Cellulite Reduction: Regular dry brushing may help reduce the appearance of cellulite by promoting circulation and breaking down fatty deposits under the skin. This can contribute to smoother-looking skin over time.

5. Stress Relief: The rhythmic motion of dry brushing can promote relaxation and reduce stress levels. It serves as a gentle self-care practice that encourages mindfulness and enhances overall well-being.

6. Enhanced Skin Tone and Texture: Continued dry brushing can improve skin tone and texture by promoting the regeneration of new skin cells and collagen production. This results in smoother, softer skin with a healthier appearance.

7. Preparation for Skincare Products: By exfoliating the skin and improving circulation, dry brushing enhances the effectiveness of skincare products. It allows moisturizers, oils, and serums to penetrate more deeply into the skin, maximizing their benefits.

8. Easy to Incorporate: Dry brushing is simple to incorporate into a daily routine and typically takes only a few minutes before showering. It can be done on dry skin in gentle, upward strokes towards the heart, starting from the feet and moving upwards.

Dry brushing offers a holistic approach to skin care and detoxification, supporting overall health and well-being. Incorporating this practice into your skincare routine, as recommended by health experts, including Barbara O'Neill, can provide numerous benefits for skin health, circulation, and detoxification processes.

6.3 Detox Baths and Topical Applications

Detox baths and topical applications are popular methods for supporting the body's natural detoxification processes through the skin. These practices involve using various ingredients and techniques to promote relaxation, detoxification, and skin health.

1. Epsom Salt Baths: Epsom salt, composed of magnesium sulfate, is a common ingredient in detox baths. Adding Epsom salt to warm bathwater helps relax muscles, reduce inflammation, and draw out toxins through the skin. Magnesium, absorbed through the skin during bathing, supports detoxification and promotes overall relaxation.

2. Baking Soda Baths: Baking soda, or sodium bicarbonate, is known for its alkalizing properties. Adding baking soda to bathwater can help neutralize acidity on the skin's surface, soothe irritation, and support detoxification. It may also assist in balancing pH levels and improving skin texture.

3. Clay Baths: Clay, such as bentonite or kaolin clay, is renowned for its ability to absorb toxins and impurities from the skin. Clay baths involve adding powdered clay to bathwater to create a detoxifying soak. Clay binds to toxins and heavy metals, drawing them out through the skin's pores.

4. Apple Cider Vinegar Soaks: Apple cider vinegar (ACV) contains acetic acid, which has antimicrobial properties and may help detoxify the skin. Adding ACV to bathwater can balance skin pH, reduce odor, and support the body's detoxification processes.

5. Essential Oils: Adding essential oils like lavender, tea tree, or eucalyptus to bathwater can enhance the detoxification and relaxation benefits of baths. Essential oils have therapeutic properties that can soothe the skin, promote circulation, and support overall well-being.

6. Topical Applications: Besides baths, topical applications of detoxifying ingredients such as clay masks, herbal poultices, and detoxifying oils can support skin detoxification. These applications can draw out impurities, nourish the skin, and promote a healthy complexion.

7. Saunas and Steam Rooms: In addition to baths, saunas and steam rooms promote detoxification through sweating. The heat and humidity in saunas open pores, allowing toxins to be released through sweat. Regular sauna sessions can support overall detoxification and skin health.

8. Hydration and Rest: After detox baths or topical applications, it's essential to stay hydrated and allow the body time to rest. Drinking plenty of water helps flush out toxins released through the skin, while rest supports overall recovery and well-being.

Detox baths and topical applications offer holistic approaches to supporting the body's natural detoxification processes through the skin. These practices not only promote detoxification but also enhance relaxation, skin health, and overall well-being. Integrating detox baths and topical detoxifying applications into a regular self-care routine can provide numerous benefits for maintaining a healthy body and radiant skin.

6.4 Recipes for Detoxifying Bath Soaks and Scrubs

Creating your own detoxifying bath soaks and scrubs can be a rewarding way to enhance relaxation, promote detoxification, and support skin health. Here are some simple recipes using natural ingredients known for their detoxifying properties:

1. **Epsom Salt and Lavender Bath Soak:**

   o **Ingredients:** 1 cup Epsom salt, ½ cup baking soda, 10 drops lavender essential oil.

   o **Instructions:** Mix Epsom salt and baking soda in a bowl, then add lavender essential oil. Add the mixture to warm bathwater and soak for 20-30 minutes. The Epsom salt helps draw out toxins, while lavender essential oil promotes relaxation and soothes the senses.

2. **Clay Detox Bath:**

   o **Ingredients:** 1 cup bentonite clay, ½ cup Epsom salt, 10 drops tea tree essential oil.

   o **Instructions:** Mix bentonite clay and Epsom salt in a bowl, then add tea tree essential oil. Dissolve the mixture in warm bathwater and soak for 20-30 minutes. Bentonite clay absorbs toxins and impurities, while tea tree oil offers antimicrobial benefits.

3. **Ginger and Lemon Detox Bath:**

   o **Ingredients:** 1 cup Epsom salt, ½ cup fresh grated ginger, juice of 1 lemon.

   o **Instructions:** Combine Epsom salt, grated ginger, and lemon juice in a bowl. Add the mixture to warm bathwater and soak for 20-30 minutes. Ginger stimulates circulation and promotes sweating, aiding in detoxification, while lemon juice provides vitamin C and antioxidants.

4. **Coffee Grounds Body Scrub:**

   o **Ingredients:** 1 cup coffee grounds, ½ cup coconut oil, ¼ cup brown sugar.

   o **Instructions:** Mix coffee grounds, coconut oil, and brown sugar in a bowl to form a paste. Use the scrub to gently exfoliate the skin in circular motions before showering. Coffee grounds help improve circulation and reduce the appearance of cellulite, while coconut oil moisturizes and nourishes the skin.

5. **Himalayan Salt and Rose Petal Scrub:**

   o **Ingredients:** 1 cup Himalayan salt, ½ cup dried rose petals (crushed), ¼ cup sweet almond oil.

   o **Instructions:** Combine Himalayan salt, crushed rose petals, and sweet almond oil in a bowl. Use the scrub to gently massage the skin in circular motions, then rinse off in the shower. Himalayan salt exfoliates and detoxifies the skin, while rose petals add a luxurious fragrance and antioxidants.

6. **Oatmeal and Honey Bath Soak:**

   o **Ingredients:** 1 cup colloidal oatmeal, ½ cup raw honey, 1 tablespoon coconut oil.

   o **Instructions:** Mix colloidal oatmeal, raw honey, and coconut oil in a bowl to create a paste. Add the mixture to warm bathwater and soak for 20-30 minutes. Colloidal oatmeal soothes dry, irritated skin, while honey moisturizes and nourishes.

These recipes use natural ingredients known for their detoxifying and skin-nourishing properties. Incorporating these bath soaks and scrubs into your self-care routine can help promote relaxation, support detoxification, and enhance overall skin health. Adjust the ingredients based on your preferences and skin type to create personalized treatments that leave you feeling rejuvenated and refreshed.

Chapter 7: Incorporating Physical Activity

7.1 Role of Exercise in Detoxification

Understanding how exercise supports the body's natural detoxification processes empowers you to take control of your health. By promoting circulation, sweating, and lymphatic drainage, physical activity plays a crucial role in detoxification. Here's how it works:

Enhanced Circulation: Exercise increases blood flow, delivering oxygen and nutrients to cells while carrying away metabolic waste products and toxins. Improved circulation supports efficient detoxification by enhancing the function of organs such as the liver and kidneys.

Stimulation of Lymphatic System: The lymphatic system removes toxins and waste from tissues. Exercise stimulates lymphatic circulation, especially activities involving rhythmic movement like walking, jogging, or rebounding. These activities involve continuous and repetitive movements, which help lymph nodes filter and remove cellular waste, toxins, and pathogens.

Promotion of Sweating: Physical activity increases body temperature, prompting the sweat glands to release sweat. Sweating is a natural mechanism through which the body eliminates toxins, heavy metals, and other harmful substances. Regular exercise promotes sweating, aiding in the detoxification process.

Support for Liver Function: The liver is the body's primary detoxification organ, breaking down toxins into less harmful substances that can be excreted. Exercise supports liver function by improving blood flow and aiding in the processing and eliminating toxins.

Reduction of Chronic Inflammation: Chronic inflammation can hinder detoxification and contribute to various health issues. Regular exercise helps reduce inflammation by promoting a healthy immune response and supporting tissue repair, which in turn supports overall detoxification.

Mental and Emotional Benefits: Exercise is known to reduce stress, anxiety, and depression, which can have a positive impact on overall health and detoxification. Stress reduction enhances the body's detoxification by optimizing hormonal balance and immune function.

Types of Exercise for Detoxification: Incorporating various exercises into your routine can inspire and motivate you to maximize detoxification benefits. Cardiovascular exercises like running, cycling, and swimming promote sweating and circulation. Strength training enhances muscle tone and metabolism, supporting overall detoxification. Yoga and tai chi promote relaxation, stress reduction, and lymphatic drainage.

Hydration and Recovery: It's essential to stay informed and prepared by staying hydrated before, during, and after exercise to support detoxification. Drinking water helps flush out toxins released during physical activity. Adequate rest and recovery are also crucial for allowing the body to repair tissues and eliminate waste products effectively.

By incorporating regular exercise into your routine, you can optimize your body's natural detoxification processes, support overall health, and enhance your well-being. Whether through cardiovascular activities, strength training, or mind-body exercises, staying active is vital in maintaining a healthy body and promoting detoxification.

7.2 Recommended Activities for Supporting Detox

Several activities can effectively support the body's detoxification processes by promoting circulation, lymphatic drainage, and overall well-being:

Cardiovascular Exercise: Activities such as running, cycling, brisk walking, and swimming increase heart rate and circulation, promoting the transport of oxygen and nutrients throughout the body. Cardiovascular exercise also stimulates sweating, helping to eliminate toxins through the skin.

Strength Training: Resistance exercises like weightlifting, bodyweight exercises, and resistance bands improve muscle tone and metabolism. Muscle contraction during strength training enhances blood flow and lymphatic drainage, supporting the removal of toxins and metabolic waste.

Yoga and Stretching: Yoga poses and stretching routines promote flexibility, relaxation, and lymphatic circulation. Certain yoga poses, such as twists and inversions, stimulate detoxification by compressing and releasing internal organs, improving digestion, and promoting lymphatic flow.

Pilates: Pilates exercises focus on core strength, flexibility, and posture. The controlled movements in Pilates enhance circulation and support organ function, including the liver and kidneys, which play key roles in detoxification.

Swimming: Swimming is a low-impact aerobic exercise that engages multiple muscle groups while supporting joint health. The buoyancy of water reduces impact on joints and enhances circulation, making it an excellent choice for those looking to support detoxification through gentle movement.

Sauna or Steam Room Sessions: Heat therapy in saunas or steam rooms promotes sweating, which helps eliminate toxins through the skin. Sauna sessions also improve circulation and relaxation, supporting overall detoxification and stress reduction.

Deep Breathing Exercises: Techniques such as diaphragmatic breathing, pranayama in yoga, or deep belly breathing can enhance oxygenation and promote relaxation. Deep breathing stimulates the lymphatic system and supports detoxification by enhancing the exchange of gases in the lungs.

Mindfulness Practices: Practices like meditation, tai chi, and qigong promote relaxation, reduce stress, and support overall well-being. Stress reduction is crucial for detoxification as chronic stress can impair immune function and hinder toxin elimination.

Hydration and Nutrition: Drinking plenty of water throughout the day supports kidney function and helps flush out toxins. Consuming a balanced diet rich in fruits, vegetables, and whole grains provides essential nutrients that support detoxification pathways in the liver and digestive system.

Chapter 8: Creating a Long-Term Detox Plan

8.1 Developing Sustainable Detox Practices

Creating sustainable detox practices involves adopting habits that support long-term health and well-being without extreme measures. Here are key strategies to develop sustainable detox practices:

Consistent Hydration: Drink plenty of water throughout the day to support kidney function and aid in the elimination of toxins. Adding lemon or cucumber to water can enhance detoxification and promote hydration.

Nutrient-Rich Diet: Focus on a balanced diet rich in fruits, vegetables, whole grains, lean proteins, and healthy fats. To enhance natural detoxification processes, incorporate foods that support liver function, such as leafy greens, beets, garlic, and turmeric.

Regular Physical Activity: Engage in regular exercise to support circulation, lymphatic drainage, and sweat production. Include a variety of activities, such as cardiovascular exercise, strength training, yoga, or swimming, to promote overall detoxification and well-being.

Mindful Eating: Practice mindful eating by paying attention to hunger and satiety cues and choosing whole, unprocessed foods. Avoiding processed foods, excessive sugar, and alcohol can reduce the burden on detoxification pathways.

Stress Management: Incorporate stress-reducing practices such as meditation, deep breathing, yoga, or tai chi into your daily routine. Chronic stress can impair detoxification processes, so prioritizing relaxation is essential for sustainable detox practices.

Quality Sleep: Aim for adequate and restful sleep each night to support cellular repair and detoxification. Create a bedtime routine and environment conducive to quality sleep, such as limiting screen time before bed and keeping the bedroom cool and dark.

Natural Skincare: To reduce the body's overall toxic burden, use natural skincare products free from harmful chemicals and toxins. Choose clean ingredients that support skin health and avoid unnecessary exposure to synthetic chemicals.

Gentle Detox Practices: Incorporate gentle detox practices like herbal teas, occasional fasting, or periodic cleansing diets into your routine. Avoid extreme detox methods that may disrupt normal bodily functions or lead to nutrient deficiencies.

Regular Detox Maintenance: Implement regular maintenance practices such as dry brushing, sauna sessions, or occasional detox baths to support ongoing detoxification. These practices help eliminate toxins in the skin and support overall well-being.

Consultation with Healthcare Professionals: If considering more intensive detoxification protocols or experiencing health concerns, consult a healthcare professional or registered dietitian. They can provide personalized guidance based on your individual health needs and goals.

Adopting these sustainable detox practices into your lifestyle can support your body's natural detoxification processes, improve overall health, and promote long-term well-being. Consistency and balance are key to achieving sustainable detoxification goals while maintaining vitality and resilience.

8.2 Seasonal Detox Programs

Seasonal detox programs are designed to align with the body's natural rhythms and environmental changes throughout the year, offering targeted support for detoxification and overall health. Here's how seasonal detox programs can be beneficial:

1. **Spring Renewal:** Spring is often associated with renewal and rejuvenation. A spring detox program may focus on supporting liver function, clearing out toxins accumulated over the winter months, and enhancing digestion. Incorporating bitter greens, dandelion greens, and artichokes can support liver detoxification pathways, while fresh fruits and vegetables provide essential vitamins and minerals.

2. **Summer Cleanse:** In summer, detox programs may emphasize hydration, cooling foods, and light cleansing. Fresh fruits like watermelon and berries, along with cooling herbs such as mint and cilantro, can aid in detoxification while keeping the body hydrated and refreshed. Including activities like swimming, hiking, or outdoor yoga can support sweat production and toxin elimination.

3. **Fall Transition:** Fall detox programs often focus on preparing the body for the colder months ahead. Incorporating warming foods like soups, stews, and root vegetables can support digestion and boost immune function. Detoxifying herbs such as ginger, turmeric, and cinnamon may be included to support circulation and immunity.

4. **Winter Nourishment:** Winter detox programs prioritize nourishment and immune support during colder months. Including warming spices like ginger and cloves in meals can aid digestion and circulation. Herbal teas with elderberry, echinacea, and chamomile can provide immune support and relaxation. Practices like gentle yoga, indoor exercises, or sauna sessions can support detoxification while staying warm.

5. **Year-Round Principles:** While seasonal detox programs offer focused support, incorporating year-round detox principles is essential for maintaining overall health. This includes staying hydrated, consuming a nutrient-rich diet, engaging in regular physical activity, and managing stress effectively. Adapt detox practices to individual needs and preferences to promote sustainable health benefits throughout the year.

By aligning with seasonal changes and incorporating targeted detoxification practices, seasonal detox programs can help optimize health, support detoxification pathways, and enhance overall well-being. Consult with a healthcare professional or registered dietitian before starting any detox program, especially if you have specific health concerns or medical conditions.

8.3 Integrating Detox Practices into Daily Life

Integrating detox practices into daily life can support overall health and well-being by promoting the body's natural detoxification processes on a regular basis. Here are practical ways to incorporate detox practices into your daily routine:

1. **Hydration:** Start your day with a glass of warm water with lemon to hydrate the body and stimulate digestion. Throughout the day, aim to drink plenty of water to support kidney function and flush out toxins.

2. **Nutrient-Dense Diet:** Focus on whole, unprocessed foods rich in vitamins, minerals, and antioxidants. Include plenty of fruits, vegetables, whole grains, lean proteins, and healthy fats to support liver function and overall detoxification.

3. **Herbal Teas:** Incorporate herbal teas such as dandelion root, ginger, green tea, or milk thistle into your daily routine. These teas can support liver health, digestion, and overall detoxification processes.

4. **Daily Movement:** Engage in regular physical activity to support circulation, lymphatic drainage, and sweat production. Choose activities you enjoy, such as walking, jogging, yoga, or dancing, to promote overall well-being and detoxification.

5. **Mindful Eating:** Practice mindful eating by chewing food thoroughly, eating slowly, and paying attention to hunger and satiety cues. Avoid processed foods, excessive sugar, and alcohol, which can burden the body's detoxification pathways.

6. **Stress Management:** Incorporate stress-reducing practices such as deep breathing exercises, meditation, yoga, or tai chi into your daily routine. Chronic stress can impair detoxification processes, so prioritizing relaxation is crucial for overall health.

7. **Skin Brushing:** Dry brushing the skin before showering can stimulate lymphatic drainage, improve circulation, and exfoliate dead skin cells. Use a natural bristle brush and gentle strokes towards the heart to enhance detoxification.

8. **Detox Baths:** Take occasional detox baths using Epsom salts, baking soda, or essential oils like lavender or eucalyptus. Soaking in a warm bath can relax muscles, promote sweating, and aid in toxin elimination through the skin.

9. **Sleep Hygiene:** Establish a regular sleep routine and aim for seven to nine hours of quality sleep each night. Sleep allows the body to repair and regenerate, supporting overall detoxification and immune function.

10. **Personal Care Products:** Choose natural and organic personal care products free from harsh chemicals, synthetic fragrances, and toxins. This reduces the body's exposure to harmful substances and supports skin health and detoxification.

By integrating these detox practices into your daily life, you can support your body's natural detoxification processes, enhance overall health, and promote a sense of well-being. Consistency and balance are key to achieving sustainable health benefits and maintaining vitality over time.

Book 14: Nutrition and Wellness the Barbara O'Neill Way

Transform Your Health with Expert Guidance on Holistic Nutrition and Natural Living

Chapter 1: Foundations of Nutritional Health

1.1 Understanding the Basics of Nutrition

Nutrition forms the foundation of health, providing the body with essential nutrients for growth, repair, and maintenance of tissues and organs. Here are key aspects to understanding the basics of nutrition:

Macronutrients: These are the powerhouses of your diet, including carbohydrates, proteins, and fats. They are the fuel for your body, essential for energy production and various bodily functions. Carbohydrates are your primary energy source, proteins are the builders, crucial for tissue repair and muscle growth, and fats are the supporters, aiding in cell structure and hormone production. Understanding their roles empowers you to make informed dietary choices.

Micronutrients: These are vitamins and minerals that play critical roles in enzymatic reactions, immune function, and overall health. Examples include vitamin C, iron, calcium, and zinc, obtained through a balanced diet of fruits, vegetables, whole grains, and lean proteins.

Water: Often overlooked but essential, water is vital for hydration, digestion, nutrient transport, and temperature regulation. Drinking adequate water daily is crucial for overall health and well-being.

Whole Foods vs. Processed Foods: Whole foods such as fruits, vegetables, whole grains, nuts, and seeds are rich in nutrients and fiber, promoting optimal health. Processed foods, high in added sugars, unhealthy fats, and preservatives, offer little nutritional value and can contribute to health problems if consumed excessively.

Balanced Diet: A balanced diet consists of various foods from different food groups, providing a mix of macronutrients, micronutrients, and fiber. Aim to include colorful fruits and vegetables, lean proteins, whole grains, and healthy fats in your daily meals to support overall health and well-being.

Portion Control: Understanding portion sizes and practicing mindful eating can help prevent overeating and maintain a healthy weight. Pay attention to hunger and satiety cues, and avoid eating large portions of calorie-dense foods that may contribute to weight gain and health issues.

Nutritional Labels: They are your secret weapon in making informed food choices. By reading and understanding nutritional labels, you can decode the nutritional content of your food. Pay attention to serving sizes, calories, macronutrient content (carbohydrates, proteins, fats), and added sugars or unhealthy fats. This knowledge equips you to make healthier food choices that support your overall health and well-being.

Nutritional Needs Across Lifespan: Nutritional needs vary based on age, gender, activity level, and health status. Children, adolescents, pregnant or breastfeeding women, and older adults may have specific nutritional requirements that should be met through a balanced diet or dietary supplements if necessary.

Personalized Nutrition: Personal preferences, cultural influences, and dietary restrictions should be considered when planning meals. Tailor your diet to meet individual needs while ensuring it provides essential nutrients and supports overall health goals.

Consultation with a Registered Dietitian: For personalized nutrition advice or to address specific health concerns, consult a registered dietitian or healthcare professional. They can guide on creating a balanced meal plan, managing dietary restrictions, and making sustainable lifestyle changes to support optimal health.

1.2 The Role of Macronutrients and Micronutrients

Macronutrients and micronutrients are essential components of a balanced diet, each playing distinct roles in supporting overall health and well-being.

- **Macronutrients:**

  o **Carbohydrates:** Carbohydrates are the body's primary source of energy, providing fuel for daily activities and bodily functions. They include simple carbohydrates found in sugars and complex carbohydrates found in whole grains, fruits, and vegetables.

  o **Proteins:** Proteins are vital for building and repairing tissues, including muscles, skin, and organs. They also serve as enzymes, hormones, and antibodies essential for various biochemical processes.

  o **Fats:** Fats are crucial for energy storage, insulation, and the absorption of fat-soluble vitamins (A, D, E, K). Healthy fats, such as those found in nuts, seeds, avocados, and fatty fish, provide essential fatty acids that support brain function and cardiovascular health.

- **Micronutrients:**

  o **Vitamins:** Vitamins are organic compounds essential for metabolic processes, immune function, and overall health. Examples include vitamin C (antioxidant, immune support), vitamin D (bone health, immune function), and vitamin B complex (energy production, nerve function).

  o **Minerals:** Minerals are inorganic nutrients critical for bone health, muscle function, and enzyme activity. Important minerals include calcium (bone health), iron (oxygen transport), potassium (muscle function), and zinc (immune support, wound healing).

Balancing macronutrients and micronutrients in your diet ensures you receive adequate nutrition to support cellular function, energy metabolism, and overall health. A varied diet rich in whole foods such as fruits, vegetables, lean proteins, and healthy fats provides essential nutrients while minimizing the consumption of processed foods high in added sugars and unhealthy fats. Consulting with a registered dietitian can provide personalized guidance on optimizing your nutrient intake to support optimal health and well-being.

1.3 The Impact of Nutrition on Physical and Mental Health

Nutrition plays a crucial role in both physical and mental health, influencing various aspects of well-being and overall quality of life.

1. **Physical Health:**

   o **Energy and Vitality:** A balanced diet rich in macronutrients (carbohydrates, proteins, fats) and micronutrients (vitamins, minerals) provides the energy needed for daily activities and supports optimal bodily functions.

   o **Weight Management:** Proper nutrition contributes to maintaining a healthy weight, reducing the risk of obesity and associated health conditions such as diabetes, cardiovascular diseases, and joint problems.

   o **Immune Function:** Essential nutrients, particularly vitamins C, D, and zinc, support immune function and help the body defend against infections and illnesses.

   o **Bone Health:** Calcium, vitamin D, and magnesium are essential for bone health and reducing the risk of osteoporosis and fractures.

   o **Heart Health:** Consuming a diet low in saturated fats and high in fiber, fruits, and vegetables can lower blood pressure, reduce cholesterol levels, and support cardiovascular health.

2. **Mental Health:**

   o **Brain Function:** Nutrients such as omega-3 fatty acids (found in fish), antioxidants (found in fruits and vegetables), and vitamins B6 and B12 play a crucial role in brain function, memory, and cognitive abilities.

   o **Mood Regulation:** The gut-brain connection highlights the impact of nutrition on mood and mental health. Foods rich in omega-3 fatty acids, complex carbohydrates, and protein can help regulate mood and reduce the risk of depression and anxiety.

   o **Focus and Concentration:** Consuming balanced meals that provide steady energy levels throughout the day supports concentration, focus, and overall cognitive performance.

   o **Sleep Quality:** Certain nutrients, such as magnesium and tryptophan (found in nuts, seeds, and turkey), promote relaxation and improve sleep quality, contributing to mental well-being.

3. **Overall Well-Being:**

   o **Digestive Health:** A diet high in fiber, whole grains, and probiotics supports gut health, enhances digestion, and promotes the absorption of essential nutrients.

   o **Longevity and Aging:** Proper nutrition contributes to healthy aging by reducing the risk of chronic diseases, maintaining muscle mass and bone density, and supporting overall vitality and longevity.

Chapter 2: Whole Foods for Whole Health

2.1 Benefits of a Whole Food Diet

A whole-food diet emphasizes consuming minimally processed foods and as close to their natural state as possible. Here are several benefits associated with adopting a whole-food diet:

Nutrient Density: Whole foods, such as fruits, vegetables, whole grains, nuts, seeds, and lean proteins, are rich in essential nutrients, including vitamins, minerals, antioxidants, and fiber. These nutrients support overall health, immune function, and disease prevention.

Improved Digestion: Whole foods are typically higher in fiber compared to processed foods. Fiber promotes healthy digestion, prevents constipation, and supports a diverse gut microbiome essential for optimal digestion and nutrient absorption.

Weight Management: Whole foods tend to be lower in added sugars, unhealthy fats, and calories compared to processed foods. Consuming a diet rich in whole foods can support weight management goals by providing satiety and reducing cravings for less nutritious foods.

Reduced Risk of Chronic Diseases: A diet rich in whole foods is associated with a lower risk of chronic diseases such as cardiovascular disease, type 2 diabetes, and certain cancers. Whole foods provide antioxidants and phytochemicals that help protect cells from damage and inflammation.

Stable Blood Sugar Levels: Whole foods, especially complex carbohydrates in whole grains and vegetables, are digested more slowly than refined carbohydrates. This helps stabilize blood sugar levels, preventing spikes and crashes that can lead to fatigue and cravings.

Supports Mental Health: Nutrient-rich whole foods, particularly those high in omega-3 fatty acids (found in fatty fish), B vitamins (found in whole grains and leafy greens), and antioxidants (found in berries and dark leafy greens), support brain function and mood regulation.

Environmental Sustainability: Choosing whole foods often means supporting sustainable farming practices and reducing environmental impact. Whole-food diets typically involve fewer resources and less packaging than processed and packaged foods.

Enhanced Flavor and Satisfaction: Whole foods are known for their natural flavors and textures, providing a more satisfying eating experience. Incorporating a variety of whole foods into meals can enhance culinary creativity and enjoyment of food.

Promotes Longevity: The combination of nutrient-dense foods, reduced risk of chronic diseases, and overall health benefits associated with a whole food diet contributes to longevity and healthy aging.

Educational and Empowering: Adopting a whole-food diet encourages learning about food sources, cooking methods, and nutrition labels. This knowledge empowers individuals to make informed decisions about their food choices and health.

Incorporating more whole foods into your diet can yield numerous health benefits and improve overall well-being. Individuals can support optimal health, longevity, and sustainable dietary practices by prioritizing nutrient-rich foods in their natural state.

2.2 Identifying Whole Foods

Whole foods are minimally processed and retain their natural nutrients, offering numerous health benefits compared to processed alternatives. Here's how to identify and incorporate whole foods into your diet:

1. Fresh Produce: Whole fruits and vegetables are excellent sources of vitamins, minerals, fiber, and antioxidants. Choose a variety of colors and types to ensure a broad range of nutrients.

2. Whole Grains: Opt for intact grains like quinoa, brown rice, oats, and whole wheat over refined grains. Whole grains provide fiber, B vitamins, and minerals essential for energy and overall health.

3. Legumes and Pulses: Beans, lentils, chickpeas, and peas are nutrient-dense sources of plant-based protein, fiber, and essential minerals. They can be incorporated into soups, salads, and main dishes.

4. Nuts and Seeds: Almonds, walnuts, chia seeds, and flaxseeds are rich in healthy fats, protein, fiber, vitamins, and minerals. They make nutritious snacks and add crunch and flavor to meals.

5. Lean Proteins: Choose lean cuts of meat, poultry, and fish, or plant-based proteins like tofu and tempeh. These provide essential amino acids for muscle repair, immune function, and overall health.

6. Dairy and Alternatives: Opt for plain yogurt, milk, and cheese without added sugars or flavors. Non-dairy alternatives like almond milk or soy yogurt can be nutrient-rich options for those avoiding dairy.

7. Herbs and Spices: Fresh and dried herbs, as well as spices like turmeric, ginger, and cinnamon, not only add flavor but also provide antioxidants and other health-promoting compounds.

8. Healthy Fats: Avocados, olives, and cold-pressed oils (such as olive, coconut, and avocado oil) are rich in monounsaturated and polyunsaturated fats, essential for heart health and nutrient absorption.

9. Minimally Processed Foods: Choose foods with minimal ingredients and avoid those with added sugars, artificial flavors, and preservatives. This includes sauces, dressings, and snacks.

10. Reading Labels: When purchasing packaged foods, read labels carefully. Look for whole food ingredients at the top of the list and avoid products with lengthy ingredient lists or unfamiliar additives.

Incorporating a variety of whole foods into your diet provides essential nutrients and promotes overall health. By prioritizing whole foods over processed options, you can enhance your diet's nutritional value and support long-term well-being.

2.3 Transitioning from Processed Foods to Whole Foods

Transitioning from a diet heavy in processed foods to one centered around whole foods can significantly improve overall health and well-being. Here are steps to make this transition effectively:

1. Gradual Changes: Start by gradually replacing processed foods with whole foods. For example, swap sugary breakfast cereals for whole grain oats topped with fresh fruits and nuts.

2. Increase Fresh Produce: Incorporate more fresh fruits and vegetables into your meals and snacks. Aim for a variety of colors to ensure a wide range of nutrients.

3. Choose Whole Grains: Replace refined grains (white bread, white rice) with whole grains such as whole wheat bread, brown rice, quinoa, and whole grain pasta.

4. Read Labels: When shopping, read food labels carefully. Choose products with fewer ingredients, avoiding those with added sugars, artificial flavors, and preservatives.

5. Cook at Home: Prepare meals at home using whole ingredients. Cooking allows you to control what goes into your meals, ensuring they are nutritious and free from unhealthy additives.

6. Healthy Snacks: Replace processed snacks (chips, cookies) with whole food options like nuts, seeds, fresh fruit, yogurt, or homemade energy bars.

7. Limit Sugary Drinks: Cut back on sugary sodas, juices, and energy drinks. Opt for water, herbal teas, or infused water with fresh fruits and herbs.

8. Explore New Foods: Experiment with new whole foods, herbs, and spices to diversify your diet and discover new flavors and textures.

9. Meal Planning: Plan meals ahead of time to ensure you have nutritious options available. This can help prevent reliance on convenience foods when hunger strikes.

10. Educate Yourself: Learn about the benefits of whole foods and how they contribute to overall health. Understanding the importance of nutrition can motivate and empower you to make healthier choices.

Transitioning to a whole food diet may take time and effort, but the benefits—such as improved energy levels, better digestion, and reduced risk of chronic diseases—are well worth it. Start small, set achievable goals, and gradually incorporate more whole foods into your daily routine for long-term health benefits.

Chapter 3: Plant-Based Nutrition

3.1 Advantages of a Plant-Based Diet

A plant-based diet, which primarily consists of plant-derived foods and minimizes or excludes animal products, offers a multitude of health benefits. These include:

Rich in Nutrients: Plant-based diets are abundant in vitamins, minerals, antioxidants, and phytochemicals found in fruits, vegetables, whole grains, nuts, seeds, and legumes. These nutrients support overall health and reduce the risk of chronic diseases.

Lower in Saturated Fats: Plant-based diets typically contain lower levels of saturated fats than animal-based diets. This can help reduce cholesterol levels and lower the risk of heart disease.

High in Fiber: Whole plant foods are rich in dietary fiber, which promotes digestive health, regulates blood sugar levels, and supports a healthy weight by increasing satiety.

Reduced Risk of Chronic Diseases: Research indicates that plant-based diets are associated with a lower risk of developing conditions such as cardiovascular disease, type 2 diabetes, hypertension, and certain cancers.

Weight Management: Plant-based diets are often lower in calories and higher in fiber compared to omnivorous diets, which can support weight loss and weight management goals.

Environmental Sustainability: Plant-based diets generally have a lower environmental impact, requiring fewer natural resources such as water and land than animal agriculture. They contribute to reducing greenhouse gas emissions and preserving biodiversity.

Plant-based diets are a boon for your gut health. The consumption of fiber-rich foods promotes a diverse microbiome, bolstering your immune function and ensuring your digestive system is in top shape.

Anti-Inflammatory Properties: Many plant-based foods, such as berries, leafy greens, nuts, and seeds, contain anti-inflammatory compounds that can help reduce inflammation and support overall wellness.

Choosing a plant-based diet can be a smart financial decision. Staples like beans, lentils, whole grains, and seasonal vegetables are often more affordable than animal products, giving you the power to prioritize your health without breaking the bank.

Plant-based diets offer a rich tapestry of flavors, textures, and culinary possibilities. With creativity and exploration, you can savor a diverse and satisfying array of meals and snacks.

Adopting a plant-based diet, whether entirely or partially, can contribute to improved health outcomes and sustainable lifestyle choices. Individuals can enjoy the health benefits of this dietary pattern by prioritizing whole plant foods and reducing reliance on animal products.

3.2 Essential Nutrients in Plant-Based Foods

Plant-based diets provide a wealth of essential nutrients for overall health and well-being. Here are key nutrients commonly found in plant-based foods:

Protein: Legumes (beans, lentils, chickpeas), tofu, tempeh, quinoa, nuts, and seeds are excellent sources of plant-based protein. These foods provide essential amino acids necessary for muscle repair, immune function, and hormone production.

Omega-3 Fatty Acids: Flaxseeds, chia seeds, walnuts, hemp seeds, and algae-derived supplements (like spirulina and chlorella) are rich sources of alpha-linolenic acid (ALA), a precursor to omega-3 fatty acids. These fats support heart health and brain function and reduce inflammation.

Calcium: Leafy greens (such as kale, collard greens, and bok choy), broccoli, fortified plant-based milk (like almond or soy milk), tofu made with calcium sulfate, and almonds are calcium-rich options. Calcium is essential for bone health, muscle function, and nerve transmission.

Iron: Legumes, lentils, tofu, quinoa, spinach, fortified cereals, and pumpkin seeds are plant-based sources of iron. Pairing these foods with sources of vitamin C (like citrus fruits or bell peppers) enhances iron absorption, which is crucial for oxygen transport and energy production.

Vitamin B12: Fortified foods such as nutritional yeast, plant-based milk, and breakfast cereals, as well as B12 supplements, are essential for those following a vegan diet. Vitamin B12 supports nerve function, red blood cell production, and DNA synthesis.

Vitamin D: Fortified plant-based milk, orange juice, and cereals, as well as exposure to sunlight, are sources of vitamin D. This vitamin is crucial for calcium absorption, immune function, and bone health.

Fiber: Fruits, vegetables, whole grains (like oats, brown rice, and quinoa), legumes, nuts, and seeds are rich in dietary fiber. Fiber supports digestive health regulates blood sugar levels and promotes satiety.

Antioxidants: Berries (such as blueberries, strawberries, and raspberries), leafy greens, nuts, seeds, and colorful vegetables (like bell peppers and carrots) are rich in antioxidants like vitamins A, C, and E, as well as phytochemicals. These compounds protect cells from damage, reduce inflammation, and support overall health.

Magnesium: Leafy greens, nuts, seeds, whole grains, legumes, and avocados are sources of magnesium. This mineral supports muscle and nerve function, regulates blood sugar levels, and contributes to bone health.

Zinc: Legumes, nuts, seeds, whole grains, and tofu are plant-based sources of zinc. This mineral supports immune function, wound healing, and protein synthesis.

By incorporating a variety of nutrient-dense plant-based foods into your diet, you can ensure you receive essential vitamins, minerals, and antioxidants necessary for optimal health. With proper planning and a balanced approach, plant-based diets can meet nutritional needs and support long-term well-being.

3.3 Practical Tips for Incorporating More Plants into Your Diet

Transitioning to a more plant-based diet can be enjoyable and rewarding with the right strategies. Here are practical tips to help you incorporate more plants into your meals.

Begin by replacing one or two meat-based meals per week with plant-based alternatives. For example, try a lentil soup or a vegetable stir-fry instead of a meat dish.

Experiment with plant-based protein sources such as beans, lentils, chickpeas, tofu, tempeh, quinoa, and nuts. These foods can be incorporated into salads, soups, casseroles, and wraps.

Choose brown rice, quinoa, oats, barley, and whole wheat bread over refined grains. These grains provide fiber, vitamins, and minerals that promote satiety and digestive health.

Incorporate vegetables into every meal. Add leafy greens, bell peppers, tomatoes, carrots, cucumbers, and broccoli to salads, sandwiches, wraps, and stir-fries.

Blend leafy greens like spinach or kale with fruits, nut milk, and seeds for a nutrient-packed breakfast or snack. Smoothies are a convenient way to increase fruit and vegetable intake.

Keep a variety of nuts and seeds (like almonds, walnuts, chia seeds, and pumpkin seeds) on hand for a quick and nutritious snack. Pair them with fruit or yogurt for added flavor and nutrients.

Explore plant-based meat substitutes like veggie burgers, plant-based sausages, and meatless meatballs. These products can be grilled, baked, or sautéed and used instead of meat in your favorite dishes.

Use fresh herbs and spices to enhance the flavor of plant-based meals. Experiment with basil, cilantro, parsley, turmeric, cumin, and ginger to add depth and variety to your cooking.

Plan your weekly meals and snacks to ensure you have various plant-based options. To streamline meal preparation, prepare ingredients in advance, such as chopping vegetables or cooking grains.

Explore new recipes and cuisines that focus on plant-based ingredients. Look for inspiration from cookbooks, websites, and social media platforms dedicated to vegetarian and vegan cooking.

Incorporating more plants into your diet can improve overall health, support sustainable eating habits, and introduce you to diverse flavors and textures. By taking small steps and experimenting with different plant-based foods, you can create delicious and nutritious meals that nourish both body and mind.

Chapter 4: Superfoods and Their Benefits

4.1 What Are Superfoods?

Superfoods are nutrient-dense foods that are particularly rich in vitamins, minerals, antioxidants, and other beneficial compounds. They are often touted for their potential health benefits and are believed to contribute to overall well-being and vitality. While there is no official definition of what constitutes a superfood, these foods typically possess exceptional nutritional profiles that support various aspects of health.

Superfoods can include a wide range of plant-based foods, as well as some fish and dairy products. Some common examples of superfoods include:

1. **Berries:** Blueberries, strawberries, raspberries, and acai berries are rich in antioxidants like anthocyanins and vitamin C, which help protect cells from oxidative stress and inflammation.

2. **Leafy Greens:** Kale, spinach, Swiss chard, and collard greens are packed with vitamins A, C, K, and minerals such as iron and calcium. They are also rich in fiber, which supports digestive health.

3. **Nuts and Seeds:** Almonds, walnuts, chia seeds, and flaxseeds are sources of healthy fats, protein, fiber, vitamins, and minerals. They promote heart health and help regulate cholesterol levels.

4. **Whole Grains:** Quinoa, oats, brown rice, and barley are whole grains rich in fiber, B vitamins, and minerals like iron and magnesium. They provide sustained energy and support digestive health.

5. **Fatty Fish:** Salmon, sardines, and mackerel are high in omega-3 fatty acids, which are beneficial for heart health, brain function, and reducing inflammation.

6. **Legumes:** Beans, lentils, and chickpeas are excellent sources of plant-based protein, fiber, vitamins, and minerals. They support satiety, regulate blood sugar levels, and promote digestive health.

7. **Turmeric:** Known for its anti-inflammatory properties, turmeric contains curcumin, a compound with potential health benefits, including reducing inflammation and supporting joint health.

8. **Green Tea:** Rich in antioxidants called catechins, green tea may boost metabolism, promote fat burning, and provide protection against oxidative stress.

9. **Greek Yogurt:** High in protein and probiotics, Greek yogurt supports gut health, digestion, and immune function. Choose plain varieties without added sugars for optimal benefits.

10. **Dark Chocolate:** Dark chocolate with high cocoa content (70% or more) is rich in antioxidants, flavonoids, and minerals like iron, magnesium, and zinc. It may improve heart health and cognitive function.

Incorporating superfoods into your diet can provide a variety of nutrients that support overall health and well-being. While superfoods offer numerous health benefits, it's essential to consume a balanced diet that includes a variety of foods to ensure you receive a wide range of nutrients necessary for optimal health.

4.2 Top Superfoods to Include in Your Diet

Including superfoods in your diet can boost your intake of essential nutrients and support overall health. Here are some top superfoods to consider incorporating into your meals:

1. **Berries:** Blueberries, strawberries, raspberries, and blackberries are rich in antioxidants, vitamins (like vitamin C), and fiber. They support brain health, immune function, and may help reduce inflammation.

2. **Leafy Greens:** Kale, spinach, Swiss chard, and arugula are nutrient powerhouses packed with vitamins A, C, K, and minerals such as iron and calcium. They promote bone health, support vision, and contribute to a healthy immune system.

3. **Nuts and Seeds:** Almonds, walnuts, chia seeds, and flaxseeds are sources of healthy fats, protein, and fiber. They support heart health, help regulate cholesterol levels, and provide essential omega-3 fatty acids.

4. **Whole Grains:** Quinoa, oats, brown rice, and barley are whole grains rich in fiber, B vitamins, and minerals like iron and magnesium. They provide sustained energy, promote digestive health, and support weight management.

5. **Fatty Fish:** Salmon, sardines, and trout are rich in omega-3 fatty acids, which are essential for heart health, brain function, and reducing inflammation. Aim for fatty fish at least twice a week for optimal benefits.

6. **Legumes:** Beans, lentils, and chickpeas are excellent plant-based sources of protein, fiber, vitamins, and minerals. They promote satiety, regulate blood sugar levels, and support digestive health.

7. **Turmeric:** Known for its anti-inflammatory properties, turmeric contains curcumin, a compound with potential health benefits such as reducing inflammation, supporting joint health, and boosting immunity.

8. **Green Tea:** Rich in antioxidants called catechins, green tea may boost metabolism, promote fat burning, and provide protection against oxidative stress. Enjoy green tea as a refreshing beverage or as part of a smoothie.

9. **Greek Yogurt:** High in protein and probiotics, Greek yogurt supports gut health, digestion, and immune function. Choose plain varieties without added sugars for optimal benefits.

10. **Dark Chocolate:** Dark chocolate with high cocoa content (70% or more) is rich in antioxidants, flavonoids, and minerals like iron, magnesium, and zinc. It may improve heart health, cognitive function, and mood.

Chapter 5: Balancing Macronutrients

5.1 Carbohydrates, Proteins, and Fats

Carbohydrates, proteins, and fats are macronutrients essential for energy production, cellular function, and overall health. Here's a breakdown of each:

1. **Carbohydrates:** Carbohydrates are the body's primary source of energy. They can be classified into two main types:

   o **Simple Carbohydrates:** Found in fruits, vegetables, and refined sugars, simple carbohydrates are quickly digested and provide rapid energy. However, they can cause blood sugar spikes if consumed in excess.

   o **Complex Carbohydrates:** Found in whole grains, legumes, and starchy vegetables, complex carbohydrates contain longer chains of sugars. They provide sustained energy, promote satiety, and support digestive health due to their high fiber content.

2. **Proteins:** Proteins are vital for building and repairing tissues, producing enzymes and hormones, and supporting immune function. Sources of protein include:

   o **Animal Sources:** Meat, poultry, fish, eggs, and dairy products provide complete proteins containing all essential amino acids.

   o **Plant Sources:** Legumes (beans, lentils), nuts, seeds, tofu, tempeh, and whole grains provide protein. While some plant sources may lack certain amino acids, combining different plant proteins throughout the day can ensure adequate intake.

3. **Fats:** Fats play a crucial role in hormone production, nutrient absorption (like fat-soluble vitamins A, D, E, and K), and providing a concentrated source of energy. Healthy fats include:

   o **Monounsaturated Fats:** Found in olive oil, avocados, and nuts, monounsaturated fats can improve heart health by lowering LDL (bad) cholesterol levels.

   o **Polyunsaturated Fats:** Omega-3 and Omega-6 fatty acids are essential polyunsaturated fats found in fatty fish, flaxseeds, and walnuts. They support brain function, reduce inflammation, and maintain heart health.

   o **Saturated Fats:** Found in animal products and some plant oils, saturated fats should be consumed in moderation to prevent cardiovascular disease.

   o **Trans Fats:** Artificial trans fats found in processed foods and fried foods should be avoided due to their negative impact on heart health.

Balancing these macronutrients in your diet is essential for overall health and well-being. Choose whole, nutrient-dense foods and avoid processed and refined products to optimize your intake of carbohydrates, proteins, and fats. Adjusting your macronutrient intake based on your individual needs, activity level, and health goals can support a balanced diet and promote long-term health.

5.2 Finding the Right Balance for Your Body

Achieving a balanced diet involves understanding your body's unique nutritional needs and finding the right combination of carbohydrates, proteins, and fats to support overall health and well-being. Here are essential tips to help you find the optimal balance:

1. Assess Your Needs: Consider your age, gender, activity level, and overall health when determining your nutritional requirements. Athletes and individuals with high activity levels may need more carbohydrates for energy, while those focusing on muscle repair may require additional protein.

2. Focus on Whole Foods: Choose nutrient-dense whole foods over processed and refined options. Whole grains, fruits, vegetables, lean proteins, and healthy fats provide essential vitamins, minerals, and antioxidants without added sugars, salts, or preservatives.

3. Balance Carbohydrates: Opt for complex carbohydrates like whole grains (brown rice, quinoa, oats), legumes (beans, lentils), and starchy vegetables (sweet potatoes, squash). These foods provide sustained energy, fiber for digestive health, and essential nutrients.

4. Prioritize Proteins: Include lean protein sources such as poultry, fish, tofu, tempeh, eggs, and legumes in your diet. Protein supports muscle repair and growth, hormone production, and immune function. Ensure a variety of protein sources throughout the day.

5. Choose Healthy Fats: Incorporate sources of monounsaturated fats (olive oil, avocados, nuts) and polyunsaturated fats (fatty fish, flaxseeds, chia seeds) into your meals. These fats support heart health, brain function, and nutrient absorption.

6. Moderation is Key: Be mindful of portion sizes and moderation, especially with foods higher in saturated fats and sugars. Enjoy treats occasionally while focusing on nutrient-dense options for the majority of your meals.

7. Listen to Your Body: Pay attention to how different foods make you feel. Adjust your diet based on your energy levels, digestion, and overall well-being. Experiment with different foods and meal combinations to find what works best for you.

8. Stay Hydrated: Water is essential for digestion, nutrient absorption, and overall hydration. Aim to drink plenty of water throughout the day and limit sugary drinks and excessive caffeine.

9. Seek Professional Guidance: Consult with a registered dietitian or healthcare provider to create a personalized nutrition plan based on your health goals, medical conditions, and dietary preferences.

Finding the right balance of carbohydrates, proteins, and fats can help you maintain energy levels, support physical and mental health, and achieve overall wellness. By prioritizing whole foods, moderation, and listening to your body's cues, you can create a sustainable and nourishing diet that meets your nutritional needs and promotes long-term health.

5.3 Sample Meal Plans and Recipes

Creating balanced meal plans and incorporating nutritious recipes can help you achieve a well-rounded diet that supports your health goals. Here are some sample meal ideas and recipes to inspire healthy eating:

Breakfast:

- Avocado Toast with Poached Eggs: Whole grain toast topped with mashed avocado, poached eggs, and a sprinkle of salt and pepper. Serve with a side of fresh fruit.

- Greek Yogurt Parfait: Layer Greek yogurt with fresh berries, granola, and a drizzle of honey or maple syrup. Add nuts or seeds for extra crunch and protein.

Lunch:

- Quinoa Salad with Chickpeas and Vegetables: Cooked quinoa mixed with chickpeas, cherry tomatoes, cucumbers, red onion, and fresh herbs. Toss with olive oil and lemon juice dressing.

- Grilled Chicken Wrap: Whole wheat wrap filled with grilled chicken breast, lettuce, tomato, cucumber, and hummus. Serve with a side of carrot sticks or a small salad.

Dinner:

- Baked Salmon with Roasted Vegetables: Seasoned salmon fillet baked with olive oil, garlic, and herbs. Serve with a side of roasted sweet potatoes, broccoli, and cauliflower.

- Vegetarian Stir-Fry: Stir-fried tofu or tempeh with bell peppers, snap peas, carrots, and broccoli in a soy sauce and ginger marinade. Serve over brown rice or quinoa.

Snacks:

- Mixed Nuts and Fruit: A handful of almonds, walnuts, and dried apricots or cranberries.

- Apple Slices with Almond Butter: Fresh apple slices dipped in almond butter for a satisfying and nutritious snack.

Recipes:

1. **Quinoa Salad with Chickpeas and Vegetables:**

   o Ingredients: Cooked quinoa, chickpeas, cherry tomatoes, cucumber, red onion, fresh parsley, olive oil, lemon juice, salt, and pepper.

   o Directions: Combine quinoa, chickpeas, tomatoes, cucumber, red onion, and parsley in a bowl. In a separate bowl, whisk olive oil, lemon juice, salt, and pepper. Pour dressing over salad and toss to combine. Serve chilled.

2. **Baked Salmon with Roasted Vegetables:**

   o Ingredients: Salmon fillet, olive oil, garlic powder, dried herbs (such as thyme or rosemary), sweet potatoes, broccoli, cauliflower.

   o Directions: Preheat oven to 400°F (200°C). Place salmon on a baking sheet lined with parchment paper. Drizzle with olive oil and sprinkle with garlic powder and herbs. Arrange chopped vegetables around the salmon. Bake for 15-20 minutes or until salmon is cooked through and vegetables are tender.

Chapter 6: Gut Health and Digestion

6.1 The Importance of a Healthy Gut

The gut, often referred to as the "second brain," plays a crucial role in overall health and well-being. A healthy gut not only ensures efficient digestion and nutrient absorption but also significantly impacts the immune system, mental health, and disease prevention. Here's why maintaining a healthy gut is essential:

1. **Digestive Efficiency and Nutrient Absorption:** The primary function of the gut is to digest food and absorb nutrients. A balanced gut microbiome, composed of beneficial bacteria, helps break down complex carbohydrates, proteins, and fats, allowing the body to extract essential vitamins and minerals. When the gut is healthy, digestion is smooth, and nutrients are readily absorbed, providing the body with the necessary building blocks for energy, growth, and repair.

2. **Immune System Support:** Approximately 70% of the immune system resides in the gut. The gut-associated lymphoid tissue (GALT) is integral to the body's defense mechanisms, identifying and neutralizing pathogens. A healthy gut microbiome helps maintain the integrity of the gut barrier, preventing harmful bacteria and toxins from entering the bloodstream. Probiotics and beneficial gut bacteria also produce antimicrobial substances and compete with pathogens, reducing the risk of infections.

3. **Mental Health and Mood Regulation:** The gut-brain axis is a complex communication network linking the gut and the brain. This bidirectional relationship means that gut health can influence mental health and vice versa. The gut produces neurotransmitters such as serotonin, which regulate mood, sleep, and appetite. Dysbiosis, or an imbalance in gut bacteria, has been linked to conditions like anxiety, depression, and stress. Maintaining a healthy gut can thus support better mental health and emotional well-being.

4. **Inflammation and Chronic Diseases:** An unhealthy gut can lead to chronic inflammation, a key factor in the development of various diseases, including autoimmune disorders, heart disease, and diabetes. Beneficial gut bacteria produce short-chain fatty acids (SCFAs) like butyrate, which have anti-inflammatory properties and help regulate the immune response. A balanced gut microbiome helps control systemic inflammation and lowers the risk of chronic diseases.

5. **Weight Management:** The gut microbiome influences metabolism and body weight. Certain gut bacteria are associated with obesity, while others promote leanness. A healthy gut helps regulate appetite, energy expenditure, and fat storage. High-fiber diets, rich in prebiotics, support the growth of beneficial bacteria that aid in weight management and reduce the risk of obesity-related complications.

6. **Detoxification and Waste Elimination:** The gut plays a vital role in detoxifying the body and eliminating waste. The liver processes toxins, which are then excreted into the gut for elimination. A healthy gut ensures efficient waste removal, preventing the reabsorption of toxins. Regular bowel movements facilitated by a balanced gut flora help maintain this detoxification process.

7. **Skin Health:** The gut-skin axis highlights the connection between gut health and skin conditions. Imbalances in the gut microbiome can manifest as skin issues like acne, eczema, and psoriasis. A healthy gut promotes clear and healthy skin by reducing inflammation and supporting detoxification.

Maintaining a Healthy Gut:

- **Diet:** Consume a diet rich in fiber, fruits, vegetables, whole grains, and fermented foods like yogurt, kefir, sauerkraut, and kimchi to support beneficial gut bacteria.

- **Probiotics and Prebiotics:** Include probiotics (live beneficial bacteria) and prebiotics (non-digestible fibers that feed beneficial bacteria) in your diet to promote a balanced microbiome.

- **Hydration:** Drink plenty of water to aid digestion and nutrient absorption.

- **Stress Management:** Practice stress-reducing activities such as meditation, exercise, and adequate sleep to support gut health.

- **Limit Antibiotics:** Use antibiotics only when necessary, as they can disrupt the gut microbiome.

Prioritizing gut health is foundational for overall wellness. By understanding its importance and adopting gut-friendly practices, you can enhance your digestive efficiency, boost immunity, improve mental health, and reduce the risk of chronic diseases.

6.2 Probiotics, Prebiotics, and Fermented Foods

Maintaining a healthy gut is essential for overall well-being, and one of the most effective ways to support gut health is through the consumption of probiotics, prebiotics, and fermented foods. These components play distinct but complementary roles in promoting a balanced and diverse gut microbiome.

1. **Probiotics:** Probiotics are live beneficial bacteria that naturally inhabit the gut and provide numerous health benefits when consumed in adequate amounts. These microorganisms help maintain a healthy balance of gut flora, enhance the gut barrier function, and support the immune system. Common probiotic strains include Lactobacillus, Bifidobacterium, and Saccharomyces boulardii.

    o **Sources of Probiotics:**

        ▪ **Yogurt:** Contains live cultures of beneficial bacteria, making it one of the most popular probiotic foods.

        ▪ **Kefir:** A fermented milk drink rich in diverse probiotic strains.

        ▪ **Sauerkraut:** Fermented cabbage that offers a variety of probiotics.

        ▪ **Kimchi:** A spicy Korean dish made from fermented vegetables, often cabbage and radishes.

        ▪ **Miso:** A fermented soybean paste used in Japanese cuisine, particularly in soups.

        ▪ **Tempeh:** A fermented soybean product that serves as a good source of probiotics and protein.

2. **Prebiotics:** Prebiotics are non-digestible fibers that serve as food for beneficial gut bacteria. They promote the growth and activity of probiotics in the gut, helping to maintain a balanced microbiome. Unlike probiotics, prebiotics are not live bacteria; rather, they are found in certain types of fiber that pass through the digestive system undigested until they reach the colon.

   o **Sources of Prebiotics:**

      ▪ **Chicory Root:** A rich source of inulin, a type of prebiotic fiber.

      ▪ **Garlic:** Contains prebiotic fibers that support beneficial bacteria.

      ▪ **Onions:** High in inulin and fructooligosaccharides, both prebiotics.

      ▪ **Asparagus:** Provides prebiotic fibers that help feed healthy gut bacteria.

      ▪ **Bananas:** Particularly when underripe, they contain resistant starch, a prebiotic fiber.

      ▪ **Oats:** Contain beta-glucan, a type of fiber with prebiotic properties.

3. **Fermented Foods:** Fermented foods are produced through controlled microbial growth and enzymatic processes, which transform food components into beneficial products. Fermentation enhances the nutrient content of foods, improves digestion, and introduces a variety of beneficial bacteria into the gut. These foods often contain both probiotics and prebiotics, making them powerful allies for gut health.

   o **Benefits of Fermented Foods:**

      ▪ **Improved Digestion:** Fermentation breaks down nutrients, making them easier to digest.

      ▪ **Enhanced Nutrient Absorption:** Fermentation can increase the bioavailability of vitamins and minerals.

      ▪ **Gut Microbiome Diversity:** Regular consumption of fermented foods can increase the diversity of beneficial bacteria in the gut.

4. **Incorporating Probiotics, Prebiotics, and Fermented Foods into Your Diet:**

   o **Start Slowly:** If you're new to fermented foods, introduce them gradually to allow your gut to adjust.

   o **Diverse Sources:** Consume a variety of probiotic and prebiotic foods to support a broad range of beneficial bacteria.

   o **Consistency is Key:** Regular consumption is essential for maintaining a healthy gut microbiome.

   o **Homemade Options:** Making your own fermented foods at home can be a fun and cost-effective way to ensure they are free of additives and preservatives.

5. **Practical Tips:**

   o **Daily Probiotics:** Include a serving of probiotic-rich foods like yogurt or kefir with breakfast.

   o **Prebiotic Snacks:** Snack on raw garlic hummus, onion slices, or a banana.

   o **Fermented Sides:** Add a side of sauerkraut or kimchi to your lunch or dinner.

   o **Hydration:** Drink plenty of water to help the prebiotic fibers move through the digestive system effectively.

Incorporating probiotics, prebiotics, and fermented foods into your diet can significantly improve gut health, enhance digestion, and boost overall wellness. By understanding their roles and benefits, you can make informed choices that support a healthy and balanced gut microbiome.

6.3 Foods and Habits that Support Digestive Health

Maintaining optimal digestive health is essential for overall well-being. The digestive system not only breaks down food and absorbs nutrients but also plays a critical role in the immune system. Certain foods and lifestyle habits can significantly support and enhance digestive health, ensuring that the gut functions smoothly and efficiently.

Foods that Support Digestive Health

1. **High-Fiber Foods:** Fiber is crucial for healthy digestion. It adds bulk to stool, aiding in regular bowel movements and preventing constipation.

    o **Whole Grains:** Brown rice, oats, quinoa, and whole wheat bread are excellent sources of fiber.

    o **Fruits and Vegetables:** Apples, pears, berries, leafy greens, carrots, and broccoli are rich in fiber.

    o **Legumes:** Beans, lentils, and chickpeas provide a substantial amount of dietary fiber.

2. **Probiotic Foods:** Probiotics are live beneficial bacteria that support gut health by maintaining a balanced microbiome.

    o **Yogurt and Kefir:** These dairy products contain live cultures that enhance gut flora.

    o **Fermented Vegetables:** Sauerkraut, kimchi, and pickles are rich in probiotics.

    o **Kombucha:** This fermented tea is a good source of probiotics and can aid digestion.

3. **Prebiotic Foods:** Prebiotics are non-digestible fibers that feed beneficial gut bacteria, promoting their growth and activity.

    o **Garlic and Onions:** Both contain inulin, a type of prebiotic fiber.

    o **Bananas:** Particularly green bananas, which contain resistant starch.

    o **Asparagus and Artichokes:** These vegetables are high in prebiotic fibers.

4. **Healthy Fats:** Healthy fats can aid digestion by supporting the absorption of fat-soluble vitamins.

    o **Avocados:** Rich in healthy monounsaturated fats and fiber.

    o **Nuts and Seeds:** Almonds, chia seeds, and flaxseeds provide essential fatty acids and fiber.

    o **Olive Oil:** A source of monounsaturated fats that can help reduce inflammation in the gut.

5. **Hydrating Foods:** Staying hydrated is essential for digestive health as water helps dissolve fats and soluble fiber, allowing these substances to pass through the intestines more easily.

    o **Cucumbers and Watermelon:** High in water content and help keep the digestive system hydrated.

    o **Broths and Soups:** Provide hydration and are easy to digest.

o **Herbal Teas:** Chamomile, ginger, and peppermint teas can soothe the digestive tract and aid in digestion.

Habits that Support Digestive Health

1. **Eating Mindfully:**

   o **Chew Thoroughly:** Properly chewing food breaks it down into smaller pieces, making it easier for the stomach to digest.

   o **Eat Slowly:** Taking time to eat can prevent overeating and improve digestion by allowing the stomach to signal when it's full.

2. **Regular Exercise:**

   o **Daily Activity:** Regular physical activity stimulates the muscles of the digestive tract, helping to move food through the digestive system.

   o **Low-Impact Exercises:** Walking, yoga, and swimming can promote digestive health without putting too much strain on the body.

3. **Staying Hydrated:**

   o **Drink Water Throughout the Day:** Adequate hydration is vital for digestion as it helps dissolve nutrients and soluble fiber, making them easier to pass through the intestines.

   o **Avoid Excessive Caffeine and Alcohol:** Both can dehydrate the body and irritate the digestive system.

4. **Managing Stress:**

   o **Stress Reduction Techniques:** Practices such as meditation, deep breathing exercises, and mindfulness can help reduce stress, which is often linked to digestive issues.

   o **Adequate Sleep:** Ensuring sufficient rest can help regulate digestion and reduce stress on the body.

5. **Routine and Regularity:**

   o **Consistent Meal Times:** Eating at the same times each day can help regulate the digestive system.

   o **Balanced Meals:** Ensure each meal includes a balance of macronutrients (proteins, fats, and carbohydrates) and is rich in fiber.

6. **Avoiding Bad Habits:**

   o **Limit Processed Foods:** These often contain high levels of unhealthy fats, sugars, and additives that can disrupt digestive health.

   o **Avoid Overeating:** Eating large meals can overwhelm the digestive system, leading to discomfort and digestive issues.

Integrating These Practices

To support digestive health, aim to incorporate a variety of the mentioned foods into your daily diet and adopt the beneficial habits consistently. Start by making small changes, such as including a serving of probiotic-rich yogurt with breakfast or taking a short walk after meals to stimulate digestion. Gradually, these small changes can lead to significant improvements in digestive health and overall well-being.

Chapter 7: Hydration and Its Role in Wellness

7.1 The Importance of Staying Hydrated

Staying hydrated is essential for maintaining overall health and well-being. Water is a critical component of the human body, making up about 60% of an adult's body weight. It plays a vital role in numerous bodily functions, including digestion, nutrient absorption, temperature regulation, and the maintenance of cellular health. Understanding the importance of hydration and ensuring adequate water intake can significantly impact physical and mental health.

Hydration and Physical Health

1. **Digestive Health:**

   o **Aids Digestion:** Water is crucial for the digestive process. It helps break down food, enabling the body to absorb nutrients more efficiently. Adequate hydration prevents constipation by softening stools and promoting regular bowel movements.

   o **Supports Enzyme Function:** Digestive enzymes, which are necessary for breaking down food, function optimally in a well-hydrated environment. Without sufficient water, these enzymes cannot perform effectively, leading to digestive issues.

2. **Nutrient Transportation:**

   o **Facilitates Absorption:** Water is essential for the absorption of nutrients from food. It dissolves vitamins, minerals, and other nutrients, making them accessible for transport to various parts of the body.

   o **Circulatory Support:** Adequate hydration ensures efficient blood circulation, which is necessary for delivering nutrients and oxygen to cells and removing waste products.

3. **Temperature Regulation:**

   o **Thermoregulation:** The body relies on water to regulate its temperature through processes such as sweating and respiration. Proper hydration helps maintain a stable internal temperature, preventing overheating during physical activity or in hot environments.

4. **Joint and Muscle Health:**

   o **Lubrication:** Water acts as a lubricant for joints and muscles, reducing friction and preventing discomfort or injury. It is also a major component of the synovial fluid that cushions joints.

   o **Muscle Function:** Hydration is essential for maintaining muscle function. Dehydration can lead to muscle cramps, fatigue, and impaired performance.

Hydration and Mental Health

1. **Cognitive Function:**

- o **Brain Performance:** The brain is highly sensitive to changes in hydration levels. Even mild dehydration can impair cognitive functions such as concentration, alertness, and short-term memory. Staying hydrated helps maintain optimal brain function.

- o **Mood Regulation:** Hydration also affects mood and mental well-being. Dehydration can lead to irritability, anxiety, and overall mood disturbances. Drinking enough water can help stabilize mood and improve emotional health.

2. **Energy Levels:**

- o **Prevents Fatigue:** Dehydration is a common cause of fatigue. When the body lacks sufficient water, it has to work harder to perform basic functions, leading to feelings of tiredness and lethargy. Adequate hydration boosts energy levels and improves overall vitality.

How to Stay Hydrated

1. **Drink Plenty of Water:**

- o **Daily Intake:** The general recommendation is to drink at least 8 cups (about 2 liters) of water per day, but individual needs may vary based on factors such as age, gender, weight, and activity level.

- o **Listen to Your Body:** Thirst is a natural indicator of the body's hydration needs. Drink water regularly throughout the day, especially before, during, and after physical activity.

2. **Eat Hydrating Foods:**

- o **Water-Rich Fruits and Vegetables:** Foods like cucumbers, watermelon, oranges, strawberries, and lettuce have high water content and contribute to overall hydration.

- o **Soups and Broths:** Including soups and broths in your diet can also help maintain hydration levels.

3. **Monitor Your Hydration:**

- o **Urine Color:** A simple way to monitor hydration is by checking the color of your urine. Light yellow or clear urine typically indicates adequate hydration, while dark yellow or amber-colored urine may suggest dehydration.

- o **Hydration Reminders:** Use reminders or apps to keep track of your water intake and ensure you're drinking enough throughout the day.

4. **Limit Dehydrating Beverages:**

- o **Caffeine and Alcohol:** Both caffeine and alcohol have diuretic effects, which can lead to increased urine production and dehydration. Limit intake of these beverages and balance them with additional water.

Benefits of Staying Hydrated

1. **Enhanced Physical Performance:**

- o **Improved Endurance:** Proper hydration can enhance physical performance by reducing fatigue and increasing stamina. Athletes and active individuals benefit significantly from staying well-hydrated.

- o **Quicker Recovery:** Hydration aids in quicker recovery from physical exertion by supporting muscle repair and reducing the risk of cramps and strains.

2. **Skin Health:**

   o **Hydrated Skin:** Drinking sufficient water helps maintain skin elasticity and prevents dryness. Proper hydration can lead to a clearer, more radiant complexion and reduce the appearance of wrinkles.

3. **Detoxification:**

   o **Waste Removal:** Water is essential for the kidneys to filter waste products from the blood and excrete them through urine. Staying hydrated supports the body's natural detoxification processes and helps prevent kidney stones.

4. **Weight Management:**

   o **Appetite Control:** Sometimes, the body can confuse thirst with hunger, leading to unnecessary snacking. Drinking water before meals can help control appetite and support weight management efforts.

In conclusion, staying hydrated is fundamental for maintaining optimal health. It supports a wide range of bodily functions, from digestion and nutrient absorption to cognitive performance and mood regulation. By prioritizing adequate water intake and incorporating hydrating foods into your diet, you can enhance your physical and mental well-being, ensuring your body operates at its best.

7.2 Hydrating Foods and Beverages

Incorporating hydrating foods and beverages into your diet is an effective and enjoyable way to ensure your body receives the water it needs. While drinking water is the most straightforward method of staying hydrated, consuming foods and beverages with high water content can significantly contribute to your overall hydration. This approach not only helps in maintaining fluid balance but also provides essential nutrients and supports overall health.

Hydrating Foods

1. **Fruits:**

   o **Watermelon:** Composed of about 92% water, watermelon is one of the most hydrating fruits. It is also rich in vitamins A, C, and antioxidants like lycopene, which contribute to skin health and reduce inflammation.

   o **Strawberries:** These berries contain around 91% water and are packed with vitamins, fiber, and antioxidants. They help keep you hydrated while supporting heart health and boosting the immune system.

   o **Cucumbers:** With a water content of approximately 95%, cucumbers are extremely hydrating. They are also a good source of vitamins K and B, as well as minerals like potassium and magnesium.

   o **Oranges:** Oranges are about 86% water and are an excellent source of vitamin C, which supports immune function and skin health. Their natural sugars and fiber content also help maintain energy levels.

2. **Vegetables:**

- **Lettuce:** Certain types of lettuce, such as iceberg, are composed of about 95% water. Lettuce is low in calories and provides fiber, vitamin A, and vitamin K.

- **Celery:** Celery has a water content of about 95% and is a great source of fiber and essential nutrients like vitamin K and potassium. Its natural salt content can also help replenish electrolytes.

- **Zucchini:** With about 94% water content, zucchini is not only hydrating but also versatile in cooking. It is rich in vitamins C and A, as well as fiber and antioxidants.

- **Tomatoes:** Tomatoes consist of around 94% water and are rich in vitamins A and C, potassium, and the antioxidant lycopene. They support hydration while promoting heart health and reducing the risk of chronic diseases.

Hydrating Beverages

1. **Infused Water:**

   - **Fruit and Herb-Infused Water:** Adding slices of fruits such as lemon, lime, cucumber, or berries to water can enhance its flavor and make it more appealing. Herbs like mint, basil, and rosemary not only add a refreshing taste but also provide additional nutrients and antioxidants.

   - **Coconut Water:** Coconut water is a natural electrolyte-rich beverage that helps maintain hydration, especially after physical activity. It contains potassium, magnesium, and sodium, which aid in restoring electrolyte balance.

2. **Herbal Teas:**

   - **Peppermint Tea:** Peppermint tea is hydrating and has a cooling effect that can help soothe digestion and reduce stress. It is caffeine-free, making it a great choice for hydration without the diuretic effects of caffeine.

   - **Chamomile Tea:** Chamomile tea, known for its calming properties, is also a good hydrating beverage. It can help promote relaxation and improve sleep quality, contributing to overall well-being.

3. **Soups and Broths:**

   - **Vegetable Broth:** Broths made from vegetables or bones are hydrating and provide essential nutrients like vitamins, minerals, and amino acids. They can be consumed as a warm beverage or used as a base for soups and stews.

   - **Gazpacho:** This cold soup made from blended raw vegetables, such as tomatoes, cucumbers, and bell peppers, is a hydrating and nutritious option, especially during hot weather.

Incorporating Hydrating Foods and Beverages into Your Diet

Plan Your Meals:

Balanced Diet: Incorporate a variety of hydrating fruits and vegetables into your meals. Aim to include a mix of different colors and types to ensure you receive a broad range of nutrients.

Healthy Snacks: Choose hydrating snacks such as cucumber slices, watermelon cubes, or a handful of strawberries. These can be refreshing and nutritious options between meals.

Be Creative:

Smoothies and Juices: Blend hydrating fruits and vegetables into smoothies or juices for a delicious and nutrient-packed beverage. Adding a handful of greens, such as spinach or kale, can boost the nutrient content even further.

Hydrating Recipes: Experiment with recipes that include hydrating ingredients, such as salads, soups, and fruit-based desserts. This can make staying hydrated more enjoyable and flavorful.

Stay Consistent:

Hydration Routine: Develop a hydration routine that includes both drinking water and consuming hydrating foods and beverages. Carry a water bottle and keep hydrating snacks accessible throughout the day.

Monitor Your Intake: Pay attention to your body's signals and ensure you're consuming enough fluids and hydrating foods, especially during hot weather or periods of increased physical activity.

Book 15: Detoxifying Your Diet

A Holistic Approach to Cleansing and Nourishing Your Body Naturally

Chapter 1: Identifying and Eliminating Toxins in Your Diet

Toxins in the diet can come from various sources, including processed foods, environmental contaminants, and even some naturally occurring substances in food. Identifying and eliminating these toxins is crucial for maintaining optimal health, preventing chronic diseases, and supporting the body's natural detoxification processes. Here's how to recognize and remove dietary toxins effectively:

Identifying Common Dietary Toxins

1. **Processed Foods:**

   o **Additives and Preservatives:** Many processed foods contain artificial additives, preservatives, and colorings that can be harmful to health. These chemicals can disrupt bodily functions, contribute to inflammation, and may even have carcinogenic effects.

   o **Trans Fats:** Found in partially hydrogenated oils, trans fats are linked to increased risk of heart disease, inflammation, and other health issues. They are often present in fried foods, baked goods, and margarine.

   o **High-Fructose Corn Syrup:** Commonly used as a sweetener in sodas, candies, and many processed snacks, high-fructose corn syrup has been associated with obesity, insulin resistance, and metabolic disorders.

2. **Pesticides and Herbicides:**

   o **Residue on Produce:** Non-organic fruits and vegetables can carry residues of pesticides and herbicides, which are used to protect crops from pests and weeds. Long-term exposure to these chemicals has been linked to various health problems, including hormone disruption and cancer.

   o **Contaminated Water:** Pesticides and herbicides can also contaminate water sources, leading to indirect ingestion through drinking water and irrigation of crops.

3. **Heavy Metals:**

   o **Mercury:** Found in some types of fish, such as tuna, swordfish, and shark, mercury can accumulate in the body and affect the nervous system, leading to cognitive impairments and developmental issues.

   o **Lead:** While lead contamination in food has decreased, it can still be present in water, certain imported foods, and old pipes, posing risks to brain development and kidney function.

4. **Natural Toxins:**

   o **Mycotoxins:** Produced by certain molds found on grains, nuts, and some fruits, mycotoxins can be harmful if ingested in large amounts. They have been linked to liver damage, immune suppression, and cancer.

- Lectins: Found in some raw legumes and grains, lectins can cause digestive distress and interfere with nutrient absorption if consumed in large quantities without proper preparation (e.g., soaking or cooking).

Steps to Eliminate Dietary Toxins

1. **Choose Whole Foods:**

   - **Minimize Processed Foods:** Opt for whole, unprocessed foods as the foundation of your diet. This includes fresh fruits and vegetables, whole grains, lean proteins, and healthy fats. Whole foods are less likely to contain harmful additives and preservatives.

   - **Read Labels:** When purchasing packaged foods, read labels carefully to avoid products with artificial additives, preservatives, and trans fats. Look for short ingredient lists with recognizable, natural components.

2. **Buy Organic When Possible:**

   - **Organic Produce:** Purchase organic fruits and vegetables to reduce exposure to pesticides and herbicides. Organic farming practices avoid synthetic chemicals, making organic produce a safer option.

   - **Organic Animal Products:** Choose organic meat, dairy, and eggs, as these products are produced without the use of antibiotics, synthetic hormones, and feed grown with pesticides.

3. **Filter Water:**

   - **Use Water Filters:** Install water filters to reduce contaminants such as pesticides, heavy metals, and chlorine in your drinking water. Ensure the filter is certified to remove specific toxins of concern.

   - **Avoid Bottled Water:** Choose filtered tap water over bottled water to avoid potential contaminants from plastic packaging and to reduce environmental impact.

4. **Proper Food Preparation:**

   - **Rinse and Peel:** Wash fruits and vegetables thoroughly to remove pesticide residues. Peeling can also help reduce exposure, but it may also remove some nutrients, so balance this practice based on the type of produce.

   - **Cook Legumes and Grains:** Soak and cook legumes and grains properly to reduce natural toxins like lectins. This not only improves digestibility but also enhances nutrient absorption.

5. **Select Safe Seafood:**

   - **Low-Mercury Fish:** Choose fish with lower mercury levels, such as salmon, sardines, and trout. Limit consumption of high-mercury fish like tuna and swordfish, especially for pregnant women and young children.

   - **Sustainable Sources:** Opt for sustainably sourced seafood to ensure it is free from harmful contaminants and to support environmentally responsible fishing practices.

6. **Limit Exposure to Mycotoxins:**

   - **Store Food Properly:** Store grains, nuts, and dried fruits in cool, dry conditions to prevent mold growth. Use airtight containers and check for signs of mold before consumption.

o **Diversify Diet:** Incorporate a variety of foods into your diet to minimize the risk of consuming high levels of mycotoxins from any single source.

Benefits of Eliminating Toxins

1. **Improved Health and Vitality:**

   o **Reduced Inflammation:** By eliminating harmful additives and chemicals, you can reduce chronic inflammation, which is linked to numerous health issues, including heart disease and autoimmune disorders.

   o **Enhanced Immune Function:** Reducing toxin intake supports the immune system, helping the body better fight off infections and illnesses.

2. **Better Digestive Health:**

   o **Fewer Digestive Issues:** Minimizing toxins can alleviate digestive problems such as bloating, gas, and constipation, leading to improved gut health and overall comfort.

   o **Optimal Nutrient Absorption:** A toxin-free diet enhances nutrient absorption, ensuring that your body gets the vitamins and minerals it needs to function optimally.

3. **Increased Energy Levels:**

   o **Stable Blood Sugar:** Avoiding processed foods and high-fructose corn syrup helps maintain stable blood sugar levels, preventing energy crashes and promoting sustained energy throughout the day.

   o **Detoxification Support:** A cleaner diet supports the body's natural detoxification processes, reducing the burden on organs like the liver and kidneys and boosting overall energy levels.

By identifying and eliminating toxins in your diet, you can significantly improve your health and well-being. This proactive approach not only reduces your risk of chronic diseases but also supports your body's natural ability to detoxify and thrive.

Chapter 2: Clean Eating Principles

Clean eating is a lifestyle approach that focuses on consuming whole, unprocessed foods that are as close to their natural state as possible. The principles of clean eating emphasize the importance of nutrition, balance, and mindful eating, aiming to nourish the body and promote overall health. Here are the core principles of clean eating and how they can be incorporated into your daily routine.

Emphasize Whole, Unprocessed Foods

1. **Fruits and Vegetables:**

    o **Variety and Color:** Aim to include a wide variety of fruits and vegetables in your diet. Different colors often indicate different nutrients, so eating a rainbow of produce ensures a broad range of vitamins, minerals, and antioxidants.

    o **Fresh and Seasonal:** Choose fresh, seasonal produce whenever possible. Seasonal fruits and vegetables are often more nutrient-dense and flavorful, and they support local farming practices.

2. **Whole Grains:**

    o **Unrefined Choices:** Opt for whole grains like brown rice, quinoa, oats, and whole wheat products. These grains retain their nutrient-rich bran and germ, providing more fiber, vitamins, and minerals compared to refined grains.

    o **Minimal Processing:** Choose grains that have undergone minimal processing. For example, steel-cut oats are less processed than instant oats and retain more nutrients.

3. **Lean Proteins:**

    o **Quality Sources:** Include lean protein sources such as poultry, fish, beans, lentils, tofu, and eggs. These provide essential amino acids needed for muscle repair and overall health.

    o **Plant-Based Proteins:** Incorporate plant-based proteins, which are often lower in saturated fat and can be rich in fiber and other nutrients. Examples include lentils, chickpeas, and quinoa.

4. **Healthy Fats:**

    o **Unsaturated Fats:** Focus on healthy fats from sources like avocados, nuts, seeds, and olive oil. These fats support heart health and provide essential fatty acids.

    o **Avoid Trans Fats:** Steer clear of trans fats and hydrogenated oils found in many processed foods. These unhealthy fats are linked to inflammation and various chronic diseases.

Minimize Processed and Refined Foods

1. **Read Labels:**

    o **Ingredients List:** Pay attention to food labels and avoid products with long lists of ingredients, especially those you cannot pronounce. Simpler ingredient lists typically indicate less processing.

- **Hidden Sugars:** Be aware of added sugars hidden in processed foods. Common names for added sugars include high-fructose corn syrup, cane sugar, and malt syrup. Opt for natural sweeteners like honey or maple syrup in moderation.

2. **Home Cooking:**

- **Control Ingredients:** Cooking at home allows you to control the ingredients and preparation methods, ensuring meals are made from whole, nutritious foods without unnecessary additives.

- **Batch Cooking:** Prepare meals in batches to save time and ensure you have healthy, homemade options readily available throughout the week.

Balanced Nutrition

1. **Macronutrient Balance:**

- **Carbohydrates, Proteins, and Fats:** Aim for a balanced intake of carbohydrates, proteins, and fats at each meal. This balance supports sustained energy levels and overall health.

- **Portion Control:** Be mindful of portion sizes to maintain a healthy weight and avoid overeating. Use visual cues, like filling half your plate with vegetables, a quarter with protein, and a quarter with whole grains.

2. **Micronutrient Richness:**

- **Vitamins and Minerals:** Ensure your diet is rich in vitamins and minerals by eating a diverse array of foods. Nutrient-dense foods include leafy greens, nuts, seeds, and colorful vegetables.

- **Supplements:** While whole foods should be your primary nutrient source, supplements can help fill gaps in your diet. Consult with a healthcare provider before starting any new supplements.

Mindful Eating Practices

1. **Eat Slowly and Savor:**

- **Mindful Chewing:** Chew food thoroughly and eat slowly to aid digestion and help recognize fullness cues. This practice can prevent overeating and promote better nutrient absorption.

- **Appreciate Flavors:** Take time to appreciate the flavors, textures, and aromas of your food. This mindfulness can enhance your eating experience and satisfaction.

2. **Listen to Your Body:**

- **Hunger and Fullness Cues:** Pay attention to your body's hunger and fullness signals. Eat when you are hungry and stop when you feel comfortably full, rather than eating out of habit or emotion.

- **Emotional Eating:** Recognize emotional eating patterns and find alternative ways to cope with stress or boredom, such as exercise, hobbies, or talking to a friend.

Hydration

1. **Water Intake:**

- **Adequate Hydration:** Drink plenty of water throughout the day to stay hydrated. Water is essential for digestion, nutrient absorption, and overall bodily functions.

- **Limit Sugary Drinks:** Avoid sugary beverages like sodas and energy drinks. Instead, opt for water, herbal teas, and natural fruit-infused waters.

2. **Electrolyte Balance:**

   o **Hydrating Foods:** Include hydrating foods in your diet, such as cucumbers, watermelon, and oranges. These foods not only provide water but also supply essential electrolytes like potassium and magnesium.

Sustainable and Ethical Choices

1. **Organic and Non-GMO:**

   o **Organic Produce:** Choose organic produce to reduce exposure to pesticides and support sustainable farming practices. Organic foods are grown without synthetic pesticides and fertilizers.

   o **Non-GMO Foods:** Select non-GMO (genetically modified organism) foods when possible. Non-GMO choices are considered more natural and environmentally friendly.

2. **Local and Seasonal Foods:**

   o **Support Local Farmers:** Buying local foods supports local economies and reduces the environmental impact of transporting food long distances.

   o **Seasonal Eating:** Eating seasonally ensures that you are consuming fresh, nutrient-dense foods that are at their peak in flavor and nutrition.

By adhering to these clean eating principles, you can foster a healthier, more balanced lifestyle. This approach not only benefits your physical health but also promotes mindful eating habits and supports sustainable and ethical food choices.

Chapter 3: Recipes for Detoxifying Meals

Detoxifying meals are designed to support the body's natural detoxification processes, nourish your system with essential nutrients, and help eliminate toxins. These meals emphasize whole, unprocessed foods rich in antioxidants, fiber, and hydration. Here are some easy-to-follow recipes that can be incorporated into your daily diet to promote detoxification.

Green Detox Smoothie

A green detox smoothie is a refreshing way to start your day, packed with vitamins, minerals, and antioxidants. This smoothie helps cleanse the digestive system and provides a boost of energy.

Ingredients:

- 1 cup kale or spinach
- 1 small cucumber, chopped
- 1 green apple, cored and chopped
- 1/2 avocado
- 1 tablespoon chia seeds
- 1 tablespoon fresh lemon juice
- 1 cup coconut water or filtered water
- Ice cubes (optional)

Instructions:

- Combine all ingredients in a blender.
- Blend until smooth and creamy.
- Adjust the consistency by adding more water if needed.
- Pour into a glass and enjoy immediately.

Quinoa and Vegetable Salad

This quinoa and vegetable salad is a nutrient-dense dish that provides a great source of plant-based protein, fiber, and antioxidants. It's perfect for a light lunch or as a side dish.

Ingredients:

- 1 cup quinoa, rinsed
- 2 cups water or vegetable broth
- 1 cup cherry tomatoes, halved
- 1 cup cucumber, diced
- 1/2 red bell pepper, diced

- 1/4 cup red onion, finely chopped
- 1/4 cup fresh parsley, chopped
- 1/4 cup fresh mint, chopped
- 1/4 cup fresh lemon juice
- 2 tablespoons extra-virgin olive oil
- Salt and pepper to taste

Instructions:

- In a medium saucepan, bring water or vegetable broth to a boil. Add quinoa, reduce heat to low, cover, and simmer for 15 minutes or until water is absorbed.
- Remove from heat and let quinoa cool to room temperature.
- In a large bowl, combine cherry tomatoes, cucumber, red bell pepper, red onion, parsley, and mint.
- Add the cooked quinoa to the bowl and mix well.
- In a small bowl, whisk together lemon juice, olive oil, salt, and pepper.
- Pour the dressing over the salad and toss to combine.
- Serve immediately or refrigerate for up to 2 days.

Roasted Root Vegetables with Turmeric

Roasted root vegetables are a comforting and detoxifying meal that helps support liver function and reduce inflammation. Turmeric, known for its anti-inflammatory properties, adds a warming flavor to the dish.

Ingredients:

- 2 large carrots, peeled and chopped
- 2 medium sweet potatoes, peeled and chopped
- 1 large beet, peeled and chopped
- 1 tablespoon olive oil
- 1 teaspoon ground turmeric
- 1/2 teaspoon ground cumin
- 1/2 teaspoon ground cinnamon
- Salt and pepper to taste
- Fresh parsley for garnish

Instructions:

- Preheat the oven to 400°F (200°C).
- In a large bowl, combine carrots, sweet potatoes, and beets.
- Drizzle olive oil over the vegetables and sprinkle with turmeric, cumin, cinnamon, salt, and pepper. Toss to coat evenly.
- Spread the vegetables in a single layer on a baking sheet lined with parchment paper.
- Roast for 25-30 minutes or until vegetables are tender and slightly crispy.
- Remove from the oven and let cool for a few minutes.
- Garnish with fresh parsley and serve.

Detoxifying Miso Soup

Miso soup is a traditional Japanese dish known for its gut-healing properties. This version includes detoxifying ingredients like seaweed, ginger, and garlic to enhance its cleansing effects.

Ingredients:

- 4 cups vegetable broth
- 2 tablespoons miso paste
- 1 cup sliced shiitake mushrooms
- 1 cup chopped bok choy
- 1/4 cup chopped scallions
- 1 sheet nori (seaweed), cut into strips
- 1 tablespoon fresh ginger, grated
- 2 cloves garlic, minced
- 1 tablespoon tamari or soy sauce
- 1 teaspoon sesame oil
- Fresh cilantro for garnish

Instructions:

- In a large pot, bring vegetable broth to a simmer over medium heat.
- In a small bowl, whisk miso paste with a bit of hot broth until smooth, then add back to the pot.
- Add shiitake mushrooms, bok choy, scallions, nori, ginger, garlic, tamari, and sesame oil to the pot.
- Simmer for 10-15 minutes until vegetables are tender.
- Remove from heat and let cool slightly.
- Garnish with fresh cilantro and serve hot.

Detoxifying Beet and Carrot Juice

This vibrant juice is packed with nutrients that support liver detoxification and improve digestion. Beets and carrots are high in antioxidants, vitamins, and minerals, making this juice a perfect detoxifying drink.

Ingredients:

- 2 medium beets, peeled and chopped
- 3 large carrots, peeled and chopped
- 1 green apple, cored and chopped
- 1-inch piece of fresh ginger, peeled
- 1 tablespoon fresh lemon juice

Instructions:

- Run beets, carrots, apple, and ginger through a juicer.
- Stir in fresh lemon juice.
- Pour into a glass and enjoy immediately.

These detoxifying recipes are not only delicious but also easy to prepare. Incorporating them into your diet can help support your body's natural detoxification processes and promote overall health and wellness.

Chapter 4: Nutrition for Specific Health Concerns

4.1 Managing Weight with Nutritional Choices

Empower yourself by understanding the intricate relationship between what we consume and how our bodies respond. Managing weight effectively through nutritional choices is not solely about counting calories, but about choosing the right foods that nourish the body, boost metabolism, and support overall health. Here are some essential principles and strategies to manage weight through nutrition.

Emphasize Whole, Unprocessed Foods

Whole foods, such as fruits, vegetables, whole grains, lean proteins, and healthy fats, should form the foundation of your diet. These foods are not only rich in essential nutrients, fiber, and antioxidants, but they also provide a satisfying eating experience. By focusing on whole foods, you naturally reduce the intake of processed foods often high in added sugars, unhealthy fats, and empty calories.

Balance Macronutrients

A balanced intake of macronutrients—carbohydrates, proteins, and fats—is crucial for weight management. Each macronutrient plays a specific role in the body:

Carbohydrates: Choose complex carbohydrates like whole grains, legumes, and vegetables over simple sugars. Complex carbs provide sustained energy and help keep you full longer.

Proteins: Lean proteins from sources like poultry, fish, beans, and legumes are essential for muscle repair and growth. Protein also has a higher thermic effect, meaning it requires more energy for digestion, which can boost metabolism.

Fats: Healthy fats from sources like avocados, nuts, seeds, and olive oil are important for satiety and hormone regulation. Avoid trans fats and limit saturated fats.

Monitor Portion Sizes

Even healthy foods can contribute to weight gain if consumed in large quantities. Being mindful of portion sizes helps manage calorie intake without requiring strict calorie counting. For example, a serving of protein should be about the size of your palm, a serving of carbohydrates should be about the size of your fist, and a serving of fats should be about the size of your thumb. Using smaller plates, measuring servings, and being aware of hunger and fullness cues can aid in controlling portions.

Include Fiber-Rich Foods

Fiber is a key component in weight management as it aids in digestion, promotes a feeling of fullness, and helps control blood sugar levels. High-fiber foods like vegetables, fruits, whole grains, and legumes can reduce overall calorie intake by making you feel fuller longer.

Hydrate Adequately

Staying hydrated is essential for weight management. Often, thirst can be mistaken for hunger, leading to unnecessary calorie consumption. Drinking water before meals can also promote a sense of fullness, reducing the likelihood of overeating. Aim for at least eight glasses of water a day, and incorporate hydrating foods like cucumbers, watermelon, and leafy greens.

Plan and Prepare Meals

Planning and preparing meals in advance can help ensure that you make healthy choices consistently. It reduces the temptation to opt for convenience foods often high in calories and low in nutritional value. Meal prepping also allows you to control ingredients and portion sizes, making sticking to your dietary goals easier.

Be Mindful of Eating Habits

Mindful eating involves paying full attention to the eating experience, from the sensory pleasure of food to recognizing hunger and satiety signals. It's about being present in the moment and fully enjoying your meal. Avoiding distractions like TV or smartphones during meals can help you appreciate the food more and recognize when you are full, preventing overeating.

Limit Added Sugars and Refined Carbs

Foods high in added sugars and refined carbohydrates can lead to spikes in blood sugar levels, followed by crashes, increasing hunger and cravings. Reducing the intake of sugary snacks, sodas, and refined grains can help maintain stable blood sugar levels and reduce overall calorie intake.

Incorporate Healthy Snacks

Choosing healthy snacks can liberate you from the guilt of overeating at main meals and keep your metabolism active. Opt for snacks that combine protein, fiber, and healthy fats, such as nuts, seeds, yogurt, or fruit with nut butter. These snacks can provide sustained energy and help keep hunger at bay.

Consistency Over Perfection

Weight management is a long-term commitment and should focus on consistent, healthy habits rather than perfection. Allowing occasional indulgences without guilt can prevent feelings of deprivation and help maintain a balanced approach to eating.

Incorporating these nutritional principles into your daily routine allows you to manage your weight effectively while promoting overall health and well-being. Remember, sustainable weight management is about making lasting changes that you can maintain over time rather than quick fixes or extreme diets.

4.2 Nutrition for Heart Health

Maintaining a healthy heart is essential for overall well-being, and nutrition plays a crucial role in supporting cardiovascular health. By making mindful dietary choices, you can significantly reduce the risk of heart disease and promote a strong, efficient heart. Here are key principles and strategies for nutrition that supports heart health:

Prioritize Whole, Unprocessed Foods

Eating a diet rich in whole, unprocessed foods provides essential nutrients that benefit heart health. Whole foods include fresh fruits, vegetables, whole grains, nuts, seeds, legumes, lean proteins, and healthy fats. These foods are packed with vitamins, minerals, antioxidants, and fiber that support cardiovascular function and reduce inflammation.

Focus on Healthy Fats

Not all fats are created equal when it comes to heart health. It's important to incorporate healthy fats while limiting unhealthy ones:

Healthy Fats: Include sources of unsaturated fats such as avocados, nuts, seeds, and olive oil. Omega-3 fatty acids, found in fatty fish like salmon, mackerel, and sardines, as well as flaxseeds and walnuts, are particularly beneficial for heart health. Omega-3s help reduce inflammation, lower triglyceride levels, and improve overall cardiovascular function.

Unhealthy Fats: Limit saturated fats found in red meat, full-fat dairy products, and processed foods. Avoid trans fats, which are often present in fried foods, baked goods, and processed snacks, as they raise LDL (bad) cholesterol and lower HDL (good) cholesterol, increasing the risk of heart disease.

Incorporate Fiber-Rich Foods

Fiber, particularly soluble fiber, plays a significant role in maintaining heart health. Soluble fiber helps reduce cholesterol levels by binding to cholesterol particles and removing them from the body. Foods high in soluble fiber include oats, barley, beans, lentils, fruits (such as apples, berries, and citrus fruits), and vegetables (like carrots and Brussels sprouts).

Reduce Sodium Intake

High sodium intake is linked to high blood pressure, a major risk factor for heart disease. To reduce sodium intake, avoid adding salt to meals, and limit consumption of processed foods, canned soups, deli meats, and salty snacks. Instead, use herbs and spices to flavor your meals. Reading food labels and choosing low-sodium or no-salt-added options can also help manage sodium intake.

Emphasize Plant-Based Proteins

Including plant-based proteins in your diet can benefit heart health. Legumes (such as beans, lentils, and chickpeas), nuts, seeds, tofu, and tempeh are excellent sources of plant-based proteins. These foods are low in saturated fat and high in fiber, vitamins, and minerals, making them heart-friendly options.

Include Heart-Healthy Nutrients

Certain nutrients are particularly beneficial for heart health:

- Potassium: Helps balance sodium levels and supports healthy blood pressure. Potassium-rich foods include bananas, oranges, sweet potatoes, spinach, and tomatoes.

- Magnesium: Supports heart rhythm and blood vessel health. Sources of magnesium include leafy green vegetables, nuts, seeds, and whole grains.

- Antioxidants: Protect the heart from oxidative stress and inflammation. Antioxidant-rich foods include berries, dark chocolate, green tea, and brightly colored fruits and vegetables.

Maintain a Healthy Weight

Achieving and maintaining a healthy weight is crucial for heart health. Excess weight, particularly around the abdomen, can increase the risk of heart disease. Focus on a balanced diet that provides adequate nutrients without excessive calories. Regular physical activity, in combination with healthy eating, supports weight management and cardiovascular health.

Monitor Blood Sugar Levels

High blood sugar levels can damage blood vessels and increase the risk of heart disease. Consuming a diet that stabilizes blood sugar can help protect your heart. Choose whole grains over refined grains, limit added sugars, and include protein and healthy fats in your meals to prevent spikes in blood sugar levels.

<u>Stay Hydrated</u>

Proper hydration supports overall health, including heart function. Water is essential for maintaining blood volume and ensuring efficient circulation. Aim to drink plenty of water throughout the day and limit sugary drinks, which can contribute to weight gain and increased heart disease risk.

<u>Avoid Excessive Alcohol</u>

Moderate alcohol consumption may have some heart benefits, but excessive alcohol intake can lead to high blood pressure, heart failure, and other cardiovascular problems. If you choose to drink alcohol, do so in moderation— up to one drink per day for women and up to two drinks per day for men.

By adhering to these nutritional guidelines, you can significantly improve your heart health and reduce the risk of cardiovascular disease. Consistent, heart-healthy eating habits contribute to long-term well-being and enhance the quality of life.

4.3 Other Common Health Issues and Nutritional Solutions

Nutrition plays a pivotal role in addressing and managing various common health issues beyond heart health. Here are several health concerns and the nutritional strategies that can help mitigate their impact:

4.3.1 Diabetes Management

For individuals managing diabetes, maintaining stable blood sugar levels is paramount. Key nutritional strategies include:

- Carbohydrate Management: Monitoring carbohydrate intake and choosing complex carbohydrates with low glycemic index values.

- Fiber-Rich Foods: Consuming fiber-rich foods like whole grains, fruits, and vegetables to slow down glucose absorption.

- Lean Proteins and Healthy Fats: Balancing meals with lean proteins and healthy fats to help stabilize blood sugar levels.

4.3.2 Bone Health and Osteoporosis Prevention

To promote bone health and prevent osteoporosis, focus on:

- Calcium and Vitamin D: Consuming foods rich in calcium (e.g., dairy products, leafy greens, fortified foods) and ensuring adequate vitamin D intake (through sunlight exposure and fortified foods).

- Magnesium and Vitamin K: Including foods rich in magnesium (e.g., nuts, seeds, whole grains) and vitamin K (e.g., leafy greens, broccoli) to support bone density.

4.3.3 Digestive Issues and Gut Health

To support digestive health and alleviate digestive issues such as bloating and constipation:

- Fiber-Rich Foods: Including ample fiber from fruits, vegetables, whole grains, and legumes to promote regular bowel movements.

- Probiotics: Consuming probiotic-rich foods like yogurt, kefir, sauerkraut, and kimchi to support gut flora balance.

- Hydration: Drinking adequate water and avoiding dehydration, which can contribute to digestive discomfort.

4.3.4 Cognitive Function and Brain Health

Nutrition can play a role in maintaining cognitive function and brain health:

- Omega-3 Fatty Acids: Consuming fatty fish (e.g., salmon, mackerel) or plant-based sources of omega-3s (e.g., flaxseeds, walnuts) to support brain structure and function.

- Antioxidants: Eating a diet rich in antioxidants from colorful fruits and vegetables to protect brain cells from oxidative stress.

- B Vitamins: Ensuring sufficient intake of B vitamins (found in whole grains, leafy greens, eggs) to support cognitive processes.

4.3.5 Immune System Support

To bolster immune function and resilience against infections:

- Vitamin C: Consuming citrus fruits, strawberries, bell peppers, and broccoli for immune-boosting vitamin C.

- Zinc: Including zinc-rich foods like lean meats, poultry, seafood, beans, and nuts to support immune cell function.

- Protein: Ensuring adequate protein intake for immune system function and tissue repair.

4.3.6 Skin Health and Aging

Nutrition can contribute to skin health and combat signs of aging:

- Antioxidants: Eating foods rich in antioxidants (e.g., berries, dark chocolate, green tea) to protect skin cells from damage caused by free radicals.

- Omega-3 Fatty Acids: Including omega-3s from fish, flaxseeds, and chia seeds to support skin hydration and elasticity.

- Hydration: Drinking plenty of water and consuming hydrating foods like cucumbers and watermelon to maintain skin moisture.

4.3.7 Energy Levels and Fatigue Management

For sustained energy levels throughout the day:

- Complex Carbohydrates: Choosing whole grains, fruits, and vegetables for steady energy release.

- Iron-Rich Foods: Consuming iron-rich foods like lean meats, beans, and dark leafy greens to prevent fatigue due to iron deficiency anemia.

- Hydration: Staying adequately hydrated to support metabolic processes and prevent dehydration-related fatigue.

By integrating these nutritional strategies into your daily diet, you can effectively address common health issues and support overall well-being. Consulting with a healthcare provider or registered dietitian can provide personalized guidance tailored to your specific health needs and goals.

Book 16: Essential Oils and Aromatherapy by Barbara O'Neill

A Comprehensive Guide to Natural Healing, Emotional Balance, and Holistic Wellness

Chapter 1: Introduction to Aromatherapy

Aromatherapy is a holistic healing practice that utilizes natural plant extracts, known as essential oils, to promote physical, emotional, and psychological well-being. These essential oils are highly concentrated extracts obtained from various parts of aromatic plants, including flowers, leaves, bark, and roots. Aromatherapy harnesses the therapeutic properties of these oils through inhalation, topical application, or ingestion (in some cases under professional guidance).

1.1 History and Origins of Aromatherapy

The use of aromatic plants and their oils dates back thousands of years across different cultures worldwide. Ancient civilizations, including the Egyptians, Greeks, Romans, and Chinese, utilized aromatic plants for medicinal, spiritual, and cosmetic purposes. The Egyptians were pioneers in distillation techniques, extracting essential oils such as cedarwood, frankincense, and myrrh for embalming practices and rituals. In Greece, renowned physician Hippocrates documented the medicinal properties of aromatic oils and herbs, laying the foundation for their therapeutic use in Western medicine.

During the Middle Ages, aromatics gained popularity in Europe for their perceived healing properties during outbreaks of plague and other diseases. The term "aromatherapy" was coined in the early 20th century by French chemist René-Maurice Gattefossé, who discovered the healing effects of lavender oil after burning his hand and found that lavender accelerated the healing process and minimized scarring.

Today, aromatherapy is practiced worldwide and has evolved into a recognized complementary therapy. It is employed in various settings, including spas, hospitals, and homes, to enhance physical health, alleviate stress, improve mood, and support overall well-being.

1.2 Benefits of Aromatherapy for Physical and Emotional Health

Aromatherapy offers a myriad of benefits for both physical and emotional health:

- Stress Relief and Relaxation: Certain essential oils, such as lavender, chamomile, and bergamot, have calming properties that help reduce stress, anxiety, and tension. Inhalation of these oils or their application through massage promotes relaxation and induces a sense of tranquility.

- Enhanced Mood: Essential oils like citrus oils (e.g., orange, lemon) and floral oils (e.g., rose, jasmine) are known for their uplifting and mood-enhancing effects. They stimulate the production of neurotransmitters like serotonin and dopamine, promoting feelings of happiness and well-being.

- Pain Management: Some essential oils possess analgesic properties that can alleviate pain and inflammation. Peppermint oil, for example, is effective in relieving headaches and muscle aches when applied topically or inhaled.

- Improved Sleep Quality: Lavender and chamomile oils are popular choices for promoting sleep and combating insomnia. These oils have sedative properties that can induce relaxation and facilitate a restful night's sleep.

- Skin Care: Essential oils like tea tree, rosehip, and geranium have antibacterial, anti-inflammatory, and antioxidant properties beneficial for skincare. They are used in natural skincare products to cleanse, moisturize, and rejuvenate the skin.

- Respiratory Support: Inhalation of essential oils such as eucalyptus, peppermint, and tea tree can help clear congestion, alleviate sinusitis, and support respiratory health by reducing inflammation and promoting easier breathing.

- Cognitive Function: Some essential oils, such as rosemary and peppermint, are known for their cognitive-enhancing properties. They can improve concentration, memory retention, and mental clarity when used aromatically.

Aromatherapy is a versatile and gentle healing modality that complements conventional medicine and promotes holistic well-being. When used mindfully and safely, essential oils can provide numerous therapeutic benefits for physical ailments, emotional balance, and overall quality of life.

1.3 What Are Essential Oils?

Essential oils are highly concentrated aromatic compounds extracted from various parts of plants, including flowers, leaves, stems, bark, and roots. These oils capture the plant's scent and beneficial properties through a process of steam distillation, cold pressing, or solvent extraction. Each essential oil contains volatile compounds that give it its distinctive fragrance and therapeutic characteristics.

Essential oils are renowned for their potent healing properties and have been used for centuries in traditional medicine, aromatherapy, perfumery, and cosmetics. They are prized for their ability to support physical health, emotional well-being, and spiritual practices. Due to their concentrated nature, essential oils are typically diluted in carrier oils or used sparingly in diffusers and topical applications to ensure safe and effective use.

1.3.1 Methods of Extracting Essential Oils

The extraction of essential oils involves several methods, each tailored to the specific plant material and desired constituents:

- Steam Distillation: This is the most common method for extracting essential oils from aromatic plants. Steam is passed through the plant material, causing the volatile compounds to evaporate. The steam-oil mixture is then condensed and separated, with the essential oil floating on top of the distilled water (hydrosol).

- Cold Pressing: This method is used primarily for extracting essential oils from citrus fruits like lemon, orange, and grapefruit. The fruit peel is mechanically pressed to release the essential oil, which is then separated from the juice and peel.

- Solvent Extraction: This method is employed for delicate plant materials that cannot withstand the heat of steam distillation or cold pressing. A solvent, such as hexane or ethanol, is used to extract the essential oil from the plant material. The solvent is then evaporated to leave behind the concentrated essential oil.

- CO2 Extraction: This advanced extraction method uses carbon dioxide under high pressure and low temperature to extract essential oils without altering their chemical composition. CO2 extraction yields high-quality oils that retain more of the plant's volatile compounds compared to other methods.

The choice of extraction method depends on factors such as the plant species, part of the plant used, desired constituents, and intended applications of the essential oil.

1.4 Quality and Purity Considerations

The quality and purity of essential oils are crucial factors that impact their efficacy and safety. Here are key considerations:

Ensure the essential oil is 100% pure and free from synthetic additives, diluents, or contaminants. Pure essential oils contain only the volatile aromatic compounds extracted from the plant without alteration or adulteration.

Choose essential oils from reputable suppliers known for their commitment to quality, sustainability, and ethical practices. Oils derived from organically grown plants are preferred to avoid pesticide residues.

It's crucial to look for essential oils that have undergone third-party testing for purity, authenticity, and potency. Certifications such as USDA Organic, ECOCERT, or ISO standards provide assurance of quality and safety, making them a reliable choice for your needs.

Proper storage of essential oils is key to maintaining their stability and shelf life. Storing them in dark glass bottles helps prevent light degradation, ensuring that the oils retain their potency and effectiveness over time.

Following dilution guidelines and usage recommendations provided by aromatherapy experts is crucial. This practice helps prevent skin sensitization, irritation, or adverse reactions, ensuring a safe and enjoyable experience with essential oils.

By mastering the selection of high-quality essential oils and comprehending their extraction methods and purity considerations, you can unlock the full therapeutic potential of these natural botanical extracts. This knowledge empowers you, instilling a sense of confidence and control, to use them effectively for health, wellness, and enjoyment.

1.5 Safety Guidelines for Using Essential Oils

While essential oils offer numerous health benefits, they are potent substances that require careful handling to ensure safe and effective use. Here are crucial safety guidelines to consider:

Essential oils are highly concentrated and should almost always be diluted before applying to the skin. This is because undiluted oils can cause skin irritation or sensitization. Exceptions include oils like lavender and tea tree, which can sometimes be applied neat (undiluted) in small quantities for spot treatments. Always follow recommended dilution ratios (typically 1-5%) to avoid these skin issues.

Keep essential oils away from sensitive areas such as eyes, ears, mucous membranes, and broken or irritated skin. If accidental contact occurs, rinse thoroughly with a carrier oil, not water, to dilute the oil and minimize discomfort.

Some citrus oils, such as bergamot and grapefruit, can cause skin sensitivity when exposed to sunlight. This condition, known as phototoxicity, can lead to skin reactions like redness or blistering. To prevent these issues, avoid sun exposure for 12-24 hours after applying these oils topically.

While some essential oils are safe for ingestion under professional guidance, most should not be taken internally without proper knowledge and supervision. Internal use can lead to toxicity, especially in high doses or prolonged use.

Exercise caution when using essential oils around children and pets. Some oils are unsafe for young children or animals, and diffusing oils in poorly ventilated areas can pose respiratory risks. For instance, some oils can cause breathing difficulties in pets or allergic reactions in children. Always research the safety of an oil before using it around these vulnerable individuals.

It's crucial to consult a healthcare professional before using essential oils during pregnancy, breastfeeding, or if you have underlying health conditions, including epilepsy, asthma, or allergies. This step ensures that you are being cared for and considered in your use of essential oils, making you feel valued and looked after.

Essential oils should be stored in dark glass bottles in a cool, dry place away from direct sunlight and heat. Bottles should be kept tightly closed and out of the reach of children and pets.

By adhering to these safety guidelines, you can minimize risks and ensure a positive experience when using essential oils for aromatherapy, massage, skin care, and other therapeutic purposes. This adherence provides a sense of security and confidence in your use of essential oils, making you feel reassured and protected.

1.5.1 Dilution Ratios and Carrier Oils

Proper dilution is essential for safe and effective use of essential oils. Diluting essential oils with a carrier oil not only reduces the risk of skin irritation but also helps spread the oil evenly over the skin surface. Here are common dilution ratios and carrier oils used:

For most adults, a safe dilution ratio is 1-2% essential oil to carrier oil. This translates to approximately 1-2 drops of essential oil per teaspoon (5 mL) of carrier oil. For children, elderly individuals, or those with sensitive skin, a lower dilution ratio (0.5-1%) is recommended.

Popular carrier oils include jojoba, sweet almond, coconut, grapeseed, and avocado oil. These oils are gentle on the skin and provide additional nourishment and hydration.

Select a carrier oil based on your skin type and the desired therapeutic effects. For example, jojoba oil closely resembles the skin's natural sebum and is suitable for all skin types, while coconut oil is rich in antioxidants and has antibacterial properties.

Mix essential oils and carrier oils thoroughly before applying them to the skin. Use gentle massage techniques to promote absorption and enhance the oil's therapeutic benefits.

Using a carrier oil not only dilutes essential oils but also helps carry their aromatic molecules into the skin, ensuring a safe and effective application for aromatherapy and skincare routines.

1.5.2 Patch Testing and Allergy Considerations

Patch testing is a crucial step to assess skin sensitivity and potential allergic reactions before using a new essential oil or blend. Here's how to conduct a patch test:

- Dilute: Mix 1-2 drops of essential oil with 1 teaspoon (5 mL) of carrier oil.

- Apply: Dab a small amount of the diluted oil on the inside of your forearm or wrist.

- Wait: Allow the oil to absorb into the skin and wait for 24-48 hours. Monitor the area for any signs of redness, irritation, itching, or swelling.

- Evaluate: If you experience any adverse reactions during this period, discontinue use and cleanse the area with a carrier oil or mild soap and water. Seek medical advice if symptoms persist or worsen.

Patch testing helps identify potential sensitivities and ensures that essential oils are used safely and effectively in your aromatherapy and skincare regimen. It's particularly important when trying new oils, blends, or using oils on sensitive skin or individuals prone to allergies.

Chapter 2: Popular Essential Oils and Their Benefits

2.1 Lavender

Lavender (Lavandula angustifolia) is one of the most versatile and beloved essential oils in aromatherapy. Known for its delicate floral scent and myriad therapeutic properties, lavender has been cherished for centuries for its calming and healing effects.

2.1.1 Calming and Healing Properties

Lavender essential oil is renowned for its ability to promote relaxation and reduce stress and anxiety. Inhalation of lavender oil vapors or its application on the skin can elicit a calming response by soothing the nervous system. This makes it an excellent choice for promoting restful sleep and managing symptoms of anxiety disorders.

Beyond its emotional benefits, lavender oil possesses potent healing properties. It has natural antibacterial, antifungal, and anti-inflammatory characteristics, making it effective in treating minor skin irritations, cuts, burns, and insect bites. Its gentle nature and soothing aroma also contribute to its popularity in skincare products, where it helps to promote skin healing and reduce inflammation.

2.1.2 Uses in Aromatherapy

In aromatherapy, lavender essential oil is widely used for its therapeutic effects on both the mind and body. Here are some common uses:

- Stress Reduction: Diffuse lavender oil in your home or workplace to create a calming atmosphere and alleviate stress and tension.

- Sleep Aid: Add a few drops of lavender oil to your pillow or bedding to promote relaxation and improve sleep quality.

- Skincare: Diluted lavender oil can be applied topically to soothe sunburns, minor cuts, and insect bites. It is also used in facial oils, creams, and lotions for its gentle moisturizing and healing properties.

- Massage: Blend lavender oil with a carrier oil for a relaxing massage that eases muscle tension and promotes relaxation.

- Bath: Add a few drops of lavender oil to your bathwater for a soothing and aromatic bath experience that helps unwind after a long day.

- Air Freshener: Create a natural air freshener by mixing lavender oil with water in a spray bottle. Use it to freshen up rooms or linens with its pleasant scent.

Lavender essential oil's versatility and gentle nature make it a staple in aromatherapy practices worldwide. Whether used for its calming effects, healing properties, or aromatic qualities, lavender remains a beloved essential oil cherished for its ability to promote overall well-being and relaxation.

2.2 Peppermint

Peppermint (Mentha piperita) essential oil is prized for its invigorating aroma and versatile therapeutic properties. It is extracted through steam distillation from the leaves of the peppermint plant, a hybrid of water mint and spearmint, and is widely used in aromatherapy for its refreshing and stimulating effects.

2.2.1 Invigorating and Refreshing Effects

Peppermint essential oil is renowned for its ability to uplift and energize both the mind and body. Its refreshing aroma can help combat mental fatigue, increase alertness, and promote focus and concentration. Inhalation of peppermint oil vapor or its application on the skin can provide a cooling sensation that revitalizes and refreshes.

Beyond its mental and emotional benefits, peppermint oil has potent analgesic and anti-inflammatory properties. When applied topically in a diluted form, it can help alleviate muscle aches, joint pain, and tension headaches. Its cooling effect also makes it effective for soothing sunburns and minor skin irritations.

2.2.2 Applications in Aromatherapy

Peppermint essential oil is versatile and can be used in various ways in aromatherapy:

- Mental Clarity: Diffuse peppermint oil in your workspace or study area to enhance mental clarity, concentration, and memory retention.

- Respiratory Support: Inhale peppermint oil vapor to relieve congestion and support respiratory function during colds or allergies. Its expectorant properties can help loosen phlegm and clear the airways.

- Digestive Aid: Massage diluted peppermint oil onto the abdomen in a clockwise direction to alleviate digestive discomfort, bloating, and gas. It can also be inhaled to ease nausea.

- Hair and Scalp Health: Add a few drops of peppermint oil to your shampoo or conditioner to promote scalp health, stimulate hair growth, and impart a cooling sensation.

- DIY Recipes: Incorporate peppermint oil into homemade cleaning products, room sprays, and natural insect repellents for its fresh and clean scent.

Peppermint essential oil's stimulating and therapeutic properties make it a popular choice in aromatherapy for promoting physical, mental, and emotional well-being. Whether used for its invigorating effects, pain-relieving properties, or aromatic qualities, peppermint oil remains a versatile and cherished essential oil in holistic health practices.

2.3 Tea Tree

Tea tree (Melaleuca alternifolia) essential oil is renowned for its potent antiseptic and antibacterial properties, making it a popular choice in natural medicine and skincare. It is extracted from the leaves of the tea tree native to Australia through steam distillation.

2.3.1 Antiseptic and Antibacterial Uses

Tea tree essential oil is highly valued for its ability to combat bacteria, fungi, and viruses. Its natural antiseptic and antimicrobial properties make it effective in treating various skin conditions, including acne, fungal infections (such as athlete's foot and nail fungus), and minor cuts and wounds. It can help cleanse and disinfect the skin without causing dryness or irritation, making it suitable for sensitive skin types.

2.3.2 Practical Applications

Tea tree oil offers a wide range of practical applications in both aromatherapy and skincare:

- Acne Treatment: Diluted tea tree oil can be applied topically to acne-prone areas to help reduce inflammation, fight acne-causing bacteria, and promote clearer skin. It can also be added to facial cleansers and toners.

- Skin Care: Use tea tree oil in diluted form as a natural remedy for minor skin irritations, cuts, and insect bites. Its soothing and disinfecting properties help promote healing and prevent infection.

- Hair Care: Add a few drops of tea tree oil to your shampoo to help alleviate dandruff, dry scalp, and itchiness. It can also help control excess oil production on the scalp.

- Household Cleaner: Mix tea tree oil with water and vinegar to create a natural disinfectant spray for cleaning surfaces, floors, and bathrooms. Its antibacterial properties make it effective against household germs.

- Air Purification: Diffuse tea tree oil in your home or workplace to cleanse the air and create a fresh, invigorating atmosphere. Its purifying properties can help eliminate odors and airborne pathogens.

- Foot Care: Soak feet in a warm water bath with a few drops of tea tree oil to help treat fungal infections like athlete's foot and toenail fungus. Its antifungal properties can help alleviate itching and discomfort.

Tea tree essential oil's versatile uses and powerful healing properties make it a valuable addition to any natural medicine cabinet. Whether used for its antiseptic benefits, skincare applications, or household cleaning purposes, tea tree oil provides effective and natural solutions for promoting overall health and well-being.

Chapter 3: Creating Aromatherapy Blends

3.1 Basics of Aromatherapy Blending

Aromatherapy blending is both an art and a science, involving the skillful combination of essential oils to create harmonious and effective aromas for therapeutic purposes. When blending essential oils, several factors should be considered to achieve desired results.

Each essential oil has unique aromatic notes, therapeutic properties, and intensity levels. Familiarize yourself with the characteristics of each oil, including its top, middle, and base notes. This understanding helps in creating balanced blends that unfold over time.

Determine the purpose of your blend—whether it's for relaxation, energy, focus, or skincare. Select essential oils known for their specific therapeutic benefits related to your desired outcome.

Essential oils are categorized into top, middle, and base notes based on their volatility and evaporation rates. Top notes are light, refreshing oils that evaporate quickly (e.g., citrus oils), middle notes are balancing and harmonizing (e.g., lavender), and base notes are deep, grounding oils that linger (e.g., cedarwood). A well-rounded blend includes oils from each category.

Use a ratio of essential oils that complements each other's aromas and therapeutic properties. Typically, a blend might consist of 20-30% top notes, 50-70% middle notes, and 10-20% base notes. Dilute essential oils in a carrier oil or alcohol to ensure safe application and to enhance absorption into the skin.

Blend small quantities of essential oils at a time and experiment with different combinations. Keep notes on your blends' compositions and effects to refine your skills and create personalized blends for specific needs.

Pay attention to safety guidelines when blending essential oils, particularly regarding skin sensitivities, allergies, and contraindications. Perform a patch test before applying a new blend to larger areas of the skin.

Allow blends to mature for a few days to a few weeks to allow the aromas to meld together harmoniously. Store blends in dark glass bottles in a cool, dark place to preserve their potency and aromatic qualities.

Aromatherapy blending offers a creative and therapeutic approach to enhancing physical, emotional, and mental well-being. By mastering the basics of blending and understanding the characteristics of essential oils, you can create customized blends that cater to individual preferences and therapeutic needs.

3.2 Methods for Blending Essential Oils

Blending essential oils is a nuanced process that can be approached in several effective ways, depending on the desired outcome and personal preference:

1. Dilution in Carrier Oils: One of the most common methods is diluting essential oils in carrier oils like jojoba, almond, or coconut oil. This method not only helps in safely applying essential oils to the skin but also aids in slowing down the evaporation rate of the oils, allowing for a longer-lasting aroma.

2. Diffusion: Using an aromatherapy diffuser is another popular method for blending essential oils. Diffusers disperse micro-particles of essential oils into the air, allowing for inhalation and absorption through the respiratory system. This method is effective for creating a therapeutic atmosphere in homes, offices, or therapeutic spaces.

3. Massage Blending: Essential oils can be blended into massage oils or lotions for topical application. This method combines the benefits of aromatherapy with the therapeutic effects of massage, promoting relaxation, muscle relief, and improved circulation.

4. Sprays and Mists: Creating essential oil sprays or mists by blending oils with distilled water or alcohol is ideal for refreshing rooms, linens, or personal spaces. These sprays can also be used as natural air fresheners or to promote focus and mental clarity.

5. Baths and Soaks: Adding essential oils to bathwater or foot soaks allows for absorption through the skin and inhalation of aromatic vapors. This method is beneficial for relaxation, stress relief, and soothing muscle aches.

6. Personal Inhalers: Inhalers designed for essential oils allow for portable aromatherapy. Blending oils for inhalers is useful for on-the-go use, such as managing anxiety, boosting energy, or supporting respiratory health.

7. Custom Blends: Tailoring blends to specific needs and preferences involves combining essential oils based on their aromatic profiles, therapeutic properties, and intended effects. Experimenting with different combinations and ratios allows for the creation of unique and personalized blends.

Each method of blending essential oils offers its own benefits and applications, contributing to the versatility and effectiveness of aromatherapy in promoting overall well-being. Whether used for relaxation, skin care, emotional support, or physical wellness, mastering these blending methods allows individuals to harness the full potential of essential oils in their daily lives.

3.3 Recipes for Common Ailments and Purposes

Creating blends of essential oils can be highly effective for addressing common ailments and promoting various health purposes:

1. Relaxation Blend: Combine 3 drops of lavender, 2 drops of chamomile, and 1 drop of ylang-ylang essential oils in a diffuser to promote relaxation and reduce stress after a long day.

2. Immune Support: Create an immune-boosting blend by mixing 2 drops of tea tree, 2 drops of eucalyptus, and 1 drop of lemon essential oils in a carrier oil. Apply to the chest or diffuse in the air to support respiratory health.

3. Muscle Relief: Blend 3 drops of peppermint, 2 drops of marjoram, and 1 drop of ginger essential oils with a tablespoon of carrier oil for a soothing massage oil to relieve muscle tension and soreness.

4. Focus and Concentration: Enhance mental clarity and focus by diffusing a blend of 2 drops of rosemary, 2 drops of lemon, and 1 drop of frankincense essential oils during study or work sessions.

5. Sleep Aid: Mix 3 drops of lavender, 2 drops of cedarwood, and 1 drop of vetiver essential oils in a diffuser to create a calming atmosphere and promote restful sleep.

6. Skin Irritations: For minor skin irritations like insect bites or rashes, dilute 2 drops of lavender and 2 drops of tea tree essential oils in a teaspoon of carrier oil and apply topically.

7. Digestive Support: Combine 2 drops of peppermint, 2 drops of ginger, and 1 drop of fennel essential oils with a carrier oil and massage onto the abdomen in a clockwise motion to ease digestive discomfort.

8. Mood Uplift: Create a mood-enhancing blend by diffusing 2 drops of bergamot, 2 drops of grapefruit, and 1 drop of orange essential oils to uplift spirits and promote a positive atmosphere.

These recipes harness the therapeutic properties of essential oils to address specific needs and promote overall well-being. When blending oils, always consider individual sensitivities, dilution ratios, and safety guidelines to ensure safe and effective use.

Chapter 4: Aromatherapy for Emotional Wellbeing

4.1 Essential Oils for Stress Relief

Essential oils are renowned for alleviating stress and promoting relaxation through aromatherapy. Among the most effective oils for stress relief is lavender, which calms the nervous system and induces relaxation. Its soothing aroma helps reduce anxiety and improves sleep quality. Another potent oil is chamomile, prized for its gentle sedative properties that ease tension and promote a sense of calm. Bergamot is celebrated for its citrusy scent that uplifts mood and reduces stress levels, making it ideal for combating anxiety and depression. Frankincense, with its earthy and grounding aroma, helps to alleviate stress by promoting deep breathing and relaxation. Ylang-ylang is also effective due to its euphoric and calming properties, helping to reduce stress and boost emotional well-being. Whether used in diffusers, massages, or baths, these essential oils offer natural and holistic methods to manage stress and promote overall relaxation.

4.2 Mood-Enhancing Essential Oil Blends

Creating blends of essential oils can significantly enhance mood and create a positive atmosphere in your living or working space. A popular mood-enhancing blend includes equal parts of sweet orange, lemon, and grapefruit essential oils. These citrus oils are known for their uplifting properties, promoting a sense of joy and energy. Sweet orange oil, with its bright and cheerful aroma, helps uplift spirits and reduce anxiety. Lemon oil contributes a refreshing scent that enhances focus and clarity, which is ideal for boosting productivity and improving mood. Grapefruit oil adds a sweet, tangy aroma that invigorates the senses and promotes positivity. Blending these citrus oils creates a pleasant fragrance and helps alleviate stress and elevate mood levels naturally. Whether diffused throughout the room or used in personal inhalers, these mood-enhancing blends can transform your environment into a rejuvenating sanctuary.

4.3 Aromatherapy Techniques for Relaxation and Sleep

Aromatherapy offers various techniques that harness the therapeutic benefits of essential oils to promote relaxation and improve sleep quality. One effective method is diffusion, where essential oils are dispersed into the air using a diffuser. This technique allows the aromatic molecules to enter the respiratory system, influencing mood and inducing relaxation. Topical application is another approach, where essential oils are diluted in a carrier oil and applied to pulse points or massaged onto the skin. This method facilitates direct absorption of oils into the bloodstream, enhancing their calming effects. Inhalation involves adding a few drops of essential oils to a hot water or tissue bowl, allowing the aromatic vapors to be inhaled deeply for immediate relaxation benefits. Adding a few drops of essential oils to a warm bath creates a soothing and therapeutic experience, ideal for unwinding before bedtime. These aromatherapy techniques can be customized with oils such as lavender, chamomile, and sandalwood, renowned for their calming properties and ability to promote restful sleep. Incorporating these practices into your daily routine can help create a peaceful environment conducive to relaxation and rejuvenation.

Chapter 5: Aromatherapy for Physical Health

5.1 Essential Oils for Respiratory Health

Essential oils offer natural remedies to support respiratory health and alleviate symptoms of respiratory issues. Eucalyptus oil is widely recognized for clearing congestion and promoting easy breathing. Its intense aroma helps open the airways and soothe respiratory passages, effectively relieving colds and sinus congestion symptoms. Peppermint oil is another excellent choice, known for its cooling sensation and ability to reduce inflammation in the respiratory tract. It can relieve nasal congestion and sinus pressure, promoting clearer breathing. Tea tree oil possesses powerful antibacterial and antiviral properties that help combat respiratory infections and improve lung health. Its cleansing properties make it beneficial for treating bronchitis and other respiratory ailments.

Additionally, lemon oil offers antiseptic properties and helps to cleanse the respiratory system while boosting immunity. When using essential oils for respiratory health, it's important to dilute them properly in a carrier oil for topical application or use them in a diffuser to inhale their therapeutic vapors. These oils provide effective and natural alternatives to support respiratory wellness and enhance respiratory function.

5.2 Pain Relief and Anti-inflammatory Oils

Essential oils are valued for their potent properties in naturally relieving pain and reducing inflammation. Peppermint oil is among the most effective oils for pain relief, renowned for its cooling effect that soothes sore muscles and joints. Its menthol content provides a numbing sensation, making it particularly beneficial for alleviating headaches and migraines. Eucalyptus oil is another powerful choice, known for its anti-inflammatory properties that help reduce swelling and improve circulation. It can relieve muscle tension and joint pain, making it ideal for arthritis and rheumatic conditions. Lavender oil offers analgesic and anti-inflammatory benefits, helping to calm nerves and reduce discomfort associated with minor injuries or inflammation.

Additionally, rosemary oil is valued for its ability to stimulate circulation and alleviate muscle spasms, providing relief from muscular pain and stiffness. When using essential oils for pain relief, dilute them properly in a carrier oil and apply them topically to the affected area. Their natural healing properties make them practical alternatives to conventional pain medications, promoting holistic pain management and supporting overall well-being.

5.3 Skin Care and Beauty Applications

Essential oils are versatile and widely utilized in skincare and beauty routines for their therapeutic properties and ability to address various skin concerns. Tea tree oil is highly valued for its antibacterial and antimicrobial properties, effectively treating acne and blemishes. Lavender oil is renowned for its soothing and healing properties, making it beneficial for reducing redness and irritation and promoting overall skin health. Frankincense oil is prized for its anti-aging benefits, helping to reduce the appearance of wrinkles and fine lines while improving skin elasticity and tone. Rosehip oil, rich in vitamins and antioxidants, supports skin regeneration and helps to fade scars and pigmentation. When using essential oils in skincare, it's essential to dilute them properly in carrier oils to prevent skin irritation.

Chapter 6: Incorporating Aromatherapy into Daily Life

6.1 Creating a Home Aromatherapy Kit

Establishing a home aromatherapy kit is about assembling essential oils and curating a personalized collection that caters to various needs and preferences. Start with a foundation of versatile oils known for their therapeutic properties. Lavender essential oil, renowned for its calming effects, is ideal for relaxation and promoting better sleep. With its invigorating scent, Peppermint oil is excellent for boosting energy and alleviating headaches. Eucalyptus oil, valued for its respiratory benefits, can clear congestion and improve breathing.

Store your essential oils in dark glass bottles to protect them from light and heat, which can degrade their potency over time. Keep them in a cool, dry place, away from direct sunlight. Include carrier oils like jojoba, sweet almond, or coconut oil in your kit to dilute essential oils for topical use, such as in massage oils or skincare products. These carrier oils not only dilute the essential oils but also help to moisturize and nourish the skin.

Invest in accessories that facilitate the use of essential oils throughout your home. A quality diffuser disperses vital oil particles into the air, allowing you to enjoy the aromatic benefits of oils like lavender or chamomile throughout your living space. For personalized aromatherapy on the go, consider making personal inhalers filled with blends designed for specific purposes, such as stress relief or mental clarity.

6.2 Daily Aromatherapy Practices

Incorporating aromatherapy into your daily routine can enhance your overall well-being by promoting relaxation, reducing stress, and boosting mental clarity. Begin your morning with an uplifting blend of citrus oils such as lemon, grapefruit, or orange to awaken your senses and improve your mood. Diffuse these oils in your home while preparing for the day to create an energizing atmosphere.

During work or study sessions, diffuse essential oils known for their focus-enhancing properties, such as peppermint, rosemary, or basil. These oils can help sharpen concentration, stimulate mental clarity, and increase productivity. If you work from home or have a dedicated workspace, consider using an essential oil diffuser to maintain a conducive environment throughout the day.

In the evening, wind down with calming oils such as lavender, chamomile, or cedarwood to promote relaxation and prepare for a restful night's sleep. Diffusing these oils in your bedroom or a bedtime routine can signal to your body that it's time to unwind, helping you achieve deeper and more restorative sleep.

6.3 Aromatherapy for Home and Workplace Environments

Integrating aromatherapy into home and workplace environments can foster a more balanced and harmonious atmosphere. Strategically place diffusers in living areas or bedrooms at home to create a calming sanctuary. Lavender or ylang-ylang oils are particularly effective for promoting relaxation and reducing stress levels after a long day.

Essential oils like peppermint, eucalyptus, or lemon can be diffused in workplace settings to enhance focus, mental clarity, and productivity. Peppermint oil, in particular, is known for stimulating the mind and increasing alertness, making it suitable for office environments where concentration is key.

Use essential oil sprays to freshen up linens, furniture, or office spaces with pleasant scents that uplift the mood and create a welcoming environment. Aromatherapy can also be incorporated into self-care practices, such as using a personal inhaler with calming oils during breaks or a few drops of essential oil into a stress-relieving massage oil.

By integrating aromatherapy into home and workplace environments, you can harness the therapeutic benefits of essential oils to enhance your overall well-being, promote relaxation, and create a more enjoyable and productive environment for daily activities.

Chapter 7: Advanced Aromatherapy Techniques

7.1 Inhalation Methods: Diffusers and Steam Inhalation

Inhalation is a primary method for enjoying the therapeutic benefits of essential oils in aromatherapy. Diffusers, versatile devices, are popular for dispersing essential oil molecules into the air in a fine mist, allowing for easy inhalation. Ultrasonic diffusers, a type of diffuser, use water to create a gentle mist that also humidifies the air, making them ideal for adding moisture to indoor spaces while infusing the air with the aroma of essential oils. They can be used with various oils depending on the desired effect, giving you control over your aromatherapy experience. For instance, diffusing lavender oil promotes relaxation and aids in sleep, while diffusing peppermint oil can help improve focus and mental clarity.

Steam inhalation is another effective way to benefit from essential oils. It involves adding a few drops of essential oil to a bowl of hot water, covering the head with a towel, and inhaling the steam deeply. This method is excellent for clearing nasal passages, relieving sinus congestion, and supporting respiratory health. Oils such as eucalyptus, tea tree, and thyme are commonly used for steam inhalation due to their decongestant, antibacterial, and antiviral properties. Steam inhalation not only helps to open up the airways but also provides a deeply soothing effect on the respiratory system, bringing a sense of comfort and ease.

7.2 Topical Applications: Massage and Compresses

Topical application of essential oils involves applying diluted oils directly to the skin for absorption. This method allows for both localized and systemic therapeutic effects. Essential oils are diluted in carrier oils like coconut, jojoba, or almond oil before application to prevent skin irritation and enhance absorption.

Massage with essential oils is a popular therapeutic practice combining touch's benefits with aromatherapy. During a massage, essential oils are blended with carrier oils and applied to the skin through gentle massage techniques. This helps to relax muscles, reduce tension, and promote overall relaxation. For example, a blend of lavender and chamomile essential oils in a carrier oil can be used for a calming and soothing massage after a stressful day.

Compresses are another topical application method where essential oils are added to water and soaked into a cloth applied to the skin. This method is particularly useful for treating localized pain, inflammation, or skin conditions. For instance, a warm compress infused with ginger and peppermint oils can be applied to the abdomen to alleviate digestive discomfort or menstrual cramps. Alternatively, a cold compress with lavender and tea tree oils can soothe sunburn or insect bites.

7.3 Aromatherapy Baths and Spa Treatments

Aromatherapy baths provide a luxurious and therapeutic experience by combining essential oils' healing properties with warm water's relaxation. Adding a few drops of essential oils to a bath allows for inhalation and absorption through the skin, offering holistic benefits. Oils such as bergamot, geranium, or ylang-ylang can promote relaxation, reduce stress, and enhance mood during a bath, leaving you feeling rejuvenated and balanced.

For a spa-like experience at home, consider creating DIY aromatherapy spa treatments using essential oils. Body scrubs, masks, and lotions infused with essential oils can provide additional benefits for the skin and senses. For example, a sugar scrub with eucalyptus and peppermint oils can invigorate the senses while exfoliating the skin. A facial mask with lavender and rose oils can soothe and hydrate the skin, promoting a radiant complexion.

Incorporating these aromatherapy methods into your self-care routine can support overall well-being, enhance relaxation, and provide natural solutions for various health and wellness concerns. Whether you diffuse oils in your living space, enjoy a therapeutic massage, or indulge in an aromatherapy bath, essential oils offer versatile and effective ways to promote physical, emotional, and mental wellness.

Book 17: Healing Chronic Illnesses with Barbara O'Neill's Remedies

Embracing Natural Solutions for Sustainable Health and Empowerment

Chapter 1: Overview of Chronic Illnesses

1.1 What Are Chronic Illnesses?

Chronic illnesses are long-term health conditions that persist over an extended period, typically lasting over three months. These conditions often do not have a definitive cure and may require ongoing management to control symptoms and improve quality of life. Common chronic illnesses include diabetes, heart disease, arthritis, asthma, chronic obstructive pulmonary disease (COPD), and autoimmune disorders like rheumatoid arthritis and lupus.

The impact of chronic illnesses can vary widely depending on the specific condition and individual factors. Some chronic illnesses may cause mild discomfort or inconvenience, while others can significantly impair daily functioning and lead to severe complications if not managed properly. Symptoms can range from pain, fatigue, and difficulty breathing to cognitive impairment and emotional distress.

Managing chronic illnesses typically involves a combination of medical treatments, lifestyle modifications, and support from healthcare professionals. Treatment goals focus on alleviating symptoms, slowing disease progression, preventing complications, and improving overall well-being. This holistic approach may include medication, physical therapy, dietary changes, stress management techniques, and regular monitoring of health markers.

Living with a chronic illness can pose various challenges, including physical limitations, emotional strain, financial burdens, and social isolation. However, many individuals with chronic conditions lead fulfilling lives by actively participating in their care, seeking support from loved ones and healthcare providers, and adopting healthy coping strategies. By understanding the nature of chronic illnesses and implementing comprehensive management strategies, individuals can optimize their health outcomes and enhance their quality of life despite the challenges posed by these conditions.

1.2 Common Chronic Conditions and Their Impact

Common chronic conditions encompass a wide spectrum of health issues that persist over extended periods, significantly impacting individuals' lives and requiring ongoing management. Among the most prevalent chronic conditions are cardiovascular diseases, such as hypertension and coronary artery disease, which affect the heart and blood vessels. These conditions can lead to complications like heart attacks and strokes, impairing overall cardiovascular function and quality of life.

Another prevalent chronic condition is diabetes, characterized by elevated blood glucose levels due to insufficient insulin production or ineffective insulin use by the body. If left uncontrolled, diabetes can lead to serious complications, including nerve damage, kidney disease, and cardiovascular problems. Managing diabetes involves monitoring blood sugar levels, adopting a healthy diet, engaging in regular physical activity, and sometimes using insulin or other medications.

Chronic respiratory diseases, such as asthma and chronic obstructive pulmonary disease (COPD), also significantly impact individuals' respiratory function and quality of life. These conditions cause airflow obstruction, leading to symptoms like shortness of breath, coughing, and wheezing. Management strategies include bronchodilators, corticosteroids, oxygen therapy, and lifestyle modifications to reduce exposure to triggers like tobacco smoke and air pollutants.

Arthritis, a group of joint disorders, is another common chronic condition that causes joint pain, stiffness, and swelling. Osteoarthritis, the most prevalent type, results from wear and tear on joint cartilage over time, while rheumatoid arthritis is an autoimmune disorder causing joint inflammation. Treatment options for arthritis focus on pain management, improving joint function, and preventing further joint damage through medications, physical therapy, and lifestyle modifications.

Mental health disorders, including depression, anxiety disorders, and bipolar disorder, are also prevalent chronic conditions that affect individuals' emotional well-being and daily functioning. These conditions can cause persistent sadness, worry, or mood swings, impacting relationships, work productivity, and overall quality of life. Treatment approaches often involve psychotherapy, medication, support groups, and lifestyle changes to promote mental wellness and resilience.

Overall, managing chronic conditions requires a comprehensive approach that addresses medical treatment, lifestyle modifications, and emotional support. By understanding the impact of these conditions and implementing effective management strategies, individuals can minimize symptoms, prevent complications, and maintain a good quality of life despite the challenges posed by chronic illness.

1.3 Challenges in Conventional Treatment Approaches

Conventional treatment approaches for chronic conditions often face challenges impacting effectiveness and patient outcomes. One significant challenge is the reliance on symptom management rather than addressing underlying causes. Many treatments focus on alleviating symptoms such as pain, inflammation, or elevated blood sugar levels without necessarily addressing the root causes of the conditions. However, it's important to note that a shift towards addressing these root causes can lead to significant long-term health improvements, breaking the cycle of dependency on medications or interventions.

Another challenge is the potential for side effects and complications associated with pharmaceutical treatments. Medications used to manage chronic conditions, such as cardiovascular drugs, insulin for diabetes, or corticosteroids for autoimmune disorders, can cause adverse effects ranging from mild discomfort to severe complications like gastrointestinal issues, weight gain, or increased risk of infections. Balancing the benefits of these treatments with their potential risks requires careful monitoring and adjustment by healthcare providers.

Additionally, conventional treatments can be prohibitive for many individuals, especially when considering the long-term use of medications, frequent medical visits, and necessary diagnostic tests or procedures. This financial burden can limit access to essential healthcare services and medications, leading to disparities in treatment outcomes based on socioeconomic status or insurance coverage. To overcome this, patients and healthcare providers can explore options like generic medications, patient assistance programs, or telemedicine services to reduce costs and improve access to care.

Furthermore, conventional treatment approaches may sometimes neglect the importance of lifestyle factors and holistic approaches to health. While medications play a crucial role in managing symptoms and preventing complications, lifestyle modifications such as dietary changes, exercise, stress management, and complementary therapies like acupuncture or physical therapy can significantly impact disease progression and overall well-being. Integrating these approaches into treatment plans requires a collaborative effort between patients, healthcare providers, and community-supported resources, emphasizing the importance of a supportive network in holistic healthcare.

Lastly, the fragmented nature of healthcare delivery systems can pose challenges in coordinating care for individuals with multiple chronic conditions or complex medical histories. This fragmentation may result in gaps in communication between healthcare providers, inconsistent treatment plans, and delays in accessing necessary services or referrals. Improving care coordination and fostering a patient-centered approach are essential for optimizing treatment outcomes and enhancing the quality of life for individuals living with chronic conditions.

Chapter 2: Holistic Approach to Chronic Illness

2.1 Barbara O'Neill's Holistic Health Philosophy

Barbara O'Neill's holistic health philosophy emphasizes an integrated approach to well-being that encompasses the interconnectedness of body, mind, and spirit. Central to her philosophy is the belief that optimal health is achieved by balancing physical, emotional, mental, and spiritual factors. She advocates for natural healing methods that promote the body's innate ability to heal when supported with proper nutrition, lifestyle adjustments, and stress management techniques.

O'Neill emphasizes the importance of whole foods and plant-based diets as foundational elements of health, highlighting their role in providing essential nutrients, supporting immune function, and promoting overall vitality. Her philosophy encourages individuals to prioritize fresh, organic produce, whole grains, lean proteins, and healthy fats while minimizing processed foods, refined sugars, and artificial additives that can contribute to inflammation and chronic health issues.

In addition to nutrition, O'Neill stresses the significance of regular physical activity in maintaining optimal health. Exercise supports cardiovascular health, muscle strength, and flexibility, enhances mood, reduces stress levels, and supports healthy weight management. She promotes a balanced approach to exercise, encouraging activities that individuals enjoy and can sustain over time, whether it's yoga, walking, swimming, or strength training.

Beyond physical health, Barbara O'Neill's philosophy underscores the importance of mental and emotional well-being. She advocates for stress reduction techniques such as mindfulness meditation, deep breathing exercises, and adequate sleep to promote relaxation and resilience in coping with life's challenges. O'Neill believes cultivating a positive mindset and nurturing supportive relationships are integral to achieving holistic health.

Spiritual wellness is another cornerstone of O'Neill's philosophy. She acknowledges the profound impact of spiritual practices and beliefs on overall health. Whether through prayer, meditation, connection with nature, or involvement in a supportive community, she encourages individuals to explore and nurture their spiritual dimension to find inner peace, purpose, and emotional fulfillment.

Barbara O'Neill's holistic health philosophy promotes a proactive approach to health maintenance and disease prevention by empowering individuals to make informed choices that support their body's natural healing mechanisms. By addressing the interconnected aspects of health—physical, emotional, mental, and spiritual—her philosophy provides a comprehensive framework for achieving and sustaining optimal well-being throughout life.

2.2 Integrative Medicine: Bridging Conventional and Natural Approaches

Integrative medicine represents a dynamic approach to healthcare that bridges the gap between conventional medical practices and natural, holistic approaches to healing. At its core, integrative medicine combines the best of both worlds by integrating evidence-based traditional treatments with complementary therapies and practices that address the whole person—body, mind, and spirit.

One of the critical principles of integrative medicine is personalized care. Practitioners consider each patient's unique health history, lifestyle, and preferences to develop tailored treatment plans that prioritize both symptom management and addressing underlying causes. Integrative medicine seeks to optimize health outcomes and enhance overall well-being by considering the individual as a whole.

Integrative medicine emphasizes the importance of patient empowerment and active participation in health decisions. Patients are encouraged to take responsibility for their health through education, lifestyle modifications, and self-care practices. This collaborative approach fosters a therapeutic partnership between patients and healthcare providers, promoting empowerment and engagement in healing.

Another hallmark of integrative medicine is its emphasis on prevention and wellness. Beyond treating acute symptoms or managing chronic conditions, integrative practitioners focus on preventing illness and promoting health through nutrition counseling, stress management techniques, exercise prescriptions, and mind-body therapies. By addressing root causes and supporting the body's natural healing mechanisms, integrative medicine aims to enhance resilience and reduce the risk of disease.

Integrative medicine encompasses various therapies and modalities, including acupuncture, chiropractic care, herbal medicine, massage therapy, yoga, meditation, and nutritional supplements. These therapies are selected based on their safety, efficacy, and compatibility with conventional treatments, ensuring a comprehensive approach to health and healing.

Critically, integrative medicine promotes evidence-based practices and encourages ongoing research to evaluate the effectiveness and safety of integrative therapies. This commitment to scientific rigor ensures that integrative approaches are integrated into mainstream healthcare based on sound evidence and rigorous standards of practice.

In summary, integrative medicine represents a progressive approach to healthcare that blends the strengths of conventional medicine with the benefits of complementary and alternative therapies. By embracing a holistic view of health and prioritizing personalized care, integrative medicine offers patients a comprehensive toolkit to achieve optimal health, wellness, and vitality.

2.3 Importance of Lifestyle Changes and Stress Management

As individuals, we hold the key to our holistic health and well-being through lifestyle changes and stress management. Our diet, physical activity, sleep patterns, and stress levels profoundly impact our overall health, influencing everything from immune function to cardiovascular health and mental well-being.

Diet plays a pivotal role in health, providing essential nutrients that support cellular function, repair, and regeneration. A balanced diet rich in whole foods—such as fruits, vegetables, lean proteins, whole grains, and healthy fats—provides the necessary vitamins, minerals, and antioxidants that help to ward off disease and maintain optimal health. On the other hand, diets high in processed foods, sugars, and unhealthy fats can contribute to inflammation, obesity, and chronic conditions such as diabetes and heart disease. These unhealthy diets can lead to a range of health issues, from digestive problems and fatigue to more serious conditions like heart disease and cancer.

Regular physical activity is equally crucial for maintaining a healthy weight and supporting cardiovascular health, muscle strength, and flexibility. Exercise releases endorphins, which are natural mood lifters and help to reduce stress, anxiety, and symptoms of depression. Incorporating activities such as walking, jogging, swimming, or yoga into daily routines can have profound effects on physical and mental well-being.

Quality sleep is another cornerstone of a healthy lifestyle. Understanding and implementing good sleep hygiene practices, such as maintaining a consistent sleep schedule, creating a restful sleep environment, and avoiding stimulants before bedtime, can significantly improve sleep quality and overall health.

Managing stress is essential for maintaining optimal health. Chronic stress triggers the release of stress hormones like cortisol, which, when prolonged, can weaken the immune system, disrupt digestion, and contribute to inflammation and chronic disease. Effective stress management techniques, such as mindfulness meditation, deep breathing exercises, yoga, spending time in nature, or engaging in hobbies, help reduce stress levels and promote relaxation. These practices enhance mental clarity and emotional resilience and support physical health by lowering blood pressure and improving immune function.

In conclusion, making positive lifestyle changes and adopting effective stress management strategies are not just beneficial, but also empowering. By prioritizing nutritious eating habits, regular physical activity, quality sleep, and stress reduction techniques, individuals can take control of their health and empower themselves to lead healthier, more fulfilling lives. These lifestyle choices support physical health and nurture mental and emotional resilience, ultimately contributing to a balanced and vibrant quality of life.

Chapter 3: Nutrition and Chronic Illness

3.1 The Role of Nutrition in Managing Chronic Conditions

The role of nutrition in managing chronic conditions is paramount, as dietary choices can significantly impact the progression and management of various health issues. For individuals living with chronic conditions such as diabetes, cardiovascular disease, hypertension, or autoimmune disorders, adopting a balanced and nutrient-dense diet can play a crucial role in improving symptoms, preventing complications, and enhancing overall quality of life.

A key consideration in managing chronic conditions through nutrition is the impact of food choices on blood sugar, cholesterol, and blood pressure. For instance, individuals with diabetes benefit from monitoring carbohydrate intake to manage blood glucose levels effectively. Choosing complex carbohydrates with a low glycemic index, such as whole grains, legumes, and non-starchy vegetables, can help stabilize blood sugar levels and reduce the risk of insulin resistance.

Similarly, heart-healthy diets emphasizing fruits, vegetables, lean proteins, and healthy fats have lowered cholesterol levels and reduced cardiovascular risk. Foods rich in omega-3 fatty acids, such as fatty fish (salmon, mackerel, sardines), flaxseeds, and walnuts, are particularly beneficial for heart health due to their anti-inflammatory properties and ability to support cardiovascular function.

Dietary choices can also influence inflammatory conditions such as rheumatoid arthritis, Crohn's disease, or psoriasis. Anti-inflammatory diets, which include foods rich in antioxidants, such as berries, leafy greens, nuts, and omega-3 fatty acids, can help reduce inflammation and alleviate symptoms associated with these conditions. Avoiding processed foods, sugars, and trans fats, which can exacerbate inflammation, is also recommended.

Focusing on gut health is essential for individuals with autoimmune disorders, as the gut microbiome plays a critical role in immune function and inflammation regulation. Consuming probiotic-rich foods like yogurt, kefir, and fermented vegetables can support a healthy gut microbiome and may help mitigate autoimmune symptoms.

Beyond specific dietary recommendations, personalized nutrition plans tailored to individual health needs and preferences are crucial in managing chronic conditions effectively. Working with healthcare professionals, such as registered dietitians or nutritionists, can provide personalized guidance on dietary modifications, meal planning, and nutrient supplementation to optimize health outcomes and improve quality of life.

In summary, nutrition is pivotal in managing chronic conditions by influencing disease progression, symptom management, and overall well-being. By adopting a balanced diet that supports specific health needs and goals, individuals can empower themselves to actively manage their health and achieve long-term wellness. Integrating nutritious food choices with other lifestyle modifications, such as regular physical activity and stress management, forms a holistic approach to managing chronic conditions and promoting optimal health.

3.2 Anti-inflammatory Diet and Its Benefits

An anti-inflammatory diet is recognized for its potential to reduce inflammation throughout the body, which is linked to numerous chronic conditions and diseases. This dietary approach emphasizes whole, nutrient-dense foods that possess anti-inflammatory properties, while avoiding or minimizing processed and pro-inflammatory foods.

Key components of an anti-inflammatory diet include:

1. Fruits and Vegetables: Rich in antioxidants, vitamins, and minerals, fruits and vegetables are essential for combating oxidative stress and reducing inflammation. Berries, leafy greens, cruciferous vegetables (like broccoli and Brussels sprouts), and colorful peppers are particularly beneficial.

2. Healthy Fats: Omega-3 fatty acids found in fatty fish (such as salmon and sardines), flaxseeds, chia seeds, and walnuts are potent anti-inflammatory agents. Monounsaturated fats found in olive oil, avocados, and nuts also contribute to reducing inflammation.

3. Whole Grains: Whole grains like quinoa, brown rice, oats, and whole wheat provide fiber and nutrients that support digestive health and help regulate inflammation.

4. Lean Proteins: Incorporating lean sources of protein, such as poultry, beans, lentils, and tofu, into meals can help maintain muscle mass and support overall health without contributing to inflammation.

5. Herbs and Spices: Turmeric, ginger, garlic, and cinnamon are examples of herbs and spices known for their anti-inflammatory properties. They can be used generously in cooking to enhance flavor while promoting health benefits.

6. Probiotics: Fermented foods like yogurt, kefir, sauerkraut, and kimchi contain beneficial probiotics that support gut health. A healthy gut microbiome is crucial for reducing inflammation and promoting overall well-being.

The benefits of adopting an anti-inflammatory diet are manifold. Research suggests that reducing chronic inflammation can lower the risk of developing conditions such as heart disease, diabetes, arthritis, and certain cancers. Furthermore, individuals with inflammatory conditions like rheumatoid arthritis or inflammatory bowel disease may experience symptom relief and improved quality of life with this dietary approach.

By focusing on whole, natural foods and minimizing processed foods, added sugars, and unhealthy fats, individuals can support their body's natural defense mechanisms against inflammation. Combining an anti-inflammatory diet with regular exercise, stress management techniques, and adequate sleep forms a holistic approach to promoting long-term health and well-being. Consulting with a healthcare provider or registered dietitian can provide personalized guidance on implementing and maintaining an anti-inflammatory diet tailored to individual health needs and goals.

3.3 Nutritional Strategies for Specific Conditions

Nutritional strategies tailored to specific health conditions play a critical role in managing symptoms, improving outcomes, and enhancing overall well-being. These strategies are often designed to address the unique nutritional needs and challenges associated with various health conditions, promoting optimal health and quality of life.

For individuals with diabetes, maintaining stable blood sugar levels through a balanced diet is crucial. Emphasizing complex carbohydrates with a low glycemic index, such as whole grains, legumes, and non-starchy vegetables, can help regulate blood sugar levels and reduce the risk of complications. Monitoring carbohydrate intake, portion sizes, and incorporating lean proteins and healthy fats into meals can further support blood sugar management.

Heart disease prevention and management often involve adopting a heart-healthy diet that focuses on reducing cholesterol levels and blood pressure. This includes consuming foods rich in omega-3 fatty acids, such as fatty fish (salmon, mackerel, sardines), flaxseeds, and walnuts, which promote heart health by reducing inflammation and supporting cardiovascular function. Limiting saturated and trans fats, sodium, and refined sugars is also essential for maintaining heart health.

For individuals with inflammatory conditions like rheumatoid arthritis or inflammatory bowel disease, an anti-inflammatory diet can help alleviate symptoms and reduce inflammation. This diet emphasizes foods rich in antioxidants, such as berries, leafy greens, and nuts, as well as omega-3 fatty acids found in fatty fish and flaxseeds. Avoiding pro-inflammatory foods like processed foods, refined sugars, and trans fats can help manage symptoms and improve quality of life.

Nutritional strategies for managing autoimmune disorders often focus on supporting immune function and reducing inflammation. This may involve consuming foods that support gut health, such as probiotic-rich yogurt, kefir, and fermented vegetables, to maintain a healthy gut microbiome. Avoiding potential trigger foods and incorporating anti-inflammatory foods and supplements, under the guidance of a healthcare provider, can help manage symptoms and promote immune system balance.

For individuals with digestive disorders such as irritable bowel syndrome (IBS) or gastroesophageal reflux disease (GERD), dietary modifications are essential for symptom management. This may include identifying trigger foods that exacerbate symptoms and incorporating fiber-rich foods, like fruits, vegetables, and whole grains, to support digestive health. Limiting caffeine, alcohol, and fatty foods can also help alleviate symptoms and improve overall digestive function.

In summary, nutritional strategies tailored to specific health conditions aim to optimize health outcomes by addressing unique dietary needs, managing symptoms, and promoting overall well-being. Consulting with a registered dietitian or healthcare provider can provide personalized guidance and support in developing and implementing a nutrition plan that meets individual health goals and enhances quality of life.

Chapter 4: Herbal Remedies for Chronic Conditions

4.1 Using Herbs to Support Healing

Herbal medicine has a rich history spanning millennia, offering natural solutions to support healing and enhance overall well-being. Herbs are prized for their diverse bioactive compounds, including flavonoids, alkaloids, and essential oils, contributing to their therapeutic properties. These botanical remedies can be administered in various forms, such as teas, tinctures, capsules, and topical applications, each tailored to address specific health concerns.

One of the primary advantages of herbs lies in their holistic approach to health. Rather than targeting a single symptom, herbs work synergistically with the body's innate healing mechanisms to promote balance and vitality. For instance, echinacea and elderberry are well-known for their immune-boosting properties, helping to fortify the body's defenses against infections and reducing the severity and duration of colds and flu. Adaptogenic herbs like ashwagandha and rhodiola are valued for supporting the body's response to stress, enhancing resilience and overall energy levels.

Moreover, herbs are crucial in promoting digestive health and aiding detoxification. Ginger and peppermint, for example, can soothe digestive discomforts such as indigestion, bloating, and nausea, while dandelion and milk thistle support liver function and facilitate the elimination of toxins from the body. These botanical allies offer gentle yet practical solutions to common health challenges, empowering individuals to take charge of their well-being naturally.

4.2 Key Herbs for Managing Chronic Symptoms

Certain herbs have garnered attention for their efficacy in managing chronic symptoms associated with various health conditions. St. John's wort, recognized for its antidepressant properties, is often used to alleviate symptoms of mild to moderate depression and anxiety. By increasing serotonin levels in the brain, similar to conventional antidepressants but with potentially fewer side effects, this herb offers a natural alternative for mental health support.

Ginkgo biloba, celebrated for its cognitive-enhancing effects, is commonly recommended for individuals experiencing age-related cognitive decline or mild dementia. Ginkgo may help enhance memory, concentration, and overall cognitive function by improving blood circulation to the brain and providing neuroprotective benefits.

In addition, herbs like turmeric and boswellia are prized for their potent anti-inflammatory properties, making them valuable allies in managing conditions such as arthritis and inflammatory bowel diseases. These botanicals offer natural relief from pain and inflammation, supporting joint health and improving overall quality of life.

Furthermore, botanicals such as chamomile and valerian root are renowned for their calming and sleep-promoting effects, offering non-habit-forming alternatives to conventional sleep aids. These herbs help promote restful sleep and enhance overall sleep quality by addressing underlying factors contributing to sleep disturbances.

4.3 Herbal Formulations and Applications

Herbal formulations refer to carefully crafted combinations of herbs designed to address specific health concerns or achieve desired therapeutic effects. These formulations may include immune-boosting blends with echinacea, elderberry, and astragalus to support the body's defenses during cold and flu season. Digestive herbal blends combining herbs like ginger, fennel, and peppermint can help alleviate symptoms of indigestion, bloating, and gastrointestinal discomfort.

Topical applications of herbs involve using botanical extracts externally to address skin conditions, promote wound healing, or relieve muscle tension. Herbal salves and balms containing calendula, comfrey, and lavender are popular for soothing minor cuts, burns, and skin irritations. These preparations harness herbs' anti-inflammatory, antimicrobial, and healing properties to support skin health and accelerate the healing process.

Furthermore, herbal teas and tinctures offer versatile methods of herbal administration. Herbal teas, brewed by steeping dried herbs in hot water, allow for the gentle extraction of medicinal compounds that the body can readily absorb. Conversely, tinctures are concentrated herbal extracts preserved in alcohol or glycerin, providing a convenient and potent way to ingest herbs and benefit from their therapeutic effects.

Integrating herbs into daily wellness routines can profoundly benefit health and vitality. However, it is essential to approach herbal medicine with knowledge and caution, consulting with a qualified healthcare provider or herbalist, especially when managing chronic conditions or if you are pregnant, nursing, or taking medications. By harnessing the power of nature's pharmacy, individuals can support healing, manage chronic symptoms, and promote overall well-being naturally and holistically.

Chapter 5: Essential Oils and Chronic Illness

5.1 Aromatherapy for Pain Management

Aromatherapy, a therapeutic practice dating back thousands of years, utilizes essential oils extracted from aromatic plants to promote physical, emotional, and mental well-being. One of its notable applications is in pain management, where essential oils are used to alleviate discomfort, reduce inflammation, and support the body's natural healing processes.

Essential oils employed in aromatherapy for pain relief vary widely in their properties and effectiveness, offering a holistic approach to managing different types of pain. Among the most commonly used essential oils for pain management are:

1. Lavender: Known for its calming and analgesic properties, lavender essential oil is often used to relieve headaches, migraines, and general muscle tension. Its soothing aroma helps relax both the mind and body, making it a versatile option for various types of pain relief.

2. Peppermint: With its cooling sensation, peppermint essential oil provides relief from headaches, muscle aches, and joint pain. It acts as a natural analgesic and anti-inflammatory agent, helping to reduce pain intensity and improve circulation in affected areas.

3. Eucalyptus: Eucalyptus essential oil is renowned for its ability to ease respiratory issues, but it's also effective in alleviating muscle pain, arthritis, and joint stiffness. Its strong, camphoraceous scent stimulates circulation and reduces inflammation, offering relief from chronic pain conditions.

4. Rosemary: Rosemary essential oil is commonly used for its analgesic and anti-inflammatory properties. It helps alleviate muscle soreness, rheumatic pain, and headaches, making it beneficial for individuals with musculoskeletal discomfort.

5. Chamomile: Both Roman and German chamomile essential oils possess anti-inflammatory and calming properties. They are particularly useful for easing nerve pain, menstrual cramps, and tension headaches, promoting relaxation and pain relief.

6. Frankincense: Frankincense essential oil has been used for centuries for its anti-inflammatory and analgesic effects. It helps alleviate joint pain, arthritis symptoms, and muscle soreness, while its earthy aroma promotes relaxation and emotional balance.

5.1.1 Mechanisms of Action

The effectiveness of essential oils in pain management can be attributed to several mechanisms of action. Firstly, many essential oils contain compounds such as menthol (in peppermint) and eucalyptol (in eucalyptus) that interact with receptors in the skin, providing a cooling or warming sensation that distracts from pain signals. These oils also have anti-inflammatory properties, reducing swelling and pain associated with conditions like arthritis and muscle strains.

Furthermore, the aromas of essential oils can have a profound impact on the limbic system, the brain's emotional center. Inhalation of essential oils triggers responses in the brain that can alter perception of pain and promote relaxation. For instance, the scent of lavender has been shown to decrease anxiety and improve sleep quality, which can indirectly alleviate pain symptoms exacerbated by stress and poor sleep.

5.1.2 Methods of Application

Aromatherapy offers various methods of application to effectively manage pain:

- Topical Application: Diluted essential oils can be applied directly to the skin using massage oils, creams, or compresses. This method allows for direct absorption of the oils into the bloodstream and targeted relief to specific areas of pain.

- Inhalation: Inhalation of essential oils through diffusers, steam inhalation, or aromatic sprays allows for quick absorption into the bloodstream via the lungs. This method is effective for managing headaches, sinus pain, and respiratory discomfort.

- Baths: Adding a few drops of essential oils to a warm bath can provide full-body relaxation and pain relief. This method is particularly soothing for muscle aches, joint pain, and menstrual cramps.

- Compresses: Warm or cold compresses infused with diluted essential oils can be applied to painful areas to reduce inflammation and promote healing.

While essential oils offer natural pain relief, it's essential to use them safely:

- Always dilute essential oils with a carrier oil before applying to the skin to prevent irritation or sensitization.

- Perform a patch test before widespread use to check for allergic reactions or sensitivity.

- Consult with a qualified aromatherapist or healthcare provider, especially if you are pregnant, nursing, or have underlying health conditions.

Aromatherapy provides a gentle yet effective approach to managing pain through the use of aromatic essential oils. Whether used topically, through inhalation, or in baths, these oils offer versatile solutions for alleviating various types of pain while promoting relaxation and overall well-being. By harnessing the therapeutic properties of nature, individuals can complement conventional pain management strategies and enhance their quality of life naturally.

5.2 Essential Oils for Mental and Emotional Support

Essential oils have long been valued not only for their physical health benefits but also for their profound impact on mental and emotional well-being. Their therapeutic properties extend beyond physical ailments to include mood enhancement, stress reduction, and overall emotional balance. Here, we explore the diverse range of essential oils used for mental and emotional support, their mechanisms of action, and practical applications in aromatherapy.

5.2.1 Key Essential Oils for Mental and Emotional Support

1. Lavender: Widely recognized for its calming and soothing properties, lavender essential oil is a cornerstone in aromatherapy for emotional balance. It helps alleviate anxiety, stress, and nervous tension, promoting relaxation and improving sleep quality. Inhalation of lavender oil has been shown to reduce cortisol levels, the hormone associated with stress, and induce a sense of calmness and mental clarity.

2. Chamomile: Both Roman and German chamomile essential oils are renowned for their calming effects on the nervous system. They help reduce irritability, promote relaxation, and support emotional stability. Chamomile oil is particularly beneficial for easing anxiety, tension, and emotional stress, making it a valuable tool in promoting mental well-being.

3. Bergamot: With its citrusy and uplifting aroma, bergamot essential oil is known for its mood-enhancing and stress-relieving properties. It helps uplift mood, reduce feelings of depression, and promote a sense of positivity. Bergamot oil is often used in aromatherapy to combat seasonal affective disorder (SAD) and other forms of mild depression.

4. Frankincense: This resinous essential oil has been used for centuries in spiritual practices and healing rituals. Frankincense essential oil promotes deep breathing, relaxation, and inner peace. It helps alleviate anxiety, reduce stress levels, and enhance concentration and focus during meditation or mindfulness practices.

5. Ylang Ylang: Ylang ylang essential oil is prized for its ability to balance emotions and uplift mood. It has a sweet floral scent that helps reduce feelings of anger, frustration, and nervousness. Ylang ylang oil is commonly used in aromatherapy to enhance sensuality, promote relaxation, and support emotional harmony.

6. Peppermint: While peppermint is often associated with physical benefits, such as pain relief and digestion support, its refreshing aroma also has mental benefits. Peppermint essential oil helps stimulate the mind, improve focus and concentration, and reduce mental fatigue. It is particularly useful during periods of stress or when mental clarity is needed.

5.2.2 Mechanisms of Action

The therapeutic effects of essential oils on mental and emotional health can be attributed to their ability to interact with the limbic system—the part of the brain responsible for emotions, memories, and behaviors. Inhalation of essential oil vapors stimulates the olfactory system, sending signals to the limbic system where emotional responses are processed. This interaction triggers physiological and emotional responses that can influence mood, stress levels, and cognitive function.

Essential oils also exert pharmacological effects through their chemical constituents. For example, linalool and linalyl acetate, prominent compounds in lavender essential oil, have sedative and anxiolytic properties that help reduce anxiety and induce relaxation. Similarly, terpenes like limonene in citrus oils (e.g., bergamot) have mood-lifting effects by modulating neurotransmitter activity and promoting feelings of well-being.

5.2.3 Practical Applications

There are various ways to incorporate essential oils into daily routines for mental and emotional support:

- Aromatherapy Diffusion: Use an essential oil diffuser to disperse aromatic molecules into the air, creating a calming or uplifting atmosphere in homes, offices, or therapy spaces. Diffusing oils like lavender, bergamot, or frankincense can promote relaxation, improve mood, and reduce stress levels throughout the day.

- Topical Application: Dilute essential oils with a carrier oil (e.g., jojoba, sweet almond) and apply to pulse points, temples, or the back of the neck for quick absorption and immediate effects. This method allows for targeted relief from anxiety or tension and can be used as part of a calming bedtime routine.

- Inhalation: Add a few drops of essential oil to a tissue or handkerchief and inhale deeply. This portable method is useful for on-the-go stress relief or during moments of heightened anxiety. Alternatively, create a personal inhaler by adding essential oils to an inhaler tube for discreet use throughout the day.

- Baths and Massage: Incorporate essential oils into bath salts, body oils, or massage blends to promote relaxation, relieve muscle tension, and enhance emotional well-being. A warm bath with a few drops of ylang ylang or chamomile oil can be particularly soothing after a stressful day.

While essential oils are generally safe when used properly, it's essential to practice caution, especially with sensitive individuals, children, and pregnant or nursing women. Always dilute essential oils before topical application and perform a patch test to check for skin sensitivity. Consult with a qualified aromatherapist or healthcare provider for personalized recommendations, especially if you have underlying health conditions or are taking medications.

Essential oils offer a natural and effective way to support mental and emotional health through aromatherapy. By harnessing the therapeutic benefits of aromatic plant extracts, individuals can manage stress, improve mood, and enhance overall well-being in a holistic manner. Whether used for relaxation, mood enhancement, or stress reduction, incorporating essential oils into daily routines can promote emotional balance and resilience in the face of life's challenges.

5.3 Using Essential Oils Safely with Chronic Conditions

Using essential oils safely with chronic conditions requires careful consideration of individual health needs and potential interactions with existing treatments. While essential oils offer therapeutic benefits, their concentrated nature and bioactive compounds can interact with medications or exacerbate certain health conditions. Here are essential guidelines for safe use:

Consultation with Healthcare Provider: Before incorporating essential oils into a treatment plan for chronic conditions, consult with a healthcare provider, especially if you have pre-existing health concerns or are undergoing medical treatment. Some oils may interfere with medications or exacerbate symptoms.

Choosing Safe Essential Oils: Opt for essential oils known for their safety profile and mild properties, especially when dealing with chronic health issues. Lavender, chamomile, and frankincense are generally well-tolerated and offer calming and anti-inflammatory benefits suitable for many conditions.

Dilution and Application: Essential oils should always be diluted in a carrier oil before applying to the skin to minimize the risk of irritation or sensitization, which can be more pronounced in individuals with chronic skin conditions like eczema or psoriasis. A 2-5% dilution (10-25 drops of essential oil per ounce of carrier oil) is typically recommended.

Patch Testing: Perform a patch test before widespread use to check for allergic reactions or skin sensitivities, especially if you have sensitive skin or dermatological conditions. Apply a small amount of diluted essential oil to a small area of skin and observe for any adverse reactions over 24 hours.

Avoiding Photosensitive Oils: Certain essential oils, such as citrus oils like bergamot, lemon, and grapefruit, are photosensitive and can cause skin irritation or sensitivity when exposed to sunlight or UV rays. Exercise caution and apply these oils in diluted forms and in areas not exposed to direct sunlight.

Inhalation Methods: Aromatherapy diffusion and inhalation are generally safe for most individuals with chronic conditions. Diffusing essential oils in well-ventilated spaces can promote respiratory health and emotional well-being without direct skin contact.

Monitoring Symptoms: Pay attention to how your body responds to essential oil use. If you experience any adverse effects or worsening of symptoms, discontinue use and consult with a healthcare professional. It's essential to monitor changes in symptoms or reactions to ensure compatibility with ongoing treatments.

Personalized Approach: Each individual may respond differently to essential oils, depending on their health status, medications, and sensitivities. A personalized approach, guided by healthcare advice and sensitivity to individual needs, ensures safe and effective use of essential oils in managing chronic conditions.

By following these guidelines and incorporating essential oils judiciously into your wellness routine, you can harness their therapeutic benefits while prioritizing safety and compatibility with chronic health management. Always prioritize informed decisions and consult healthcare providers for personalized advice tailored to your specific health needs and conditions.

Chapter 6: Detoxification and Chronic Illness

6.1 Detox Strategies for Supporting Chronic Illness Recovery

Detox strategies empower individuals in their journey of chronic illness recovery, as they actively eliminate toxins from the body, reduce inflammation, and enhance overall wellness. Here are several practical approaches:

Nutritional Detoxification: Adopting nutrient-dense, whole-foods diet rich in antioxidants, vitamins, and minerals supports the body's natural detoxification pathways. Emphasizing organic fruits and vegetables, lean proteins, and healthy fats can provide essential nutrients while minimizing exposure to harmful chemicals and additives.

Hydration: Adequate hydration is essential for detoxification as it supports kidney function and helps flush toxins from the body. Drinking sufficient water throughout the day, preferably filtered or mineral, promotes optimal detoxification.

Herbal Support: Incorporating herbs known for their detoxifying properties, such as milk thistle, dandelion root, and burdock, can enhance liver function and support the body's detox efforts. These herbs can be consumed as teas, tinctures, or supplements under the guidance of a healthcare provider.

Colon Cleansing: Maintaining regular bowel movements is crucial for eliminating toxins and waste products from the body. Natural methods like increasing fiber intake through fruits, vegetables, and whole grains, as well as herbal laxatives and enemas, can support healthy colon function and detoxification.

Sweating: Engaging in activities that promote sweating, such as exercise, sauna sessions, or hot baths, can help eliminate toxins through the skin. Sweating aids in removing heavy metals, chemicals, and metabolic waste products, supporting overall detoxification.

Mind-Body Practices: Stress management techniques such as meditation, yoga, and deep breathing promote relaxation and support detoxification by reducing stress hormones like cortisol. Chronic stress can impair detoxification pathways, so incorporating these practices benefits overall health and recovery.

Sleep Optimization: Adequate sleep is essential for detoxification and overall wellness. During sleep, the body undergoes cellular repair and toxin removal processes. Establishing a regular sleep schedule and creating a conducive sleep environment can support detoxification and enhance recovery from chronic illness.

Environmental Toxin Reduction: Minimizing exposure to environmental toxins, such as pesticides, heavy metals, and household chemicals, supports ongoing detox efforts. Choosing organic foods, using natural cleaning products, and improving indoor air quality can reduce toxin load and support overall health.

Individualized Approach: It's crucial to tailor detox strategies to individual needs and health conditions. Consulting with a healthcare provider or a qualified practitioner provides reassurance and helps develop a personalized detoxification plan that addresses specific health goals and considerations.

By successfully incorporating these detox strategies into a comprehensive wellness plan, individuals recovering from chronic illness can feel a sense of accomplishment. They support their body's natural detoxification processes, promote healing, and enhance overall health and vitality.

6.2 Cleansing Protocols for Improved Health Outcomes

Cleansing protocols are structured approaches to improve health outcomes by enhancing the body's natural detoxification processes. These protocols typically involve dietary modifications, lifestyle changes, and sometimes specific therapies designed to eliminate toxins and support overall wellness. Here are key components and considerations for effective cleansing protocols:

Dietary Modifications: Central to most cleansing protocols is a focus on nutrient-dense, whole foods that support detoxification. This often includes increasing the intake of organic fruits and vegetables rich in antioxidants, vitamins, and minerals. Emphasizing fiber from sources like whole grains, legumes, and seeds aids in promoting regular bowel movements and removing toxins from the digestive tract.

Hydration: Adequate hydration is fundamental in any cleansing protocol as it supports kidney function and facilitates the elimination of toxins through urine. Drinking plenty of water throughout the day, preferably filtered to reduce contaminants, helps maintain optimal hydration levels and supports detoxification pathways.

Herbal Supplements: Incorporating herbs known for their detoxifying properties can enhance cleansing protocols. Examples include milk thistle, dandelion root, and turmeric, which support liver function and aid in the elimination of toxins. These herbs can be consumed as teas, tinctures, or supplements to complement dietary changes.

Intermittent Fasting: Some cleansing protocols advocate for intermittent fasting, where individuals cycle between eating and fasting. This approach can promote cellular repair, enhance metabolic processes, and support detoxification by giving the digestive system a break and allowing the body to focus on eliminating toxins.

Colon Cleansing: Supporting optimal colon health is crucial in cleansing protocols. Methods such as increasing fiber intake, using herbal laxatives, or undergoing colon hydrotherapy can help remove accumulated waste and toxins from the colon. These practices improve digestion, enhance nutrient absorption, and support overall detoxification.

Sweating: Activities that promote sweating, such as exercise, sauna sessions, or hot baths, play a role in cleansing protocols by facilitating the elimination of toxins through the skin. Sweating helps remove heavy metals, environmental pollutants, and metabolic waste products, supporting overall detoxification efforts.

Mind-Body Practices: Stress reduction techniques, including meditation, deep breathing exercises, and yoga, are often integrated into cleansing protocols. Chronic stress can impair detoxification pathways, so incorporating these practices supports overall health and enhances the body's ability to eliminate toxins.

Professional Guidance: It's essential to approach cleansing protocols under the guidance of a healthcare provider or qualified practitioner, especially for individuals with underlying health conditions or specific dietary needs. A personalized approach ensures the protocol aligns with individual health goals, supports overall wellness, and minimizes potential risks.

Implementing these cleansing protocols with careful consideration of individual needs and health status can help optimize detoxification processes, promote improved health outcomes, and support long-term wellness.

6.3 Liver and Kidney Support During Detox

Liver and kidney support are critical aspects of any detoxification process, as these organs play pivotal roles in filtering and eliminating toxins from the body. During detox, it's essential to prioritize strategies that optimize liver and kidney function to ensure effective toxin removal and overall health. Here are vital considerations for supporting the liver and kidneys during detox:

The liver is the body's primary detoxification organ, metabolizes toxins into less harmful substances that can be excreted. Supporting liver function during detox involves consuming foods rich in antioxidants and nutrients that aid in detoxification pathways. Cruciferous vegetables like broccoli, Brussels sprouts, and cabbage contain compounds that support liver detox enzymes. Additionally, incorporating herbs such as milk thistle, turmeric, and dandelion root can help protect liver cells and enhance detoxification processes.

Adequate hydration is crucial for kidney health and overall detoxification. The kidneys filter waste products and toxins from the bloodstream, excreting them through urine. Drinking plenty of water throughout the day supports optimal kidney function by ensuring a sufficient flow of urine to remove toxins effectively. Hydration also helps prevent kidney stones and urinary tract infections, common concerns during detoxification.

Maintaining electrolyte balance is essential for supporting kidney function. Electrolytes such as potassium, sodium, and magnesium play critical roles in kidney health and overall bodily functions. Consuming foods rich in electrolytes, such as bananas, leafy greens, and nuts, helps maintain balance and supports kidney function during detox.

Certain herbs are known for their kidney-supportive properties and can be beneficial during detox. For example, parsley is a natural diuretic that helps increase urine production, aiding in the elimination of toxins through the kidneys. Nettle leaf is another herb that supports kidney function by promoting healthy urinary flow and reducing inflammation.

During detox, it's crucial to avoid overwhelming the liver and kidneys with excessive toxins or aggressive detox protocols. Gradual and gentle detox approaches allow these organs time to process and eliminate toxins effectively without causing undue stress. It is important to monitor symptoms such as fatigue, headaches, or digestive discomfort, as they may indicate the need to adjust the detox protocol.

Individuals with pre-existing liver or kidney conditions should consult with a healthcare provider before beginning any detox program. A healthcare professional can provide personalized recommendations and monitor liver and kidney function throughout the detox process. This ensures the detox protocol is safe and effective for individual health needs.

Chapter 7: Mind-Body Techniques for Chronic Illness

7.1 Stress Reduction and Mindfulness Practices

Stress reduction and mindfulness practices, including detoxification programs, are not just beneficial, but empowering elements of any holistic health regimen. These practices, by supporting mental and emotional well-being, give you the power to significantly enhance your body's ability to detoxify effectively. Here's how stress reduction and mindfulness practices play a crucial role in detox:

Stress profoundly impacts the body, influencing hormone levels, immune function, and even digestion. Chronic stress can impair detoxification pathways in the liver and kidneys, compromising their ability to eliminate toxins efficiently. Mindfulness practices such as meditation, deep breathing exercises, and yoga help reduce stress levels by calming the mind and promoting relaxation. These practices support optimal liver and kidney function during detox by alleviating stress.

Mindfulness practices play a significant role in detoxification by reducing cortisol levels. High levels of the stress hormone cortisol can interfere with detoxification processes and contribute to toxin buildup in the body. Mindfulness practices have been shown to reduce cortisol levels, creating a more favorable environment for detoxification. Lower cortisol levels support liver function and enhance the body's ability to metabolize and eliminate toxins effectively.

Detoxification is not just about physical cleansing but also about emotional healing. Stress reduction techniques such as mindfulness meditation can provide a sense of relief, helping individuals process emotions and release mental toxins contributing to stress. This emotional cleansing complements physical detoxification, promoting a feeling of overall well-being and balance.

Quality sleep is a crucial but often overlooked factor in detoxification and overall health. Mindfulness practices improve sleep quality by reducing insomnia, enhancing sleep efficiency, and promoting restorative sleep patterns. Adequate sleep supports the body's natural detoxification processes, allowing organs like the liver and kidneys to perform optimally during the night.

Mindfulness practices play a key role in bolstering immune function during detoxification. Chronic stress weakens the immune system, making the body more vulnerable to infections and illnesses. Mindfulness practices reduce stress and inflammation, supporting overall health and resilience during detoxification.

Integrating stress reduction and mindfulness practices into daily life is critical to maximizing their benefits during detox. Consistent practice cultivates resilience to stressors, enhancing self-awareness, and fostering a sense of calm and clarity. These practices, like taking short breaks for deep breathing, practicing gratitude, or engaging in mindful eating, can significantly reduce stress and promote overall well-being, making you more prepared to face life's challenges.

Incorporating stress reduction and mindfulness practices into a detox program enhances its effectiveness by promoting relaxation, supporting detoxification pathways, and fostering emotional balance. By prioritizing these practices alongside dietary adjustments and herbal support, individuals can achieve a comprehensive approach to detoxification that nurtures both body and mind.

7.2 Biofeedback and Relaxation Therapies

Biofeedback and relaxation therapies are innovative techniques that play a pivotal role in holistic health practices, particularly in managing stress, enhancing relaxation, and supporting overall well-being. These therapies utilize technology and mindfulness techniques to empower individuals to gain better control over their physiological responses. Here's how biofeedback and relaxation therapies contribute to health and wellness:

Biofeedback is a process that enables individuals to learn how to control physiological functions that are typically involuntary, such as heart rate, blood pressure, muscle tension, and skin temperature. During biofeedback sessions, sensors are attached to the body to monitor these functions, providing real-time feedback through visual or auditory cues. This feedback helps individuals become aware of their body's responses to stress and learn techniques to modify these responses.

Types of Biofeedback

There are several types of biofeedback techniques used in practice, including:

- Electromyography (EMG): Measures muscle activity and tension.

- Electrodermal Activity (EDA): Monitors sweat gland activity, indicating stress levels.

- Heart Rate Variability (HRV): Assesses the variation in time intervals between heartbeats, reflecting autonomic nervous system function.

- Temperature Biofeedback: Tracks changes in skin temperature, which can indicate relaxation or stress response.

Relaxation Therapies

Complementary to biofeedback, relaxation therapies focus on inducing a state of deep relaxation and reducing stress levels. These therapies include:

- Progressive Muscle Relaxation: Involves tensing and relaxing muscle groups systematically to promote relaxation.

- Guided Imagery: Uses visualization techniques to create mental images that promote relaxation and well-being.

- Mindfulness Meditation: Cultivates present-moment awareness and acceptance, reducing stress and enhancing overall mental clarity.

- Breathwork: Techniques such as diaphragmatic breathing and paced breathing help regulate the breath, calming the nervous system and promoting relaxation.

Biofeedback and relaxation therapies are often integrated into holistic health practices and wellness programs to complement traditional medical treatments. They are used in clinical settings for conditions such as chronic pain, hypertension, anxiety disorders, and insomnia. These therapies empower individuals to take an active role in their health, promoting self-care and overall well-being.

With advancements in technology, biofeedback devices are becoming more portable and accessible for home use. Mobile apps and wearable devices offer biofeedback training, allowing individuals to practice relaxation techniques anywhere and anytime.

In summary, biofeedback and relaxation therapies are valuable tools in promoting health and well-being by teaching individuals to manage stress, enhance relaxation, and improve physiological functioning. By incorporating these therapies into daily life and wellness routines, individuals can experience lasting benefits for both body and mind.

7.3 Yoga and Tai Chi for Chronic Disease Management

Yoga and Tai Chi are ancient practices that have gained recognition in modern healthcare for their profound benefits in managing chronic diseases. These practices combine physical postures, breathing exercises, and meditation techniques to promote overall health and well-being. Here's how Yoga and Tai Chi contribute to chronic disease management:

7.3.1 Yoga for Chronic Disease Management

Yoga involves a series of postures (asanas), breathing exercises (pranayama), and meditation techniques (dhyana). It is known for its therapeutic effects on various chronic conditions, including:

- Cardiovascular Health: Yoga can help lower blood pressure, reduce heart rate variability, and improve circulation, thereby supporting heart health.

- Musculoskeletal Disorders: Yoga postures can enhance flexibility, strength, and joint mobility, benefiting individuals with conditions like arthritis and back pain.

- Mental Health: Yoga promotes relaxation, reduces stress, and improves mood, which is beneficial for managing anxiety, depression, and other mental health disorders.

- Respiratory Conditions: Breathing exercises in Yoga (pranayama) improve lung function and respiratory efficiency, aiding in conditions such as asthma and chronic obstructive pulmonary disease (COPD).

7.3.2 Tai Chi for Chronic Disease Management

Tai Chi, originating from ancient Chinese martial arts, involves slow, deliberate movements and deep breathing. It offers several benefits for chronic disease management, including:

- Balance and Fall Prevention: Tai Chi improves balance, coordination, and proprioception, reducing the risk of falls, particularly in older adults.

- Pain Management: The gentle movements of Tai Chi can alleviate chronic pain, such as that associated with osteoarthritis and fibromyalgia.

- Cognitive Function: Tai Chi enhances cognitive function, memory, and concentration, providing benefits for individuals with neurodegenerative disorders like Alzheimer's disease.

- Stress Reduction: Similar to Yoga, Tai Chi promotes relaxation, reduces stress hormones, and enhances overall mental well-being.

Numerous studies have demonstrated the efficacy of Yoga and Tai Chi in improving physical function, quality of life, and symptom management across various chronic diseases. These practices are increasingly recommended by healthcare professionals as complementary therapies to conventional treatments.

Yoga and Tai Chi are integrated into healthcare settings through specialized programs and classes tailored to specific chronic conditions. They are part of comprehensive treatment plans aimed at enhancing patient outcomes, reducing healthcare costs, and improving overall quality of life.

Both Yoga and Tai Chi can be adapted to accommodate individuals with different fitness levels, physical abilities, and health conditions. Classes range from gentle and therapeutic to more vigorous styles, ensuring accessibility for diverse populations.

In conclusion, Yoga and Tai Chi offer holistic approaches to managing chronic diseases by promoting physical health, mental well-being, and overall quality of life. These practices empower individuals to take an active role in their health, providing sustainable benefits that complement conventional medical treatments.

Chapter 8: Physical Activity and Chronic Conditions

8.1 Exercise Guidelines for Chronic Illness

Exercise is crucial for managing chronic illness as it offers numerous physical and mental health benefits. However, it's essential to follow specific guidelines tailored to individual conditions and capabilities to ensure safety and effectiveness.

Exercise guidelines for chronic illness emphasize a tailored approach based on the type and severity of the condition, overall health status, and individual fitness level. This personalized approach helps prevent exacerbation of symptoms while promoting optimal health outcomes.

Before starting any exercise program, individuals with chronic illnesses should consult healthcare providers, such as physicians, physical therapists, or exercise physiologists. These professionals can provide personalized recommendations and modify exercise plans according to medical history and current health status.

Types of Exercise

The type of exercise recommended varies depending on the chronic condition:

- Cardiovascular Exercise: Aerobic activities like walking, cycling, swimming, and dancing improve cardiovascular fitness, endurance, and circulation. They are beneficial for conditions such as heart disease, hypertension, and diabetes.

- Strength Training: Resistance exercises using weights, resistance bands, or body weight help build muscle strength, improve joint stability, and enhance bone health. This is crucial for conditions like osteoporosis, arthritis, and muscle weakness.

- Flexibility and Balance Exercises: Stretching, yoga, and Tai Chi enhance flexibility, balance, and coordination, reducing the risk of falls and injuries, particularly in older adults with conditions like osteoarthritis or Parkinson's disease.

Exercise intensity and duration should be gradually increased based on individual tolerance and fitness level. Low to moderate-intensity exercises are generally recommended for most chronic conditions to avoid fatigue and prevent overexertion.

Regular monitoring of symptoms, vital signs, and exercise tolerance is essential. Adjustments to the exercise program may be needed based on individual responses, especially during flare-ups or changes in health status.

Safety precautions include proper warm-up and cool-down routines, hydration, use of appropriate footwear and equipment, and awareness of environmental conditions. Exercise should be discontinued or modified if adverse symptoms such as chest pain, dizziness, or severe fatigue occur.

Regular physical activity improves cardiovascular health, enhances muscle strength and flexibility, promotes weight management, reduces stress, anxiety, and depression, and improves overall quality of life. It also supports immune function and helps manage chronic pain.

Exercise guidelines for chronic illness emphasize a holistic approach that integrates exercise with other aspects of healthcare, such as nutrition, medication management, and stress reduction techniques. This multidisciplinary approach optimizes health outcomes and empowers individuals to actively manage their chronic conditions.

In conclusion, adhering to tailored exercise guidelines for chronic illness promotes physical function, mental well-being, and overall quality of life. It enables individuals to maintain independence, manage symptoms effectively, and achieve long-term health benefits.

8.2 Adapted Physical Activities for Different Conditions

Adapted physical activities play a crucial role in enhancing the quality of life for individuals with various chronic conditions, ensuring they can engage in safe and effective exercise routines tailored to their specific needs and capabilities.

For individuals with cardiovascular conditions such as heart disease or hypertension, adapted activities focus on low to moderate-intensity aerobic exercises. These may include walking, stationary cycling, or water aerobics, which help improve cardiovascular health without placing excessive strain on the heart.

Respiratory conditions like asthma or chronic obstructive pulmonary disease (COPD) benefit from activities that improve lung function and respiratory endurance. Breathing exercises, gentle yoga, and swimming in a warm, humid environment are beneficial as they enhance respiratory efficiency and oxygen uptake.

Conditions affecting muscles, joints, or bones such as arthritis or osteoporosis require adapted activities that reduce joint impact and improve joint flexibility and strength. Range-of-motion exercises, gentle stretching, Tai Chi, and aquatic exercises in warm water help maintain joint mobility and reduce pain.

Neurological conditions like multiple sclerosis (MS), Parkinson's disease, or stroke require exercises that focus on improving balance, coordination, and functional mobility. Tai Chi, Pilates, dance therapy, and specific balance training exercises are beneficial as they enhance proprioception and reduce the risk of falls.

For individuals with diabetes, regular physical activity plays a critical role in improving blood sugar control and reducing the risk of complications. Aerobic exercises like brisk walking or cycling combined with resistance training to build muscle strength and improve insulin sensitivity are recommended.

Cancer survivors benefit from adapted physical activities that support recovery, reduce fatigue, and improve overall well-being. Activities such as gentle yoga, Pilates, and walking help maintain muscle mass, improve flexibility, and support emotional health during and after cancer treatment.

Cognitive conditions such as dementia or Alzheimer's disease benefit from adapted activities that stimulate cognitive function and maintain independence. Activities involving repetitive movements, music therapy, and structured exercises tailored to cognitive abilities promote brain health and emotional well-being.

Exercise during pregnancy is essential for maintaining physical fitness and preparing for childbirth. Adapted activities such as prenatal yoga, swimming, and low-impact aerobics help improve posture, reduce back pain, and promote relaxation and stress reduction.

Older adults often benefit from adapted physical activities that focus on maintaining mobility, balance, and independence. Activities such as chair yoga, gentle stretching, resistance band exercises, and group fitness classes designed for seniors improve cardiovascular health and reduce the risk of falls.

The key to adapted physical activities lies in an individualized approach that considers the person's medical history, current health status, functional abilities, and personal preferences. Working with healthcare professionals, such as physical therapists or exercise physiologists, ensures that exercise programs are safe, effective, and enjoyable.

Adapted physical activities cater to the unique needs of individuals with chronic conditions, promoting physical fitness, improving overall health outcomes, and enhancing quality of life. By incorporating tailored exercises into daily routines, individuals can maintain independence, manage symptoms effectively, and achieve long-term health benefits.

8.3 Benefits of Regular Movement and Exercise

Regular movement and exercise offer a myriad of benefits that extend beyond physical fitness, impacting overall health and well-being in profound ways. Engaging in consistent physical activity promotes cardiovascular health by strengthening the heart muscle, improving circulation, and lowering blood pressure. This reduces the risk of heart disease, stroke, and other chronic conditions associated with sedentary lifestyles.

Moreover, regular exercise plays a pivotal role in maintaining a healthy weight by burning calories and building muscle mass. This helps to manage body fat levels and prevent obesity, which is a significant risk factor for diabetes, joint problems, and certain cancers. Combined with a balanced diet, exercise supports metabolic function and enhances energy levels, contributing to a more active and fulfilling lifestyle.

Beyond physical health, regular movement and exercise have profound effects on mental and emotional well-being. Physical activity stimulates the release of endorphins, neurotransmitters that promote feelings of happiness and relaxation, effectively reducing symptoms of anxiety and depression. It also improves sleep quality, helping individuals achieve deeper and more restorative rest, which is crucial for cognitive function and emotional resilience.

Regular exercise supports bone health by increasing bone density and strength, reducing the risk of osteoporosis and fractures, especially important as people age. It also enhances flexibility, joint mobility, and balance, which are critical for preventing falls and maintaining independence in daily activities.

Furthermore, engaging in physical activity fosters social connections and enhances quality of life by participating in group exercises, sports, or recreational activities. This social interaction provides emotional support, boosts self-esteem, and reduces feelings of loneliness or isolation.

Book 18: Natural Pain Relief through Barbara O'Neill's Techniques

Natural Remedies for Pain Relief: Effective Techniques for Holistic Healing and Wellness

Chapter 1: Types and Causes of Pain

1.1 Overview of Acute and Chronic Pain

Acute and chronic pain represent distinct yet interconnected aspects of the human experience, each presenting unique challenges and considerations in healthcare management. Acute pain typically arises suddenly and is often associated with tissue damage or injury, serving as a vital warning signal that alerts the body to potential harm. It is usually short-lived and resolves as the underlying cause heals. Early intervention is crucial in acute pain, as it can prevent further complications. Common examples include post-operative pain, trauma-related injuries, and acute infections.

Conversely, chronic pain persists beyond the expected healing time and endures for weeks, months, or even years. Unlike acute pain, chronic pain may not have an identifiable cause or may persist despite adequate treatment of the underlying condition. Conditions such as arthritis, fibromyalgia, neuropathies, and chronic back pain are among the myriad causes of chronic pain, impacting millions of individuals worldwide. In fact, according to the World Health Organization, chronic pain affects an estimated 20% of the global population, making it a significant public health concern.

Both types of pain can significantly impair physical function, emotional well-being, and quality of life. Acute pain, while transient, can be severe and require immediate intervention to alleviate discomfort and facilitate recovery. Effective management strategies often involve a combination of pharmacological interventions, such as nonsteroidal anti-inflammatory drugs (NSAIDs) or opioids for severe pain, complemented by non-pharmacological approaches like physical therapy or acupuncture.

Chronic pain, on the other hand, poses more complex challenges due to its persistent nature and multifaceted impact on daily life. Treatment strategies for chronic pain typically emphasize a multimodal approach, which means using a variety of interventions from different disciplines, tailored to address both the physical and psychosocial aspects of pain. This may include a combination of medications, physical rehabilitation, cognitive-behavioral therapy, and integrative therapies such as acupuncture, massage, or mindfulness-based practices.

Importantly, chronic pain management requires a comprehensive assessment to identify contributing factors and individualize treatment plans accordingly. This thorough approach is essential in chronic pain management, as it ensures that all aspects of the condition are addressed. Healthcare providers strive to mitigate pain intensity, improve functional ability, and enhance quality of life through collaborative care approaches that empower patients to actively participate in their pain management journey.

In summary, while acute pain serves a protective function and resolves with healing, chronic pain represents a persistent condition that necessitates a holistic and personalized approach to treatment. By understanding the distinctions between acute and chronic pain and employing evidence-based interventions, healthcare providers can optimize outcomes, alleviate suffering, and improve overall well-being for individuals affected by these challenging conditions.

1.2 Common Causes of Pain

Pain, whether acute or chronic, can arise from various underlying conditions and circumstances, each influencing its management and treatment. Acute pain typically stems from injury or trauma, such as fractures, burns, cuts, or surgical procedures. These injuries activate pain receptors in the affected area, signaling the brain about potential harm and triggering protective responses.

Chronic pain, on the other hand, often persists beyond the expected healing time and may not always have a clear cause. Some of the common causes of chronic pain include:

1. Musculoskeletal Conditions: Disorders affecting bones, joints, muscles, tendons, and ligaments can lead to chronic pain. Conditions such as osteoarthritis, rheumatoid arthritis, fibromyalgia, and low back pain fall under this category.

2. Neuropathic Pain: Resulting from damage or dysfunction of the nervous system, neuropathic pain manifests as shooting, burning, or stabbing sensations. Examples include diabetic neuropathy, post-herpetic neuralgia (shingles), and nerve compression syndromes.

3. Inflammatory Conditions: Inflammation is a common source of pain and discomfort. Inflammatory disorders like inflammatory bowel disease (IBD), rheumatoid arthritis, and systemic lupus erythematosus (SLE) can cause persistent pain due to ongoing immune responses.

4. Trauma and Injury: Past injuries, especially if they have not healed properly or have led to nerve damage, can result in chronic pain. This includes whiplash injuries, sports injuries, and traumatic brain injuries.

5. Chronic Headaches and Migraines: Recurrent headaches and migraines can cause debilitating pain and are often associated with genetic predisposition, environmental triggers, and neurochemical imbalances.

6. Central Sensitization: This occurs when the central nervous system becomes hypersensitive to pain signals, amplifying the perception of pain even in the absence of ongoing tissue damage. Conditions like fibromyalgia and complex regional pain syndrome (CRPS) involve central sensitization.

7. Psychological Factors: Emotional distress, stress, anxiety, and depression can exacerbate pain perception and contribute to the development of chronic pain conditions. Addressing these factors is crucial in comprehensive pain management.

8. Cancer-related Pain: Cancer itself, as well as treatments like chemotherapy, radiation therapy, and surgery, can cause acute and chronic pain. Pain management in cancer patients often requires a multidisciplinary approach to improve quality of life.

9. Post-surgical Pain: Although acute in nature, post-operative pain can become chronic in some cases due to nerve damage or poor healing outcomes.

Understanding the underlying causes of pain is essential for developing effective treatment plans that address both the symptoms and their root causes. Healthcare providers employ a range of approaches, from medication and physical therapy to psychological support and complementary therapies, to help individuals manage and alleviate pain effectively.

1.3 Impact of Pain on Physical and Mental Health

The impact of pain on physical and mental health is profound, affecting individuals in multifaceted ways and often extending beyond the physical sensations. Physically, pain can lead to limitations in mobility, reduced flexibility, muscle tension, and overall decreased physical function. Chronic pain conditions such as arthritis, fibromyalgia, and back pain can significantly impair an individual's ability to perform daily activities, work, and engage in social interactions, thereby compromising their quality of life.

Mentally and emotionally, persistent pain can contribute to feelings of frustration, helplessness, anxiety, and depression. The constant discomfort and the challenges of managing pain on a daily basis can erode one's emotional resilience and lead to mood swings, irritability, and social withdrawal. Chronic pain may also disrupt sleep patterns, leading to fatigue and exacerbating cognitive impairments such as difficulty concentrating and memory problems.

Furthermore, the psychological impact of chronic pain can create a cycle of worsening symptoms, where stress and negative emotions amplify pain perception, leading to further emotional distress and physical discomfort. This cycle underscores the importance of addressing the emotional and psychological aspects of pain management alongside physical treatments.

Chronic pain conditions often require a comprehensive approach that integrates medical treatments with lifestyle modifications, physical therapy, psychological support, and sometimes complementary therapies such as acupuncture or mindfulness-based interventions. Effective pain management strategies aim not only to alleviate physical symptoms but also to enhance overall well-being and restore function, empowering individuals to lead fulfilling lives despite their pain.

Healthcare providers play a crucial role in helping patients navigate the complexities of chronic pain, providing education, personalized treatment plans, and ongoing support to improve both physical and mental health outcomes. By addressing the holistic impact of pain and tailoring interventions to individual needs, healthcare teams can optimize outcomes and enhance the overall quality of life for individuals living with chronic pain.

Chapter 2: Holistic Approach to Pain Management

2.1 Barbara O'Neill's Holistic Health Philosophy in Pain Relief

Barbara O'Neill's holistic health philosophy offers a comprehensive approach to pain relief that integrates natural remedies, lifestyle modifications, and emotional well-being. Central to her philosophy is the belief that addressing the root causes of pain involves treating symptoms and nurturing the body's innate ability to heal itself.

In Barbara O'Neill's approach, pain relief begins with understanding and optimizing overall health through nutrition. She emphasizes whole foods that reduce inflammation and support tissue repair. Her philosophy advocates for a diet rich in antioxidants, omega-3 fatty acids, and vitamins that can help alleviate pain and promote healing. Additionally, she emphasizes the importance of hydration and detoxification to remove toxins contributing to inflammation and pain.

Physical activity is another cornerstone of Barbara O'Neill's pain relief strategy. She promotes gentle exercises and stretches tailored to individual needs. She believes in the benefits of movement, not only for improving flexibility and strength but also for enhancing circulation, which can reduce pain and stiffness in joints and muscles.

Emphasizing the mind-body connection, Barbara O'Neill incorporates stress management techniques such as meditation, deep breathing, and relaxation exercises to alleviate tension and promote a sense of calm. By reducing stress and anxiety, these practices can help modulate pain perception and improve overall emotional well-being.

Barbara O'Neill also advocates for the use of natural therapies such as herbal remedies and essential oils, which she believes can complement conventional treatments by providing additional pain relief and promoting healing. Her approach encourages individuals to explore these natural options under healthcare professionals' guidance to ensure safety and effectiveness.

Barbara O'Neill's holistic health philosophy in pain relief is rooted in empowering individuals to take an active role in their well-being through education, lifestyle changes, and natural therapies. By addressing the physical, emotional, and spiritual aspects of pain, her approach aims to not only alleviate symptoms but also to support long-term health and vitality.

2.2 Integrative Medicine: Combining Natural and Conventional Approaches

As Barbara O'Neill advocates, integrative medicine harmoniously combines natural healing practices with conventional medical approaches to achieve optimal health outcomes. This approach recognizes the strengths of both paradigms and seeks to leverage their respective benefits while minimizing potential drawbacks.

Integrative medicine emphasizes a patient-centered approach that considers the whole person—body, mind, and spirit—rather than just isolated symptoms or diseases. It encourages collaboration between healthcare providers from various disciplines, including conventional doctors, naturopathic physicians, nutritionists, and mental health professionals, to create personalized treatment plans.

Barbara O'Neill promotes integrative medicine by integrating evidence-based natural therapies such as herbal remedies, nutritional supplements, acupuncture, and mind-body practices with conventional medical treatments like pharmaceuticals, surgery, and physical therapy. This approach aims to enhance the effectiveness of treatment while reducing side effects and promoting overall well-being.

Integrative medicine also emphasizes preventive care and lifestyle modifications to address underlying factors contributing to illness. This may include dietary changes, stress reduction techniques, regular exercise, and optimizing sleep patterns, all of which are integral to Barbara O'Neill's holistic approach.

Moreover, integrative medicine encourages patients to be actively involved in their own health management. It empowers individuals to make informed decisions about their healthcare options, fostering a sense of ownership and accountability in their healing journey.

By embracing integrative medicine, Barbara O'Neill advocates for a balanced and comprehensive approach to health that respects individual preferences and values. It acknowledges that every person is unique and may respond differently to various treatments, emphasizing the importance of personalized care plans tailored to meet specific needs and goals. Ultimately, integrative medicine seeks to optimize health outcomes by combining the best of both worlds—natural and conventional medicine—in a collaborative and holistic framework.

2.3 Importance of Lifestyle Modifications and Stress Reduction

Lifestyle modifications and stress reduction techniques are pivotal in Barbara O'Neill's holistic approach to health and well-being. These aspects are central to fostering overall vitality, resilience, and longevity by addressing the underlying factors contributing to disease and imbalance.

Firstly, Barbara O'Neill's holistic approach to health and well-being places a strong emphasis on lifestyle modifications. These encompass a wide range of choices individuals can make to support their health. A balanced and nutritious diet, rich in whole foods and low in processed and sugary foods, is a cornerstone of this approach. Coupled with regular physical activity, tailored to individual abilities and preferences, these practices are not just beneficial, but necessary for maintaining good health.

Moreover, managing stress is crucial in maintaining optimal health. Chronic stress can negatively impact the immune system, digestion, sleep patterns, and overall vitality. Barbara O'Neill advocates stress reduction techniques such as meditation, deep breathing exercises, yoga, and mindfulness practices. These techniques help individuals cultivate resilience to stressors, promote relaxation, and foster a sense of inner calm and balance.

Additionally, Barbara O'Neill encourages adequate sleep as a cornerstone of good health. Quality sleep supports immune function, cognitive performance, and mood regulation. Establishing a consistent sleep routine and creating a conducive sleep environment are essential to her holistic approach. Furthermore, Barbara O'Neill underscores the importance of maintaining healthy relationships and social connections. These positive social interactions are not just a source of support during stress or difficulty, but also a key contributor to emotional well-being. Nurturing these connections is an essential part of the holistic approach to health and well-being.

Chapter 3: Nutrition and Pain Relief

3.1 Anti-inflammatory Diet for Pain Management

An anti-inflammatory diet is a foundational aspect of Barbara O'Neill's holistic approach to managing pain effectively. This dietary approach focuses on reducing inflammation throughout the body, often associated with chronic pain conditions and various health issues. The premise behind an anti-inflammatory diet is to consume foods that help mitigate inflammation and promote overall health and well-being.

Central to an anti-inflammatory diet are whole, nutrient-dense, minimally processed foods. This includes a variety of colorful fruits and vegetables, which are rich in antioxidants, vitamins, and minerals. These nutrients help combat oxidative stress and reduce the production of inflammatory molecules in the body, potentially alleviating pain and discomfort.

Healthy fats, mainly those high in omega-3 fatty acids, are crucial in an anti-inflammatory diet. Sources such as fatty fish (salmon, mackerel, sardines), flaxseeds, chia seeds, and walnuts are known for their anti-inflammatory properties. Omega-3 fatty acids help balance the body's inflammatory response by reducing the production of inflammatory prostaglandins and cytokines.

In contrast, an anti-inflammatory diet minimizes or eliminates foods that can promote inflammation. This includes refined carbohydrates, processed foods, sugars, and trans fats, which can trigger inflammatory responses in the body. Reducing these foods' consumption helps lower inflammation levels and may alleviate pain symptoms.

Whole grains and legumes are also integral to an anti-inflammatory diet due to their fiber content and complex carbohydrates. Fiber supports gut health and a balanced microbiome, crucial for immune function and inflammation regulation. Additionally, whole grains provide sustained energy and help stabilize blood sugar levels, further supporting overall health.

Barbara O'Neill emphasizes personalized nutrition plans tailored to individual needs and health conditions. An anti-inflammatory diet is not a one-size-fits-all approach but a framework that can be adapted based on specific dietary preferences, allergies, and sensitivities. By adopting an anti-inflammatory diet, individuals may experience reduced pain levels, improved mobility, and enhanced overall quality of life.

In conjunction with dietary changes, Barbara O'Neill advocates for complementary, holistic practices such as stress management, regular physical activity, adequate sleep, and mindfulness techniques. These strategies work synergistically to support the body's natural healing processes, reduce inflammation, and optimize pain management outcomes over the long term.

3.2 Nutrients and Supplements for Pain Relief

Nutrients and supplements play a crucial role in Barbara O'Neill's holistic approach to pain relief, complementing dietary strategies and lifestyle modifications. These elements are essential for supporting the body's natural healing processes, reducing inflammation, and alleviating pain symptoms effectively.

Omega-3 fatty acids are prominent among these nutrients, known for their potent anti-inflammatory properties. Found abundantly in fatty fish like salmon, mackerel, and sardines, as well as in plant-based sources like flaxseeds and walnuts, omega-3s help regulate inflammation pathways in the body. They inhibit the production of inflammatory compounds such as prostaglandins and leukotrienes, thereby reducing pain intensity and improving joint function in conditions like arthritis.

Vitamin D is another critical nutrient that supports musculoskeletal health and pain management. Often referred to as the "sunshine vitamin," vitamin D modulates immune responses and reduces inflammation. Inadequate levels of vitamin D have been linked to increased pain sensitivity and chronic pain conditions. Barbara O'Neill emphasizes the importance of maintaining optimal vitamin D levels through sun exposure and supplementation, particularly in regions with limited sunlight.

Curcumin, the active compound in turmeric, is renowned for its potent anti-inflammatory and antioxidant properties. Used for centuries in traditional medicine, curcumin inhibits inflammatory pathways such as NF-kB and COX-2, which contribute to pain and inflammation. Supplementing with curcumin or incorporating turmeric into daily meals can help alleviate pain associated with arthritis, joint stiffness, and other inflammatory conditions.

Magnesium is another mineral crucial for pain management and muscle relaxation. It plays a vital role in over 300 enzymatic reactions in the body, including those involved in muscle function and nerve transmission. Magnesium deficiency has been associated with increased muscle cramps, tension headaches, and fibromyalgia symptoms. Barbara O'Neill recommends magnesium-rich foods such as leafy greens, nuts, seeds, and whole grains and supplementation, if necessary, to support pain relief and overall health.

In addition to these nutrients, certain herbal supplements can provide significant pain relief benefits. For example, Boswellia serrata, also known as Indian frankincense, possesses anti-inflammatory properties that can help reduce pain and improve mobility in conditions like osteoarthritis. Similarly, ginger extract has demonstrated analgesic effects and may be beneficial for managing muscle pain and soreness.

Barbara O'Neill underscores the importance of obtaining nutrients and supplements from whole foods whenever possible, as they offer a synergistic blend of vitamins, minerals, and phytonutrients. However, she acknowledges that supplementation may be necessary to address specific deficiencies or therapeutic needs. Consulting with a healthcare provider or a qualified nutritionist can help tailor a personalized regimen that effectively addresses individual health concerns and optimizes pain management outcomes.

3.3 Foods to Avoid for Pain Reduction

In Barbara O'Neill's holistic approach to pain reduction, identifying and avoiding certain foods that can exacerbate inflammation and pain is crucial. By eliminating or minimizing these dietary triggers, individuals can potentially alleviate symptoms and support overall well-being.

Refined sugars and high-glycemic carbohydrates are top contenders on the list of foods to avoid. These include sugary snacks, sodas, white bread, and pastries. These foods can spike blood sugar levels rapidly, leading to increased production of inflammatory molecules like cytokines and advanced glycation end products (AGEs). Such spikes can aggravate conditions like arthritis and contribute to chronic pain.

Processed and fried foods are also best avoided due to their high levels of trans fats, saturated fats, and unhealthy oils. These fats can promote inflammation in the body, worsening pain symptoms. Barbara O'Neill recommends opting for healthier cooking methods like baking, steaming, or grilling, and choosing foods rich in omega-3 fatty acids, such as fatty fish and nuts.

Refined grains like white rice, white pasta, and products made from refined flour can also contribute to inflammation. These foods lack fiber and essential nutrients found in whole grains and can cause blood sugar spikes similar to refined sugars. Barbara O'Neill advises substituting refined grains with whole grains like quinoa, brown rice, and whole wheat products, which provide sustained energy and help regulate blood sugar levels.

Certain nightshade vegetables, such as tomatoes, eggplants, peppers, and potatoes, contain alkaloids that may exacerbate inflammation and pain in some individuals, particularly those with arthritis or joint pain. While reactions vary among individuals, Barbara O'Neill suggests monitoring the consumption of nightshades and potentially eliminating them to determine their impact on pain levels.

Additionally, artificial additives and preservatives found in processed foods and beverages can trigger inflammatory responses in sensitive individuals. These additives include artificial sweeteners, flavor enhancers, and food colorings. Barbara O'Neill encourages choosing whole, natural foods and beverages, such as water and herbal teas, over sugary or artificially flavored drinks.

Lastly, excessive alcohol consumption can contribute to inflammation and pain, particularly in conditions like gout and fibromyalgia. Alcohol can disrupt sleep patterns, impair immune function, and deplete essential nutrients like B vitamins and magnesium. Barbara O'Neill advises moderation or avoidance of alcohol to support pain management efforts and overall health.

By identifying and minimizing these dietary triggers, individuals can help reduce inflammation, manage pain more effectively, and support their body's natural healing processes. Barbara O'Neill emphasizes the importance of adopting balanced, whole-food diet rich in nutrients and antioxidants to promote optimal health and well-being.

Chapter 4: Herbal Remedies for Pain Relief

4.1 Key Herbs for Pain Management

Key herbs play a pivotal role in Barbara O'Neill's approach to pain management, offering natural alternatives to pharmaceuticals with potential side effects. These herbs are renowned for their anti-inflammatory, analgesic, and calming properties, making them valuable additions to holistic pain relief strategies.

Turmeric: Known for its active compound curcumin, turmeric is a potent anti-inflammatory herb. It inhibits enzymes that trigger inflammation and reduces levels of inflammatory markers in the body. Barbara O'Neill recommends incorporating turmeric into daily cooking or taking it as a supplement to alleviate chronic pain conditions like arthritis.

Ginger: Ginger is celebrated for its anti-inflammatory properties, which can help alleviate joint pain and stiffness. It contains gingerol, a bioactive compound that inhibits inflammatory pathways in the body. Barbara O'Neill suggests consuming ginger tea or adding fresh ginger to meals to benefit from its pain-relieving effects.

Devil's Claw: Native to southern Africa, Devil's Claw is recognized for its anti-inflammatory and analgesic properties. It's commonly used to relieve lower back pain, arthritis, and other inflammatory conditions. Barbara O'Neill advises taking Devil's Claw as a supplement or in a tea to support pain management efforts.

White Willow Bark: White Willow Bark contains salicin, a compound similar to aspirin, which provides pain relief and reduces inflammation. It's used to alleviate acute and chronic pain, including headaches, osteoarthritis, and lower back pain. Barbara O'Neill recommends consulting with a healthcare provider before using White Willow Bark, especially for individuals sensitive to aspirin.

Boswellia: Also known as Indian frankincense, Boswellia possesses powerful anti-inflammatory properties. It helps reduce pain and inflammation by inhibiting pro-inflammatory enzymes. Barbara O'Neill suggests Boswellia supplements or topical creams for conditions like osteoarthritis and rheumatoid arthritis.

Arnica: Arnica is a traditional remedy for reducing pain and inflammation associated with bruises, sprains, and muscle soreness. Barbara O'Neill recommends Arnica gel or cream for topical application to soothe acute pain and promote healing.

Capsaicin: Found in chili peppers, Capsaicin has analgesic properties that help relieve pain by reducing substance P, a neurotransmitter involved in pain perception. Barbara O'Neill suggests using Capsaicin cream or patches for localized pain relief, such as in arthritis or neuropathic pain.

St. John's Wort: Known for its antidepressant properties, St. John's Wort also exhibits anti-inflammatory effects that can help alleviate nerve pain and muscle discomfort. Barbara O'Neill advises using St. John's Wort oil topically or taking it as a supplement under guidance for pain management.

Valerian Root: Valerian Root is prized for its sedative and muscle-relaxing properties, making it beneficial for relieving tension-related pain and promoting restful sleep. Barbara O'Neill recommends Valerian Root tea or supplements to ease muscular pain and improve sleep quality.

Chamomile: Chamomile possesses anti-inflammatory and relaxing properties that can help soothe muscle spasms, tension headaches, and digestive discomfort associated with stress-induced pain. Barbara O'Neill suggests using Chamomile tea or essential oil for pain relief and relaxation.

Incorporating these key herbs into a holistic pain management plan can provide natural relief from chronic or acute pain while supporting overall health and well-being. Barbara O'Neill emphasizes the importance of consulting with a qualified healthcare provider before starting any herbal treatment, especially when combining herbs with existing medications or for individuals with underlying health conditions.

4.2 Herbal Formulations and Applications

Herbal formulations are integral to Barbara O'Neill's holistic approach to health and wellness, offering natural solutions for various ailments and promoting overall well-being. These formulations typically combine synergistic herbs known for their therapeutic properties, creating powerful remedies that address specific health concerns. Here are some key herbal formulations and their applications in Barbara O'Neill's practice:

Herbal Tinctures

Tinctures are concentrated herbal extracts made by soaking herbs in alcohol or glycerin. They preserve the active compounds of herbs and are easily absorbed by the body. Barbara O'Neill recommends tinctures for their versatility and effectiveness in treating conditions such as digestive issues, anxiety, and insomnia. Popular herbal tinctures include Valerian Root for sleep support, Peppermint for digestive relief, and Lemon Balm for stress reduction.

Herbal Teas and Infusions

Herbal teas and infusions involve steeping dried or fresh herbs in hot water to extract their medicinal properties. This method is gentle yet effective, allowing for the extraction of vitamins, minerals, and phytochemicals. Barbara O'Neill advocates for herbal teas like Chamomile for relaxation, Ginger for digestion, and Nettle for its nutritive properties.

Herbal Capsules and Tablets

Herbal capsules and tablets provide a convenient way to consume concentrated herbal extracts. They are often standardized to contain specific amounts of active ingredients, ensuring consistent potency. Barbara O'Neill recommends capsules for herbs such as Turmeric, Boswellia, and Devil's Claw to support joint health and reduce inflammation.

Herbal Oils and Salves

Herbal oils and salves are topical formulations infused with herbs and carrier oils. They are applied directly to the skin to relieve pain, inflammation, and skin conditions. Barbara O'Neill suggests using Arnica salve for bruises and muscle soreness, Calendula oil for skin irritation, and Eucalyptus oil for respiratory congestion.

Herbal Poultices and Compresses

Herbal poultices involve applying mashed herbs directly to the skin, while compresses use herbal-infused water-soaked cloths. These applications are beneficial for treating localized pain, inflammation, and swelling. Barbara O'Neill advises using Comfrey or Plantain poultices for wound healing and inflammation reduction.

Herbal Syrups and Elixirs

Herbal syrups and elixirs combine herbs with honey or glycerin to create sweet-tasting remedies that are soothing to the throat and easy to administer. They are commonly used for respiratory health, immune support, and as general tonics. Barbara O'Neill recommends Elderberry syrup for immune boosting, Licorice root elixir for digestive relief, and Hawthorn berry syrup for heart health.

Herbal Baths and Soaks

Herbal baths and soaks involve adding herbal preparations to bathwater to promote relaxation, detoxification, and skin health. They are particularly effective for easing muscle tension and soothing the mind. Barbara O'Neill suggests using Lavender, Chamomile, and Epsom salts for calming baths that promote restful sleep and stress relief.

By incorporating these herbal formulations into daily routines, individuals can harness the healing power of plants to support their health naturally. Barbara O'Neill emphasizes the importance of selecting high-quality herbs, following recommended dosages, and consulting with a qualified healthcare practitioner, especially when using herbs alongside medications or for chronic health conditions.

4.3 Topical and Internal Use of Herbs for Pain

Topical and internal applications of herbs for pain relief are foundational in Barbara O'Neill's approach to holistic health. These methods leverage the therapeutic properties of herbs to alleviate discomfort and promote healing from within.

Barbara O'Neill advocates for the topical application of herbs through various forms such as oils, salves, and poultices. Herbal oils like Arnica and St. John's Wort are renowned for their anti-inflammatory and analgesic properties, making them effective for soothing sore muscles, joint pain, and bruises. Salves infused with herbs such as Calendula and Eucalyptus offer localized relief from arthritis, dermatitis, and minor wounds. Additionally, herbal poultices, using herbs like Comfrey or Ginger, can be applied directly to the skin to reduce inflammation and promote tissue repair.

Internally, herbs can be consumed as teas, tinctures, capsules, or incorporated into food to address pain and inflammation at a systemic level. Herbal teas such as Chamomile, Ginger, and Turmeric are consumed regularly to support digestive health, reduce inflammation, and provide overall pain relief. Tinctures made from herbs like Devil's Claw and Boswellia are highly concentrated extracts that can be added to water or taken directly under the tongue to manage chronic pain conditions such as arthritis and fibromyalgia. Herbal capsules, containing potent extracts of herbs such as Willow Bark or Turmeric, are often standardized to ensure consistent dosage and efficacy in alleviating pain and inflammation.

Barbara O'Neill emphasizes the importance of choosing herbs that are suited to individual needs and conditions, ensuring they are sourced from reputable suppliers to guarantee quality and purity. It's essential to follow recommended dosages and consult with a qualified healthcare practitioner, particularly when integrating herbal remedies with conventional treatments or for managing chronic pain conditions.

Chapter 5: Essential Oils for Pain Relief

5.1 Aromatherapy Techniques for Pain Management

Aromatherapy, using essential oils derived from plants for therapeutic purposes, has long been recognized as an effective technique for managing pain. Using these natural oils' powerful properties, aromatherapy can help alleviate various types of pain, from headaches and muscle aches to chronic conditions like arthritis. Here, we delve into specific aromatherapy techniques that can be employed for pain management.

5.1.1 Inhalation Methods

One of the simplest and most effective ways to use essential oils for pain relief is inhalation. This method can be achieved using diffusers, steam inhalation, or simply by inhaling directly from the bottle. Diffusers disperse essential oils into the air, allowing continuous inhalation that can help reduce pain and promote relaxation over time. Oils like lavender, peppermint, and eucalyptus are commonly used for their analgesic and anti-inflammatory properties. Steam inhalation involves adding a few drops of essential oil to a bowl of hot water, covering the head with a towel, and inhaling deeply. This technique is particularly beneficial for respiratory-related pain and sinus headaches.

5.1.2 Topical Applications

Applying essential oils directly to the skin is another effective method for managing pain. Essential oils must be diluted with carrier oils such as coconut, jojoba, or almond oil to prevent skin irritation. Massaging diluted essential oils into the affected area can provide localized relief from muscle aches, joint pain, and inflammation. For instance, a blend of peppermint and eucalyptus oil can help soothe sore muscles, while frankincense and myrrh are excellent for reducing inflammation associated with arthritis. Hot and cold compresses can also be infused with essential oils. A hot compress with a few drops of lavender or chamomile oil can relax tense muscles, whereas a cold compress with peppermint oil can help reduce swelling and pain from injuries.

5.1.3 Aromatherapy Baths

Aromatherapy baths are a luxurious and highly effective way to use essential oils for pain relief. Adding a few drops of essential oils like lavender, marjoram, or rosemary to a warm bath can help ease muscle tension, reduce inflammation, and promote relaxation. The combination of warm water and essential oils enhances circulation and helps the body absorb the oils' therapeutic properties more efficiently. For those with chronic pain conditions, regular aromatherapy baths can be a vital part of their pain management regimen.

5.1.4 Pain Relief Blends

Creating specific blends of essential oils tailored to individual pain conditions can maximize the effectiveness of aromatherapy. For example, a lavender, rosemary, and peppermint blend can be used for tension headaches. At the same time, a mixture of eucalyptus, ginger, and black pepper oil can be beneficial for joint and muscle pain. These blends can be used in various ways, including in diffusers, as part of a massage oil, or added to a bath.

5.1.5 Consistency and Regular Use

Regular and consistent use is the key to effective pain management with aromatherapy. Incorporating essential oils into daily routines, such as using a pain relief blend in a diffuser during work hours or applying a soothing oil blend before bedtime, can provide ongoing relief and help prevent pain flare-ups.

While aromatherapy is generally safe, it is crucial to use essential oils properly to avoid adverse effects. Always dilute essential oils before topical application and perform a patch test to check for allergies. Consult with a healthcare provider before using essential oils, especially if you are pregnant, nursing, or dealing with chronic health conditions.

Aromatherapy offers a versatile and natural approach to pain management, utilizing the potent properties of essential oils to provide relief and enhance overall well-being. By incorporating inhalation, topical applications, baths, and customized blends, individuals can effectively manage their pain and improve their quality of life.

5.2 Essential Oils for Muscle Pain, Joint Pain, and Headaches

Essential oils have long been used for their therapeutic properties, particularly in managing various types of pain such as muscle pain, joint pain, and headaches. These natural remedies offer an alternative to conventional pain relief methods, providing effective and holistic approaches to alleviating discomfort. Here, we explore the essential oils best suited for each type of pain and the ways to use them.

Muscle Pain

Muscle pain, often resulting from overexertion, injury, or stress, can significantly impact daily activities. Essential oils such as peppermint, eucalyptus, and rosemary are particularly effective for soothing sore muscles.

- Peppermint Oil: Known for its cooling effect, peppermint oil contains menthol, which helps to relax muscles and reduce inflammation. Applying a diluted blend of peppermint oil with a carrier oil like coconut or almond oil directly to the affected area can provide immediate relief. Peppermint oil can also be added to a warm bath to soothe the entire body after a strenuous workout.

- Eucalyptus Oil: Eucalyptus oil is prized for its anti-inflammatory and analgesic properties. It helps to increase blood circulation to the affected muscles, promoting faster healing. A eucalyptus oil-infused compress can be used on sore muscles, or it can be added to massage oil for a therapeutic massage.

- Rosemary Oil: Rosemary oil helps reduce muscle spasms and improves circulation, making it an excellent choice for muscle pain. It can be used in a warm compress or mixed with a carrier oil for a deep tissue massage.

Joint Pain

Joint pain, common in conditions like arthritis, can be debilitating. Essential oils such as frankincense, ginger, and marjoram are beneficial in managing joint discomfort.

- Frankincense Oil: Frankincense oil has powerful anti-inflammatory properties that help reduce joint swelling and pain. Regular application of a frankincense oil blend on the affected joints can provide significant relief. It can also be diffused to promote a calming environment, which may help reduce pain perception.

- Ginger Oil: Ginger oil is well-known for its warming and anti-inflammatory effects. It helps to increase circulation and reduce inflammation in the joints. Mixing ginger oil with a carrier oil and massaging it into the joints can alleviate stiffness and pain.

- Marjoram Oil: Marjoram oil has soothing properties that make it effective for reducing joint pain. It can be used in a bath or as a massage oil to help ease joint discomfort and improve flexibility.

Headaches

Headaches, whether caused by stress, tension, or other factors, can be effectively managed with essential oils like lavender, peppermint, and chamomile.

- Lavender Oil: Lavender oil is renowned for its calming and sedative properties, making it ideal for tension headaches. Inhaling lavender oil through a diffuser or applying a few drops to the temples and back of the neck can provide quick relief. A lavender-infused warm compress can also help relax the muscles and alleviate headache pain.

- Peppermint Oil: Peppermint oil's menthol content provides a cooling sensation that can help reduce headache symptoms. Applying diluted peppermint oil to the temples and forehead can alleviate tension headaches and migraines. Inhaling peppermint oil can also help open up the sinuses, providing relief from sinus headaches.

- Chamomile Oil: Chamomile oil is known for its anti-inflammatory and calming properties. It can help reduce the pain and stress associated with headaches. A few drops of chamomile oil added to a warm bath or diffused in the air can help relieve headache pain and promote relaxation.

Methods of Application

For effective pain relief, essential oils can be used in various ways:

- Topical Application: Always dilute essential oils with a carrier oil before applying to the skin. A 2-3% dilution is generally safe for most people.

- Inhalation: Using a diffuser or simply inhaling from the bottle can help relieve pain and promote relaxation.

- Baths: Adding a few drops of essential oil to a warm bath can provide overall relief from pain and tension.

- Compresses: Both hot and cold compresses infused with essential oils can be applied to the affected area for targeted relief.

While essential oils are generally safe, it is important to use them properly to avoid adverse effects. Always perform a patch test before using a new oil topically. Consult with a healthcare provider, especially if you are pregnant, nursing, or have underlying health conditions.

5.3 Blending Essential Oils for Pain Relief

Blending essential oils for pain relief is an art and science that combines the therapeutic properties of various oils to create powerful, synergistic mixtures. These blends can target specific types of pain such as muscle aches, joint discomfort, and headaches, providing holistic and natural relief. Understanding the properties of different essential oils and how they complement each other is key to creating effective pain relief blends.

The concept of synergy in aromatherapy is based on the idea that the combined effect of multiple essential oils is greater than the sum of their individual effects. This principle is crucial when blending oils for pain relief, as it allows for the creation of powerful, multi-faceted treatments that can address various aspects of pain and inflammation.

5.3.1 Selecting Essential Oils

When creating a blend for pain relief, it is important to select oils that have analgesic (pain-relieving), anti-inflammatory, and muscle-relaxing properties. Some of the most effective essential oils for pain relief include:

- Peppermint Oil: Known for its cooling and analgesic properties, peppermint oil is excellent for relieving muscle and joint pain.

- Lavender Oil: With its calming and anti-inflammatory effects, lavender oil helps reduce pain and promote relaxation.

- Eucalyptus Oil: This oil has strong anti-inflammatory properties and helps increase blood flow to the affected area, which can reduce pain and speed up healing.

- Rosemary Oil: Rosemary oil is beneficial for reducing muscle spasms and improving circulation, making it ideal for muscle pain.

- Frankincense Oil: Known for its powerful anti-inflammatory properties, frankincense oil is effective in reducing joint pain and swelling.

- Ginger Oil: With its warming effect and anti-inflammatory properties, ginger oil is excellent for alleviating joint and muscle pain.

5.3.2 Creating Effective Blends

To create an effective pain relief blend, follow these steps:

1. Determine the Purpose of the Blend: Identify the type of pain you are targeting (muscle pain, joint pain, headaches) and choose oils that are known to be effective for that specific condition.

2. Select Your Carrier Oil: A carrier oil is necessary to dilute the essential oils and facilitate their application. Popular carrier oils include coconut oil, jojoba oil, and sweet almond oil.

3. Calculate the Dilution Ratio: For pain relief blends, a dilution ratio of 2-3% is generally recommended. This means adding 12-18 drops of essential oil per ounce (30 ml) of carrier oil.

4. Combine the Oils: Mix the selected essential oils with the carrier oil in a clean, dark glass bottle. Ensure the bottle is tightly sealed and shake well to blend the oils thoroughly.

5.3.3 Sample Blends for Pain Relief

Here are some sample blends tailored for different types of pain:

- Muscle Pain Relief Blend:
    - 5 drops of peppermint oil
    - 5 drops of lavender oil
    - 5 drops of rosemary oil
    - 30 ml of carrier oil

- Joint Pain Relief Blend:
    - 5 drops of frankincense oil
    - 5 drops of ginger oil
    - 5 drops of eucalyptus oil
    - 30 ml of carrier oil

- Headache Relief Blend:
    - 5 drops of lavender oil
    - 5 drops of peppermint oil
    - 30 ml of carrier oil

Chapter 6: Mind-Body Techniques for Pain Management

6.1 Stress Reduction and Pain Perception

The relationship between stress and pain perception is profound and complex. Stress, both chronic and acute, can significantly heighten the perception of pain, making it more intense and challenging to manage. This connection is mediated by the body's stress response, which involves the release of hormones such as cortisol and adrenaline. These hormones prepare the body for a "fight or flight" response but also exacerbate inflammation and tension, increasing pain levels.

Stress, when experienced, can disrupt the body's innate pain-relief mechanisms. This disruption is a result of the activation of the sympathetic nervous system, leading to increased muscle tension, heart rate, and blood pressure. The heightened state of arousal can initiate or worsen pain, creating a cycle where stress and pain reinforce each other. For instance, stress-induced muscle tension in the neck and shoulders can lead to tension headaches or worsen conditions like arthritis.

Effective stress management is a key component of pain management. Techniques that reduce stress can help lower the body's pain threshold and improve overall pain perception. Regular practice of stress-reduction methods can lead to enduring benefits, including reduced frequency and intensity of pain episodes. Cognitive-behavioral therapy, mindfulness meditation, and relaxation exercises are particularly effective in breaking the cycle of stress and pain. These techniques help individuals develop coping skills, reframe negative thought patterns, and promote relaxation, all contributing to better pain management.

6.2 Meditation and Mindfulness Practices

Meditation and mindfulness practices are powerful tools for managing pain and reducing stress. These practices involve focusing the mind on the present moment, which can help break the cycle of chronic pain and anxiety. By fostering awareness and acceptance, individuals can learn to observe their pain without becoming overwhelmed, thereby decreasing their perception of pain.

Mindfulness meditation, for instance, teaches individuals to focus on their breath and bodily sensations, fostering a non-judgmental awareness of the present moment. This practice has been shown to alter how the brain processes pain signals, reducing the intensity and unpleasantness of pain. Research has demonstrated that mindfulness meditation can increase activity in areas of the brain associated with pain regulation, such as the prefrontal cortex, and decrease activity in areas linked to pain perception, such as the anterior cingulate cortex and amygdala.

Another effective technique is guided imagery, which involves visualizing calming and healing images. This method can distract the mind from pain and promote relaxation. Progressive muscle relaxation, which involves tensing and then slowly relaxing different muscle groups, can also be beneficial. It helps to release tension and reduce stress, thereby alleviating pain. When practiced regularly, these techniques can create lasting changes in the brain, enhancing an individual's ability to manage pain and stress.

In addition to these practices, integrating mindfulness into daily activities, such as mindful walking, eating, or even chores, can help maintain a state of relaxation and awareness throughout the day. This ongoing mindfulness practice can prevent stress from accumulating and exacerbating pain.

6.3 Biofeedback and Relaxation Therapies for Pain Relief

Biofeedback is a therapeutic technique that helps individuals gain control over physiological functions that are typically involuntary, such as heart rate, muscle tension, and blood pressure. By using biofeedback devices, individuals can learn to recognize and modify their body's responses to pain and stress. This self-regulation can lead to significant improvements in pain management and overall well-being.

During a biofeedback session, sensors are attached to the body to measure physiological responses. This information is then displayed on a monitor, providing real-time feedback. For example, a person can see muscle tension levels and learn relaxation techniques to reduce tension. Over time, this can help decrease pain. Biofeedback is particularly effective for conditions such as chronic migraines, fibromyalgia, and tension headaches.

Relaxation therapies, such as deep breathing exercises, are like a soothing balm for pain relief. Deep breathing involves taking slow, deep breaths to activate the body's relaxation response. This can lower stress levels, decrease muscle tension, and improve pain perception. Techniques such as diaphragmatic breathing, where the breath is drawn deep into the abdomen, can be remarkably calming, providing a sense of comfort and ease.

Combining biofeedback with relaxation techniques can provide a comprehensive approach to pain management. For instance, individuals can use biofeedback to monitor their physiological responses and practice deep breathing or progressive muscle relaxation to counteract stress and pain. Other relaxation techniques, such as yoga, tai chi, and progressive muscle relaxation, can also be integrated into a biofeedback program to enhance its effectiveness.

In addition to these techniques, regular physical activity, adequate sleep, and a healthy diet can support stress reduction and pain management. Exercise releases endorphins, the body's natural painkillers, and can improve mood and reduce stress. Adequate sleep is crucial for the body's repair processes and overall well-being. A balanced diet supports the body's health and can reduce inflammation, a common contributor to pain. By integrating these holistic approaches into daily life, individuals can create a robust pain management strategy that addresses pain's physical and psychological aspects.

Chapter 7: Physical Therapies and Pain Relief

7.1 Exercise and Movement for Pain Management

Exercise and movement play a crucial role in managing and alleviating pain. Regular physical activity can help reduce inflammation, improve mobility, and enhance overall well-being, making it an essential component of a comprehensive pain management plan. Whether dealing with chronic conditions like arthritis, back pain, or fibromyalgia, incorporating appropriate exercise routines can lead to significant improvements in pain levels and quality of life.

One of the primary benefits of exercise for pain management is its ability to reduce inflammation. Many types of chronic pain are associated with inflammation in the joints, muscles, or other tissues. Regular physical activity helps regulate the body's inflammatory response, reducing the production of pro-inflammatory cytokines and increasing anti-inflammatory markers. This can lead to decreased pain and swelling, particularly in rheumatoid arthritis and osteoarthritis.

Improving mobility and flexibility is another critical aspect of pain management through exercise. Stiffness and limited range of motion can exacerbate pain and contribute to a cycle of inactivity and worsening symptoms. Stretching exercises, yoga, and tai chi are particularly beneficial for enhancing flexibility and reducing stiffness. These activities gently stretch the muscles and connective tissues, promoting better joint function and reducing discomfort.

Strengthening exercises are also vital for managing pain, especially for conditions involving the musculoskeletal system. Building muscle strength provides better support for the joints, reducing their load and alleviating pain. Resistance training, using weights or resistance bands, can help strengthen the muscles around painful joints, such as the knees, hips, and back. For example, maintaining the quadriceps can provide better support for the knee joint, reducing pain in individuals with knee osteoarthritis.

Cardiovascular exercise, such as walking, swimming, or cycling, is essential for overall health and pain management. These activities improve cardiovascular fitness, increase endorphin levels, and enhance mood, all contributing to pain relief. Endorphins, the body's natural painkillers, are released during aerobic exercise, providing an immediate sense of well-being and reducing pain perception. Swimming is especially beneficial for individuals with joint pain, as the buoyancy of water reduces the impact on the joints while providing resistance for muscle strengthening.

Incorporating low-impact exercises is crucial for individuals with chronic pain, as high-impact activities can sometimes exacerbate pain. Activities like swimming, cycling, and using an elliptical machine provide cardiovascular benefits without putting undue stress on the joints. Additionally, practices such as Pilates can improve core strength and stability, which is beneficial for individuals with back pain.

It is essential to start slowly and gradually increase the intensity and duration of exercise to avoid overexertion and potential injury. A physical therapist or a trained exercise professional can help design a personalized exercise program tailored to an individual's needs and limitations. They can guide proper form and technique, ensuring that exercises are performed safely and effectively.

Listening to the body and pacing oneself is crucial in managing pain through exercise. It's important to recognize and respect the body's signals, taking breaks when needed and avoiding pushing through severe pain. Consistency is key, and regular, moderate exercise is more beneficial than sporadic, intense workouts.

In addition to structured exercise routines, incorporating more movement into daily activities can help manage pain. Simple changes, such as taking short walks, using the stairs, or gardening, can increase overall activity levels and relieve pain.

Exercise and movement help manage physical pain and improve mental health. Physical activity reduces stress, anxiety, and depression, all of which can exacerbate pain perception. By enhancing mood and promoting relaxation, exercise contributes to a holistic approach to pain management.

Integrating regular exercise and movement into a pain management plan offers numerous benefits, from reducing inflammation and improving mobility to enhancing mental well-being. With healthcare professionals' guidance, individuals can develop a safe and effective exercise routine that supports long-term pain relief and improved quality of life.

7.2 Stretching and Strengthening Exercises

Understanding the benefits of stretching and strengthening exercises empowers you to take control of your health. These exercises are foundational to effective pain management and an overall wellness strategy. They help alleviate pain and prevent future discomfort by enhancing flexibility, muscle strength, and joint stability. Integrating these exercises into daily routines can significantly improve physical function, mobility, and quality of life.

7.2.1 Benefits of Stretching

Stretching exercises are essential for maintaining and improving flexibility. Flexibility is crucial for a full range of motion in the joints, which is necessary for performing daily activities with ease. Regular stretching helps lengthen muscles and tendons, reducing stiffness and tension that can contribute to pain. It also increases muscle blood flow, promoting healing and reducing soreness.

One key benefit of stretching is reducing muscle tightness and preventing injuries. Tight muscles are more prone to strains and sprains, leading to acute pain and long-term issues if not addressed. Stretching before and after physical activities prepares the muscles for exertion and helps them recover more effectively afterward.

Dynamic stretching, which involves active movements that stretch the muscles through their full range of motion, is particularly beneficial before exercise. Examples include leg swings, arm circles, and torso twists. These movements help warm the body, improve circulation, and enhance neuromuscular coordination, reducing the risk of injury.

Static stretching, where you hold a stretch for a prolonged period (usually 15-60 seconds), is effective for increasing flexibility and releasing muscle tension. Common static stretches include hamstring stretches, quadriceps stretches, and shoulder stretches. Holding these positions helps elongate the muscles and improve flexibility over time.

7.2.2 Benefits of Strengthening Exercises

Strengthening exercises are equally important for pain management and overall health. Building muscle strength supports the joints, reduces their load, and enhances their stability. This is particularly beneficial for individuals with osteoarthritis, where joint support is crucial for pain reduction and improved function.

Strengthening exercises can be categorized into two main types: resistance training and bodyweight exercises. Resistance training involves using weights, resistance bands, or machines to create resistance against which the muscles must work. This type of training is effective for building muscle mass, increasing bone density, and improving overall strength.

Bodyweight exercises, such as squats, lunges, push-ups, and planks, use the individual's body weight as resistance. These versatile exercises can be performed anywhere without the need for special equipment. They are particularly effective for building functional strength, which is the ability to easily perform everyday activities without pain.

Core strengthening is critical to any exercise program, especially for individuals experiencing back pain. Strengthening the core muscles, including the abdominals, obliques, and lower back muscles, provides better support for the spine and improves posture. Exercises like planks, bridges, and abdominal crunches target these muscles and help reduce back pain and improve stability.

7.2.3 Integrating Stretching and Strengthening into Daily Routine

To maximize the benefits of stretching and strengthening exercises, it is important to integrate them into a consistent daily routine. A well-rounded exercise program should include a balance of stretching and strengthening activities to address all aspects of physical health.

A typical routine might begin with a warm-up that includes dynamic stretching to prepare the body for exercise. This could be followed by a combination of strengthening exercises targeting different muscle groups. Then, the conclusion could be made with static stretching to relax the muscles and improve flexibility.

Consistency is key to seeing long-term benefits. Even short sessions of 15-30 minutes each day can significantly improve strength, flexibility, and pain management. Listening to the body and progressing gradually, such as increasing the number of repetitions or the weight used, is essential to avoid overexertion and injury.

Seeking guidance from a physical therapist or a certified fitness trainer can be beneficial, especially for individuals with chronic pain or specific conditions. These professionals can tailor an exercise program to your individual needs and ensure that exercises are performed correctly and safely, giving you the reassurance and confidence you need in your exercise journey.

Incorporating stretching and strengthening exercises into daily life helps manage and alleviate pain and enhances overall physical health, functional ability, and quality of life. By committing to a regular routine, individuals can achieve better mobility, increased strength, and a significant reduction in pain and discomfort.

7.3 Physical Modalities: Heat, Cold, and Massage Therapies

Physical modalities such as heat, cold, and massage therapies are powerful tools in the management of pain and the promotion of overall well-being. These therapies offer non-invasive, effective ways to address a range of musculoskeletal issues, reduce inflammation, improve circulation, and enhance recovery processes.

7.3.1 Heat Therapy

Heat therapy, also known as thermotherapy, involves the application of heat to the body to alleviate pain and improve tissue function. It is particularly effective for chronic pain conditions, muscle stiffness, and joint pain. The application of heat helps to dilate blood vessels, increasing blood flow to the affected area, which promotes healing and reduces muscle spasms.

There are several methods of applying heat therapy, including:

- Hot Packs and Heating Pads: These can be applied directly to the painful area to provide immediate relief. Heating pads can be electric or microwaveable, offering convenience for home use.

- Warm Baths and Showers: Immersing the body in warm water helps to relax muscles and joints, providing widespread relief from stiffness and pain.

- Paraffin Wax Treatments: Commonly used for arthritis in the hands and feet, paraffin wax provides soothing heat and helps to improve range of motion.

Heat therapy is most effective when applied for 15-20 minutes at a time. It is important to use a moderate level of heat to avoid burns or overheating, and it should not be used on acute injuries, as it can exacerbate inflammation.

7.3.2 Cold Therapy

Cold therapy, or cryotherapy, involves the application of cold to reduce inflammation, swelling, and pain, particularly after acute injuries such as sprains, strains, or bruises. Cold therapy works by constricting blood vessels, which decreases blood flow to the injured area and helps to numb the area, providing pain relief.

Common methods of applying cold therapy include:

- Ice Packs and Gel Packs: These can be wrapped in a towel and applied to the affected area for short periods, typically 10-15 minutes, to reduce inflammation and numb the pain.

- Cold Compresses: Cloths soaked in cold water can be used to provide cooling relief to larger areas or sensitive regions of the body.

- Ice Baths: Immersing the body or a limb in ice water can be particularly effective for reducing inflammation and pain in larger muscle groups.

Cold therapy should be used with caution to avoid frostbite or nerve damage. It is recommended to limit application to intervals of 10-15 minutes and to always place a barrier, such as a cloth, between the cold source and the skin.

7.3.3 Massage Therapy

Massage therapy involves the manipulation of the body's soft tissues, including muscles, tendons, and ligaments, to relieve pain, reduce stress, and promote overall wellness. There are various types of massage techniques, each with unique benefits for different conditions:

- Swedish Massage: This is a gentle form of massage that uses long strokes, kneading, and deep circular movements to relax and energize the body. It is excellent for reducing muscle tension and improving circulation.

- Deep Tissue Massage: This technique targets deeper layers of muscle and connective tissue, using slower, more forceful strokes to alleviate chronic muscle tension and knots.

- Trigger Point Massage: Focused on areas of tight muscle fibers that can form in muscles after injuries or overuse, this technique applies pressure to specific points to relieve pain and improve function.

- Sports Massage: Designed to help athletes prevent and treat injuries, sports massage involves a combination of techniques to improve flexibility, reduce fatigue, and enhance endurance.

Massage therapy offers several benefits, including improved circulation, reduced muscle tension, enhanced flexibility, and a general sense of relaxation and well-being. It can be tailored to individual needs and preferences, making it a versatile and highly effective modality for pain management.

7.4 Integrating Physical Modalities into Pain Management

Integrating heat, cold, and massage therapies into a comprehensive pain management plan can significantly enhance their effectiveness. For example, alternating between heat and cold therapy can help manage both acute and chronic pain by leveraging the benefits of both modalities. Heat can be used to relax muscles and increase blood flow before activities, while cold therapy can be applied afterward to reduce inflammation and numb pain.

Massage therapy can be incorporated regularly to maintain muscle health, reduce stress, and prevent the recurrence of pain. It can be particularly beneficial when combined with other treatments such as stretching and strengthening exercises, physical therapy, or chiropractic care.

For those managing chronic pain conditions, it is essential to work with healthcare professionals to determine the most appropriate use of these modalities. This ensures that treatments are applied safely and effectively, tailored to the individual's specific needs and conditions.

By understanding and utilizing the benefits of heat, cold, and massage therapies, individuals can achieve significant pain relief, improve their physical function, and enhance their overall quality of life. These modalities offer accessible, non-invasive options that can be easily integrated into daily routines, providing a holistic approach to managing pain and promoting health.

Book 19: Boosting Immunity Naturally with Barbara O'Neill

Empowering Your Immunity: Natural Strategies and Insights for Optimal Health

Chapter 1: Overview of the Immune System

8.1 Understanding How the Immune System Works

The immune system is the body's defense mechanism against infections and diseases. It comprises a complex network of cells, tissues, and organs that identify and neutralize harmful invaders like bacteria, viruses, fungi, and parasites. The immune system's primary function is to distinguish between self and non-self, targeting and eliminating pathogens while sparing the body's own healthy cells.

<u>Innate Immunity</u>

The immune system operates through two main components: innate immunity and adaptive immunity. Innate immunity is the body's first line of defense. It is a non-specific response that acts quickly to prevent the spread of infection. Innate immunity includes physical barriers like the skin and mucous membranes, chemical barriers such as stomach acid and enzymes in saliva, and cellular defenses including white blood cells like neutrophils and macrophages. These cells recognize and engulf pathogens through a process called phagocytosis.

<u>Adaptive Immunity</u>

Adaptive immunity is more specialized and slower to respond compared to innate immunity. It involves the production of specific antibodies by B cells and activating T cells, which target infected cells. The adaptive immune system has a memory component, allowing it to recognize and respond more effectively to pathogens it has encountered. This memory is the principle behind vaccination, where exposure to a harmless form of a pathogen trains the immune system to respond quickly and robustly upon future encounters.

8.2 Components of the Immune System

The immune system consists of various components that work in concert to protect the body from infections and diseases. These components can be classified into physical barriers, cells, and organs.

<u>Physical Barriers</u>

Skin: Acts as a physical barrier to prevent the entry of pathogens.

Mucous Membranes: Line the respiratory, digestive, and urogenital tracts, trapping pathogens and preventing their entry.

Cilia: Hair-like structures in the respiratory tract that move mucus and trapped pathogens out of the airways.

<u>Cellular Components</u>

White Blood Cells (Leukocytes): Include various types such as neutrophils, macrophages, dendritic cells, and lymphocytes (B cells and T cells).

Neutrophils: The most abundant white blood cells that quickly respond to infection.

Macrophages: Engulf and digest pathogens and present their antigens to T cells.

Dendritic Cells: Act as messengers between the innate and adaptive immune systems by presenting antigens to T cells.

Lymphocytes: B cells produce antibodies, while T cells destroy infected cells and help regulate immune responses.

Organs and Tissues

Bone Marrow: Produces all blood cells, including immune cells.

Thymus: Where T cells mature.

Lymph Nodes: Filter lymph fluid and house immune cells that trap and destroy pathogens.

Spleen: Filters blood, removes old or damaged blood cells and helps fight infections.

Tonsils and Adenoids: Trap pathogens enter through the mouth and nose.

8.3 Factors Affecting Immune Function

Various factors, including genetics and age, lifestyle, and environmental exposures, can influence the effectiveness of the immune system.

Genetic Factors

Genetics play a pivotal role in shaping the strength of an individual's immune system. Certain genetic conditions can lead to immune deficiencies, making individuals more susceptible to infections. Conversely, genetic variations can bolster immune responses, providing better protection against certain pathogens. Understanding these genetic factors can empower individuals to make informed health decisions.

Age

The efficiency of the immune system undergoes significant changes with age. Infants and young children have immature immune systems, making them more vulnerable to infections. As people age, their immune systems typically weaken, a phenomenon known as immunosenescence, which increases susceptibility to infections, autoimmune diseases, and cancer. This understanding can inspire individuals to take proactive steps to support their immune health as they age.

Nutrition

Proper nutrition is vital for maintaining a healthy immune system. Nutrient deficiencies, especially of vitamins and minerals like vitamin C, vitamin D, zinc, and iron, can impair immune function. A balanced diet of fruits, vegetables, whole grains, lean proteins, and healthy fats supports overall immune health.

Lifestyle Factors

Exercise: Regular physical activity enhances immune function and reduces the risk of chronic diseases such as heart disease, diabetes, and obesity.

Sleep is a crucial factor in maintaining a healthy immune system. Adequate sleep is essential for the immune system to function correctly. Sleep deprivation can impair immune responses. This knowledge can encourage individuals to prioritize their sleep, thereby supporting their immune health.

Stress: Chronic stress can suppress immune function, making the body more susceptible to infections.

Smoking and Alcohol: Both smoking and excessive alcohol consumption weaken the immune system, increasing vulnerability to infections and diseases.

Environmental Factors

Exposure to Pathogens: Pathogens are disease-causing microorganisms like bacteria, viruses, and fungi. Regular exposure to these in a controlled manner, such as through vaccination, helps build immunity.

Hygiene: Good hygiene practices, such as handwashing, can prevent infections and reduce the burden on the immune system.

Pollution: Environmental pollutants and toxins can impair immune function and increase the risk of infections and autoimmune diseases.

Understanding how the immune system works, its components and the factors affecting its function is essential for maintaining health and preventing disease. By adopting a healthy lifestyle and making informed choices, individuals can support their immune system's ability to protect and heal the body effectively.

Chapter 2: Holistic Approach to Immune Support

2.1 Holistic Health Philosophy in Boosting Immunity

A holistic health philosophy emphasizes the interconnectedness of the body, mind, and spirit, recognizing that optimal health is achieved through balance and harmony in all aspects of life. This approach focuses on natural boosting of the immune system, prioritizing prevention and the body's innate healing abilities. Key elements of this philosophy include.

Nutrition: A diet rich in whole, unprocessed foods is fundamental. Emphasizing fruits, vegetables, whole grains, lean proteins, and healthy fats ensures that the body receives essential nutrients to support immune function. Specific foods, such as garlic, ginger, turmeric, and fermented foods like yogurt and kefir, are particularly beneficial for their immune-boosting properties.

Hydration: Adequate water intake is crucial for maintaining overall health and supporting the immune system. Proper hydration helps eliminate toxins and supports all bodily functions, including those of the immune system.

Sleep: Quality sleep is essential for the immune system to function effectively. During sleep, the body repairs itself and strengthens its defenses. Aiming for 7-9 hours of uninterrupted sleep per night can significantly enhance immune response.

Exercise: Regular physical activity improves circulation, reduces stress hormones, and promotes the efficient function of immune cells. Moderate exercise, such as walking, cycling, or yoga, is recommended for its overall health benefits.

Mindfulness and Stress Reduction: Chronic stress can suppress immune function. Incorporating mindfulness practices, such as meditation, deep breathing exercises, and yoga, helps manage stress and supports immune health. Reducing stress through these practices can improve the body's ability to fight off infections.

Herbal Remedies: Incorporating herbs known for their immune-boosting properties, such as echinacea, elderberry, and astragalus, can provide additional support. These herbs can be consumed as teas, tinctures, or supplements.

2.2 Integrative Medicine: Integrating Natural and Conventional Approaches

Integrative medicine combines the best of conventional and natural therapies to enhance patient care. This approach recognizes the value of modern medical treatments while also emphasizing the importance of natural and holistic methods. Fundamental principles of integrative medicine include:

Patient-Centered Care: Treating the patient as a whole person, not just addressing symptoms or diseases. This involves understanding the patient's lifestyle, preferences, and overall health goals.

Combining Modalities: Using a combination of conventional treatments (such as medications, surgeries, and medical procedures) with complementary therapies (like acupuncture, massage, and herbal medicine) to create a comprehensive treatment plan. For example, a cancer patient might receive chemotherapy while also using acupuncture and nutritional therapy to manage side effects and improve overall well-being.

Preventive Focus: Emphasizing prevention and the promotion of health through lifestyle modifications, stress management, and natural therapies. Regular screenings and early intervention are part of this preventive strategy.

Evidence-Based Practice: Integrative medicine relies on scientific evidence to support the use of complementary therapies. It involves ongoing research and clinical studies to validate the efficacy and safety of various treatments.

Collaboration: Encouraging collaboration among healthcare providers from different disciplines to ensure a coordinated and holistic approach to patient care. This team-based approach can enhance treatment outcomes and patient satisfaction.

2.3 Importance of Lifestyle Modifications and Stress Management

Lifestyle modifications and stress management are critical to maintaining a robust immune system and overall health. These strategies empower you to make conscious choices, taking control of your health by improving daily habits and reducing stress.

Healthy Diet: Adopting a balanced diet rich in vitamins, minerals, and antioxidants supports immune function. Reducing intake of processed foods, sugar, and unhealthy fats can prevent inflammation and boost the body's defenses.

Regular Exercise: Incorporating regular physical activity into daily routines is achievable for everyone. Whether it's walking, swimming, or strength training, exercise can be tailored to your individual fitness levels and preferences, making it a part of your unique health journey.

Adequate Sleep: Ensuring sufficient and quality sleep is crucial for health. Establishing a regular sleep schedule, creating a restful sleep environment, and limiting screen time before bed can improve sleep quality.

Stress Reduction Techniques: Chronic stress negatively impacts the immune system. When the body is under stress, it produces cortisol, a hormone that can suppress the immune system. Implementing stress reduction techniques such as mindfulness meditation, deep breathing exercises, yoga, and spending time in nature can help manage stress levels and thereby, support immune function.

Social Connections: Maintaining strong social ties and engaging in meaningful relationships provide emotional support and reduce stress. Social interactions can boost mood and overall well-being.

Avoiding Harmful Substances: Reducing or eliminating the use of tobacco, excessive alcohol, and other harmful substances can significantly improve health outcomes and support the immune system.

By integrating these lifestyle modifications and stress management techniques, you're not just improving your immune function and overall health. You're also taking a holistic approach that considers your emotional well-being, which is key to achieving long-term health and vitality.

Chapter 3: Nutrition and Immune Function

3.1 Nutrients Essential for Immune Health

Maintaining a robust immune system relies heavily on the intake of essential nutrients that support the body's defense mechanisms.

Known for its immune-boosting properties, vitamin C is a powerful antioxidant that helps protect cells from damage by free radicals. It enhances the production and function of white blood cells, which are crucial for fighting infections. Foods rich in vitamin C include citrus fruits, strawberries, bell peppers, and broccoli.

Vitamin D deficiency is linked to increased susceptibility to infections. It can be obtained from sun exposure, fortified foods, fatty fish, and supplements.

Essential for maintaining the integrity of mucosal barriers in the respiratory and gastrointestinal tracts, vitamin A also supports the function of immune cells like T-cells and B-cells. Sources include carrots, sweet potatoes, spinach, and liver.

Another potent antioxidant, vitamin E helps regulate and maintain immune function. It protects cell membranes from oxidative damage and supports the activities of immune cells. Nuts, seeds, spinach, and avocado are good sources.

Zinc deficiency can impair immune response and increase the risk of infections. Rich sources include meat, shellfish, legumes, and seeds.

Selenium is essential for the proper functioning of the immune system, enhancing the immune response and protecting against oxidative stress. Foods high in selenium include Brazil nuts, seafood, and eggs.

Iron is necessary for the proliferation and maturation of immune cells. It also supports the production of hemoglobin, which carries oxygen to cells. Red meat, beans, and fortified cereals are good iron sources.

Fatty acids have anti-inflammatory properties and support immune function by enhancing the activity of white blood cells. Sources include fatty fish, flaxseeds, and walnuts.

3.2 Foods that Support Immune Function

A diet rich in diverse, nutrient-dense foods can significantly boost immune function. Some of the best foods for supporting the immune system include:

1. **Citrus Fruits**: Oranges, grapefruits, lemons, and limes are packed with vitamin C, which is crucial for immune health.

2. **Berries**: Blueberries, strawberries, and raspberries are rich in antioxidants, vitamins, and fiber, which help strengthen the immune system.

3. **Leafy Greens**: Spinach, kale, and Swiss chard provide vitamins A, C, and E, as well as folate and iron, all of which support immune function.

4. **Garlic**: Known for its antimicrobial and antiviral properties, garlic contains compounds that boost the immune response.

5. **Ginger**: With its anti-inflammatory and antioxidant properties, ginger can help reduce inflammation and support immune health.

6. **Turmeric**: Curcumin, the active ingredient in turmeric, has powerful anti-inflammatory and antioxidant effects, enhancing immune function.

7. **Yogurt and Kefir**: These fermented foods contain probiotics, which are beneficial bacteria that support gut health and, in turn, boost the immune system.

8. **Nuts and Seeds**: Almonds, sunflower seeds, and pumpkin seeds provide essential nutrients like vitamin E, zinc, and healthy fats.

9. **Green Tea**: Rich in antioxidants and amino acids, green tea can enhance immune function and protect against infections.

10. **Mushrooms**: Varieties like shiitake, maitake, and reishi have immune-boosting properties due to their high content of beta-glucans and other bioactive compounds.

3.3 Supplements for Immune Support

While a balanced diet is the best way to obtain essential nutrients, supplements can help fill gaps and provide additional support. Some effective supplements for boosting immune health include:

1. **Vitamin C**: Available in various forms, vitamin C supplements can help ensure adequate intake, especially during times of increased stress or illness.

2. **Vitamin D**: For individuals with limited sun exposure or dietary intake, vitamin D supplements are essential for maintaining optimal immune function.

3. **Zinc**: Zinc supplements can support immune health, particularly during cold and flu season. They are available in lozenge, tablet, and liquid forms.

4. **Probiotics**: Supplements containing beneficial bacteria can enhance gut health and boost the immune system. Look for multi-strain probiotic supplements for broader benefits.

5. **Elderberry**: Known for its antiviral properties, elderberry supplements can help reduce the severity and duration of colds and flu.

6. **Echinacea**: This herb is available in various forms, including capsules, tinctures, and teas, and can help enhance immune function.

7. **Astragalus**: Often used in traditional Chinese medicine, astragalus supplements can support the immune system and improve overall health.

8. **Selenium**: For those with dietary deficiencies, selenium supplements can help enhance immune response and protect against oxidative damage.

9. **Curcumin**: Available as a supplement, curcumin from turmeric can provide anti-inflammatory and antioxidant benefits.

Chapter 4: Herbal Remedies for Immune Support

4.1 Nutrients Essential for Immune Health

Maintaining a robust immune system depends heavily on the intake of specific nutrients that bolster the body's defenses. Essential nutrients include:

Vitamin C: This powerful antioxidant is crucial for protecting cells against damage from free radicals. It enhances the production and function of white blood cells, which play a pivotal role in fighting infections. Foods rich in vitamin C include citrus fruits, strawberries, bell peppers, and broccoli.

Vitamin D: Vitamin D is vital for modulating the immune system and enhancing the pathogen-fighting capabilities of monocytes and macrophages. Deficiency in this vitamin is associated with a higher susceptibility to infections. It can be obtained from sun exposure, fortified foods, fatty fish, and supplements.

Vitamin A: Essential for maintaining the integrity of mucosal barriers in the respiratory and gastrointestinal tracts, vitamin A also supports the function of immune cells like T-cells and B-cells. Sources include carrots, sweet potatoes, spinach, and liver.

Vitamin E: Another potent antioxidant, vitamin E helps regulate and maintain immune function by protecting cell membranes from oxidative damage and supporting immune cell activities. Nuts, seeds, spinach, and avocado are good sources.

Zinc: Zinc is crucial for the normal development and function of immune cells. A deficiency in zinc can impair immune response and increase the risk of infections. Rich sources include meat, shellfish, legumes, and seeds.

Selenium: Selenium is essential for the proper functioning of the immune system, enhancing the immune response and protecting against oxidative stress. Foods high in selenium include Brazil nuts, seafood, and eggs.

Iron: Iron is necessary for the proliferation and maturation of immune cells and supports the production of hemoglobin, which carries oxygen to cells. Red meat, beans, and fortified cereals are good sources of iron.

Omega-3 Fatty Acids: These fatty acids possess anti-inflammatory properties and support immune function by enhancing the activity of white blood cells. Sources include fatty fish, flaxseeds, and walnuts.

4.2 Foods that Support Immune Function

A diet rich in diverse, nutrient-dense foods can significantly boost immune function. Some of the best foods for supporting the immune system include.

Citrus Fruits: Oranges, grapefruits, lemons, and limes are packed with vitamin C, which is crucial for immune health.

Berries: Blueberries, strawberries, and raspberries are rich in antioxidants, vitamins, and fiber, which help strengthen the immune system.

Leafy Greens: Spinach, kale, and Swiss chard provide vitamins A, C, and E, as well as folate and iron, all of which support immune function.

Garlic: Known for its antimicrobial and antiviral properties, garlic contains compounds that boost the immune response.

Ginger: With its anti-inflammatory and antioxidant properties, ginger can help reduce inflammation and support immune health.

Turmeric: Curcumin, the active ingredient in turmeric, has powerful anti-inflammatory and antioxidant effects, enhancing immune function.

Yogurt and Kefir: These fermented foods contain probiotics, which are beneficial bacteria that support gut health and, in turn, boost the immune system.

Nuts and Seeds: Almonds, sunflower, and pumpkin seeds provide essential nutrients like vitamin E, zinc, and healthy fats.

Green Tea: Rich in antioxidants and amino acids, green tea can enhance immune function and protect against infections.

Mushrooms: Varieties like shiitake, maitake, and reishi have immune-boosting properties due to their high content of beta-glucans and other bioactive compounds.

Chapter 5: Essential Oils for Immune Support

5.1 Aromatherapy Techniques for Immune Boosting

Aromatherapy offers several techniques to support and enhance immune function. These methods harness the potent properties of essential oils to stimulate the body's natural defenses and improve overall well-being.

Diffusion: Using a diffuser, essential oils can be dispersed into the air, allowing for continuous inhalation of the therapeutic compounds. This method is particularly effective for purifying the air and promoting respiratory health. Ultrasonic diffusers are popular as they do not use heat, preserving the integrity of the essential oils.

Steam Inhalation: This technique involves adding a few drops of essential oil to a bowl of hot water. Leaning over the bowl with a towel draped over the head, inhale deeply to allow the steam to carry the essential oils into the respiratory system. This method is excellent for easing congestion and supporting respiratory health, especially during cold and flu season.

Topical Application: Essential oils can be diluted in carrier oils (such as jojoba, almond, or coconut oil) and applied directly to the skin. This method allows the oils to be absorbed into the bloodstream. For immune support, apply diluted oils to the chest, neck, and soles of the feet.

Massage: Combining the benefits of touch therapy with essential oils, massage can be a powerful way to boost immunity. Essential oils can be blended with carrier oils and used for a full-body massage, which promotes relaxation, reduces stress, and enhances immune function.

Baths: Adding a few drops of essential oil to a warm bath can create a soothing and therapeutic experience. The warm water helps to open pores and allows the essential oils to be absorbed through the skin while also providing inhalation benefits. Epsom salts can be added to enhance detoxification.

Compresses: Essential oils can be added to warm or cold compresses and applied to specific areas of the body. This method can help relieve localized pain, reduce inflammation, and support the immune system.

5.2 Essential Oils Known for Their Immune-Enhancing Properties

Certain essential oils are particularly renowned for their immune-boosting properties due to their antimicrobial, antiviral, and anti-inflammatory effects.

1. Eucalyptus: Known for its ability to clear the respiratory tract, eucalyptus oil has strong antiviral and antibacterial properties. It is particularly effective in fighting respiratory infections and enhancing overall immune response.

2. Tea Tree: This oil is a powerful antiseptic, antibacterial, and antiviral agent. It is effective in treating a variety of infections and supporting the body's natural defenses.

3. Lavender: Lavender oil not only promotes relaxation and reduces stress but also has antimicrobial properties that support immune health. It is gentle enough for various applications, including baths and topical use.

4. Lemon: With its high vitamin C content, lemon oil is a potent immune booster. It also has strong antibacterial and antiviral properties, making it effective in fighting infections.

5. Thyme: Thyme oil is highly antimicrobial and can help protect against various pathogens. It is particularly useful during cold and flu season.

6. Frankincense: This oil has powerful anti-inflammatory and immune-boosting properties. It supports overall health and enhances the body's ability to fight off infections.

7. Oregano: Oregano oil is one of the most potent antimicrobial essential oils. It is effective against bacteria, viruses, and fungi, making it a valuable addition to any immune-boosting regimen.

5.3 Creating Immune Support Blends with Essential Oils

Combining different essential oils can create powerful blends that enhance immune function. Here are a few recipes to get started:

1. Immune Boosting Diffuser Blend:

    o   3 drops Eucalyptus

    o   3 drops Lemon

    o   2 drops Tea Tree

    o   2 drops Lavender Add these oils to a diffuser and run for 30 minutes to purify the air and boost immunity.

2. Respiratory Support Steam Inhalation:

    o   2 drops Eucalyptus

    o   2 drops Peppermint

    o   1 drop Thyme Add the oils to a bowl of hot water, cover your head with a towel, and inhale deeply for 5-10 minutes.

3. Immune Boosting Massage Oil:

    o   10 drops Lavender

    o   8 drops Frankincense

- o   6 drops Lemon

- o   4 drops Oregano

- o   2 tablespoons carrier oil (e.g., jojoba or almond oil) Mix the oils in a dark glass bottle and use for a full-body massage to enhance immune function.

4. Healing Bath Soak:

- o   5 drops Lavender

- o   5 drops Tea Tree

- o   2 drops Eucalyptus

- o   1 cup Epsom salts Mix the essential oils with Epsom salts and add to a warm bath for a relaxing and immune-boosting soak.

5. Immune Support Compress:

- o   3 drops Thyme

- o   3 drops Lemon

- o   2 drops Lavender Add the oils to a bowl of warm water, soak a cloth in the mixture, and apply to the chest or back to support respiratory health and boost immunity.

Incorporating these blends into daily routines can help maintain a robust immune system and enhance overall well-being. Remember to always dilute essential oils properly and perform a patch test to check for skin sensitivity.

Chapter 6: Lifestyle Practices for Immune Health

6.1 Importance of Sleep in Immune Function

Sleep plays a crucial role in maintaining and enhancing immune function. During sleep, the body undergoes critical restorative processes that are essential for optimal health and immunity.

Immune System Maintenance

During sleep, the immune system releases cytokines, which are proteins that help combat infections and inflammation. Certain cytokines need to increase when there is an infection, inflammation, or stress, and sleep facilitates this increase. Chronic sleep deprivation can lead to a decrease in the production of these protective cytokines, weakening the immune response.

Cellular Repair

Sleep is the time when the body repairs cells, tissues, and muscles. This repair process is vital for maintaining a strong immune system. The production of infection-fighting antibodies and cells is reduced when you don't get enough sleep, making the body more susceptible to illnesses.

Memory and Learning

The immune system also relies on memory to respond to pathogens it has encountered before. Sleep helps to consolidate memory and learning, which means it may also play a role in how the immune system remembers and responds to infections.

Hormonal Balance

Sleep helps regulate the production of hormones that are crucial for immune function. Lack of sleep disrupts the balance of these hormones, leading to increased inflammation and a reduced ability to fight infections.

Chronic Diseases

Poor sleep is linked to various chronic conditions, such as obesity, diabetes, and cardiovascular disease, which can further compromise immune function. By ensuring adequate sleep, the risk of these conditions can be reduced, indirectly supporting immune health.

6.2 Stress Reduction Techniques and Their Impact on Immunity

Chronic stress has a detrimental impact on the immune system, making it crucial to adopt stress reduction techniques to maintain and enhance immunity.

Mindfulness and Meditation: Practices such as mindfulness meditation can significantly reduce stress levels. Regular meditation helps lower cortisol levels, a stress hormone that, when elevated, suppresses the immune response. By promoting relaxation and reducing anxiety, meditation supports a healthy immune system.

Deep Breathing Exercises: Techniques such as diaphragmatic breathing can activate the body's relaxation response, decreasing stress and enhancing immune function. Deep breathing helps reduce cortisol levels and increases oxygen flow to the body, promoting overall health.

Yoga and Tai Chi: These mind-body practices combine physical movement, meditation, and breathing exercises to reduce stress and improve immune function. Regular practice can lower stress hormones, increase flexibility, and improve mental clarity, all of which contribute to a stronger immune system.

Progressive Muscle Relaxation (PMR): This technique involves tensing and then slowly relaxing different muscle groups in the body. PMR can help reduce physical tension and mental stress, supporting a healthy immune response.

Adequate Sleep: As discussed, sleep is vital for stress reduction and immune health. Ensuring a regular sleep schedule and good sleep hygiene practices can help reduce stress and bolster immune function.

Physical Activity: Regular exercise is an effective stress reliever and immune booster. Physical activity reduces levels of the body's stress hormones, such as adrenaline and cortisol, while stimulating the production of endorphins, which are natural mood lifters.

6.3 Physical Activity and Its Role in Immune Support

Engaging in regular physical activity is essential for maintaining a robust immune system. Exercise provides numerous benefits that contribute to overall immune health.

1. Enhanced Circulation: Regular physical activity improves blood circulation, which allows immune cells and substances to move through the body more efficiently. This enhanced circulation helps the immune system detect and respond to pathogens more quickly.

2. Stress Reduction: Exercise is a natural stress reliever. It lowers stress hormones and stimulates the production of endorphins, which improve mood and promote relaxation. By reducing stress, exercise indirectly supports immune function.

3. Inflammation Reduction: Regular exercise has been shown to reduce chronic inflammation, which is linked to various diseases and weakened immune function. By keeping inflammation in check, physical activity supports a healthier immune system.

4. Improved Sleep Quality: Exercise can help regulate sleep patterns and improve sleep quality. As adequate sleep is vital for immune health, regular physical activity supports the body's ability to fight off infections.

5. Weight Management: Maintaining a healthy weight through exercise is crucial for immune health. Obesity is associated with impaired immune function and increased susceptibility to infections. Regular physical activity helps manage weight, reducing the risk of obesity-related immune dysfunction.

6. Lymphatic System Support: The lymphatic system, a key component of the immune system, relies on physical movement to circulate lymph fluid throughout the body. Regular exercise helps keep the lymphatic system functioning optimally, enhancing the body's ability to remove toxins and fight infections.

Chapter 7: Hygiene and Immunity

7.1 Proper Hygiene Practices for Boosting Immunity

Maintaining proper hygiene is fundamental for boosting immunity and preventing infections. Effective hygiene practices help minimize exposure to pathogens and support overall health.

1. Hand Washing: Regular and thorough hand washing with soap and water is one of the most effective ways to prevent the spread of infections. Hands should be washed for at least 20 seconds, especially before eating, after using the restroom, and after coming into contact with potentially contaminated surfaces.

2. Hand Sanitizers: When soap and water are not available, hand sanitizers with at least 60% alcohol can be used as an alternative. These sanitizers are effective at reducing the number of germs on the hands but should not replace hand washing whenever possible.

3. Oral Hygiene: Good oral hygiene, including brushing teeth twice a day and flossing daily, helps prevent oral infections that can affect overall health. Regular dental check-ups are also essential for maintaining oral health and preventing systemic infections.

4. Personal Cleanliness: Regular bathing and showering help remove dirt, sweat, and pathogens from the skin. Keeping the skin clean reduces the risk of infections and supports the immune system's ability to function effectively.

5. Food Safety: Proper handling, cooking, and storage of food are crucial for preventing foodborne illnesses. This includes washing fruits and vegetables, cooking meats to the appropriate temperature, and storing food at safe temperatures.

6. Clean Living Environment: Regular cleaning and disinfecting of living spaces reduce the presence of pathogens. High-touch surfaces such as doorknobs, light switches, and countertops should be cleaned frequently to minimize the risk of infection.

7. Respiratory Hygiene: Covering the mouth and nose with a tissue or elbow when coughing or sneezing helps prevent the spread of respiratory infections. Proper disposal of tissues and regular hand washing after coughing or sneezing are also important.

8. Vaccinations: Staying up-to-date with recommended vaccinations helps protect against various infectious diseases. Vaccinations boost the immune system by providing it with the tools to recognize and fight specific pathogens.

7.2 Natural Cleaning Products and Their Benefits

Using natural cleaning products offers numerous benefits for health and the environment, contributing to a healthier immune system.

Reduced Chemical Exposure: Conventional cleaning products often contain harsh chemicals that can irritate the skin, eyes, and respiratory system. Natural cleaning products, made from ingredients like vinegar, baking soda, and essential oils, reduce exposure to these harmful chemicals.

Environmental Sustainability: Natural cleaning products are typically biodegradable and free from synthetic fragrances and dyes, making them less harmful to the environment. They reduce pollution and the accumulation of toxic substances in water sources.

Antimicrobial Properties: Many natural ingredients, such as tea tree oil, lemon, and vinegar, have natural antimicrobial properties. They effectively clean surfaces and reduce the presence of pathogens without the need for harsh chemicals.

Safer for Children and Pets: Natural cleaning products are safer for households with children and pets, who are more susceptible to the harmful effects of chemical cleaners. Using natural products helps create a safer living environment for the whole family.

Improved Indoor Air Quality: Natural cleaning products do not release volatile organic compounds (VOCs) that can contribute to indoor air pollution. Improved air quality supports respiratory health and overall immune function.

7.3 Environmental Factors Affecting Immune Health

The environment plays a significant role in influencing immune health. Various environmental factors can either support or weaken the immune system.

1. Air Quality: Poor air quality, caused by pollution, smoke, and allergens, can impair respiratory health and weaken the immune system. Clean air is essential for maintaining strong immune function. Using air purifiers and ensuring proper ventilation can help improve indoor air quality.

2. Water Quality: Access to clean and safe drinking water is crucial for health. Contaminated water can carry pathogens and toxins that compromise immune function. Using water filters and ensuring a clean water supply support overall health.

3. Toxin Exposure: Environmental toxins, such as pesticides, heavy metals, and industrial chemicals, can weaken the immune system. Minimizing exposure to these toxins by choosing organic produce, avoiding plastic containers, and using natural personal care products can support immune health.

4. Sunlight Exposure: Adequate sunlight exposure is essential for the production of vitamin D, a critical nutrient for immune function. Spending time outdoors and ensuring safe sun exposure can help maintain healthy vitamin D levels.

5. Green Spaces: Access to green spaces and nature can reduce stress and support mental health, which in turn positively impacts immune function. Regularly spending time in natural environments can enhance overall well-being.

6. Noise Pollution: Chronic exposure to loud noise can increase stress levels and negatively affect immune health. Reducing noise pollution and creating a quieter living environment can help support immune function.

7. Climate and Weather: Extreme weather conditions, such as very cold or hot temperatures, can stress the body and affect immune function. Maintaining a comfortable indoor climate and protecting the body from harsh weather can help support the immune system.

Chapter 8: Mind-Body Techniques for Immune Support

8.1 Meditation and Its Effect on Immune Function

Meditation, an ancient practice rooted in mindfulness and focused awareness, has been extensively studied for its numerous health benefits, including its profound impact on immune function. Engaging in regular meditation can enhance immune system performance, reduce stress-induced immune suppression, and contribute to overall well-being.

8.1.1 Reducing Stress and Immune Suppression

Chronic stress is one of the most significant factors that negatively impact immune function. When the body is under constant stress, it releases stress hormones such as cortisol and adrenaline, which can suppress the immune response and increase susceptibility to infections and illnesses. Meditation helps mitigate these effects by activating the body's relaxation response, thereby reducing the production of stress hormones.

Numerous studies have shown that meditation can lower cortisol levels, thereby enhancing immune function. For instance, a study published in the journal *Psychosomatic Medicine* found that participants who practiced mindfulness meditation experienced a significant decrease in cortisol levels compared to those who did not meditate. Lower cortisol levels correlate with a stronger and more responsive immune system.

8.1.2 Enhancing Immune Cell Activity

Meditation has been linked to improved activity of various immune cells, including natural killer (NK) cells, T-cells, and B-cells. These cells play critical roles in identifying and combating pathogens, as well as in maintaining overall immune health. A study conducted by researchers at the University of California, Los Angeles (UCLA) found that participants who engaged in an eight-week mindfulness meditation program showed increased activity of NK cells, which are essential for early defense against viruses and cancerous cells.

Similarly, another study published in the journal *Brain, Behavior, and Immunity* demonstrated that meditation could enhance the immune response by increasing the production of antibodies. Participants who practiced mindfulness meditation had higher levels of antibodies in response to the influenza vaccine compared to those in the control group, indicating a more robust immune response.

8.1.3 Reducing Inflammation

Chronic inflammation is associated with various health issues, including autoimmune diseases, cardiovascular conditions, and chronic infections. Meditation has been shown to reduce markers of inflammation in the body, thus supporting immune health. Research published in the journal *Annals of the New York Academy of Sciences* indicated that mindfulness meditation could lower levels of pro-inflammatory cytokines, which are signaling molecules that promote inflammation.

By reducing inflammation, meditation helps maintain a balanced immune system, preventing it from becoming overactive and attacking healthy tissues. This balance is crucial for individuals with autoimmune conditions, where the immune system mistakenly targets the body's own cells.

8.1.4 Improving Psychological Well-being

Mental health and immune function are closely intertwined. Depression, anxiety, and other psychological conditions can weaken the immune system, making the body more vulnerable to illness. Meditation promotes mental well-being by reducing symptoms of anxiety and depression, enhancing mood, and improving overall emotional resilience.

A study published in the *Journal of Consulting and Clinical Psychology* found that mindfulness-based stress reduction (MBSR) programs significantly reduced symptoms of anxiety and depression in participants, contributing to improved immune function. Better mental health supports a more robust immune response, enabling the body to fight off infections more effectively.

8.1.5 Enhancing Sleep Quality

Quality sleep is vital for maintaining optimal immune function. Meditation has been shown to improve sleep patterns, leading to better rest and recovery. By promoting relaxation and reducing stress, meditation helps individuals achieve deeper, more restorative sleep, which is essential for a healthy immune system.

A study published in *JAMA Internal Medicine* revealed that participants who practiced mindfulness meditation experienced significant improvements in sleep quality and reduced symptoms of insomnia. Improved sleep supports the immune system by allowing the body to repair and regenerate, enhancing overall health.

In conclusion, meditation offers a holistic approach to enhancing immune function. By reducing stress, enhancing immune cell activity, lowering inflammation, improving psychological well-being, and promoting better sleep, meditation strengthens the body's natural defenses, contributing to improved health and resilience against illnesses. Integrating regular meditation practice into daily routines can be a powerful tool for supporting long-term immune health.

8.2 Yoga and Tai Chi for Strengthening Immunity

Yoga and Tai Chi, two ancient practices with roots in Eastern traditions, offer a wealth of benefits for physical, mental, and emotional well-being. Among these benefits, their ability to bolster the immune system is particularly noteworthy. These practices combine movement, breath control, and meditation to create a holistic approach to health that enhances immune function in multiple ways.

Stress Reduction and Immune Enhancement

One of the primary ways Yoga and Tai Chi strengthen the immune system is by reducing stress. Chronic stress is known to suppress immune function, making the body more susceptible to infections and diseases. Both Yoga and Tai Chi incorporate mindfulness and deep breathing techniques that help lower stress levels.

Studies have shown that these practices can reduce the production of cortisol, a stress hormone that can inhibit immune response when present in high levels. For example, research published in *Psychoneuroendocrinology* found that participants who engaged in regular Yoga practice had significantly lower cortisol levels and improved immune function compared to those who did not practice Yoga.

Physical Movement and Circulation

Both Yoga and Tai Chi involve a series of movements and postures that enhance circulation and lymphatic drainage. The lymphatic system is a crucial component of the immune system, responsible for transporting white blood cells and removing toxins from the body. The gentle, flowing movements of Tai Chi, combined with the stretching and strengthening poses of Yoga, promote efficient circulation of blood and lymph, which helps in the optimal functioning of immune cells.

Breath Control and Respiratory Health

Pranayama, or breath control, is an integral part of Yoga, while Tai Chi emphasizes coordinated breathing with movement. Deep, mindful breathing improves respiratory efficiency and increases oxygenation of the blood, which is essential for maintaining healthy immune function. Enhanced oxygen levels support the production and activity of immune cells, enabling the body to respond more effectively to pathogens.

A study published in the *International Journal of Yoga* found that regular practice of pranayama techniques significantly improved lung function and respiratory efficiency, which are critical for immune health. Better respiratory health means a stronger first line of defense against respiratory infections.

Mind-Body Connection and Mental Health

The mind-body connection is a fundamental aspect of both Yoga and Tai Chi. These practices enhance mental clarity, reduce anxiety, and improve overall mood. Mental health plays a significant role in immune function, as psychological stress and negative emotions can weaken the immune system. By fostering a positive mental state, Yoga and Tai Chi contribute to a more resilient immune system.

A study in *Behavioral Medicine* demonstrated that Tai Chi practice reduced symptoms of depression and anxiety, leading to improved immune markers. Similarly, research in *The Journal of Alternative and Complementary Medicine* found that Yoga practitioners showed significant reductions in anxiety and depression, which correlated with better immune responses.

Anti-Inflammatory Effects

Chronic inflammation is a common underlying factor in many diseases and can compromise immune function. Both Yoga and Tai Chi have been shown to reduce markers of inflammation in the body. For instance, Yoga practices such as gentle stretches, twists, and inversions help to stimulate the parasympathetic nervous system, promoting relaxation and reducing inflammatory responses.

Tai Chi, with its slow and controlled movements, also exerts anti-inflammatory effects. A study published in *The American Journal of Chinese Medicine* found that regular Tai Chi practice reduced levels of pro-inflammatory cytokines, which are signaling molecules that drive inflammation.

Enhanced Sleep Quality

Quality sleep is vital for a robust immune system, as it allows the body to repair and regenerate. Both Yoga and Tai Chi have been shown to improve sleep quality by promoting relaxation and reducing stress. Yoga nidra, a form of guided relaxation, and Tai Chi's meditative aspects help calm the mind and prepare the body for restful sleep.

Research in *Sleep Medicine Reviews* found that individuals practicing Yoga experienced significant improvements in sleep quality and duration. Tai Chi has similarly been shown to enhance sleep, with studies in *Sleep Medicine* reporting better sleep patterns and reduced symptoms of insomnia among practitioners.

Community and Social Support

Engaging in Yoga and Tai Chi often involves being part of a community, which provides social support and a sense of belonging. Social connections are important for mental health and can positively influence immune function. Group classes or even virtual sessions can foster a supportive environment, encouraging regular practice and overall well-being.

Yoga and Tai Chi offer comprehensive benefits for immune health by reducing stress, enhancing circulation, improving respiratory function, supporting mental health, reducing inflammation, and promoting better sleep. Integrating these practices into daily life can significantly bolster the immune system, contributing to greater overall health and resilience against illnesses.

8.3 Mindfulness Practices for Immune Health

Mindfulness practices, which emphasize being present in the moment and cultivating awareness, have gained significant attention for their health benefits. These practices, which include techniques such as meditation, deep breathing, and mindful movement, can play a crucial role in enhancing immune health. The connection between the mind and body is profound, and cultivating mindfulness can have far-reaching effects on the immune system.

Reducing Stress and Boosting Immunity

One of the primary ways mindfulness practices benefit the immune system is through stress reduction. Chronic stress can lead to elevated levels of cortisol, a hormone that suppresses immune function when persistently high. By practicing mindfulness, individuals can lower their stress levels and, consequently, reduce cortisol production. This creates a more balanced hormonal environment conducive to a robust immune response.

Research published in *Health Psychology* has shown that mindfulness meditation can significantly reduce stress and anxiety, leading to improved immune function. Participants who practiced mindfulness meditation showed a decrease in inflammatory markers and an increase in immune cell activity, indicating a strengthened immune system.

Enhancing Emotional Regulation

Emotional regulation is another area where mindfulness practices exert a positive impact on immune health. Negative emotions like anger, anxiety, and depression can weaken the immune system, making the body more susceptible to infections. Mindfulness helps individuals manage and process these emotions more effectively, reducing their detrimental impact on immune function.

A study in *Psychosomatic Medicine* found that individuals who engaged in mindfulness-based stress reduction (MBSR) programs exhibited lower levels of pro-inflammatory cytokines, which are proteins involved in the inflammatory response. This suggests that by improving emotional regulation, mindfulness can help maintain a balanced immune response.

Improving Sleep Quality

Quality sleep is essential for a healthy immune system, as it allows the body to repair and regenerate. Mindfulness practices, such as meditation and mindful breathing, have been shown to improve sleep quality by promoting relaxation and reducing stress. Better sleep supports the production and function of immune cells, enhancing the body's ability to fight off pathogens.

A study in the *Journal of the American Medical Association (JAMA) Internal Medicine* found that mindfulness meditation significantly improved sleep quality among older adults with moderate sleep disturbances. Improved sleep patterns were associated with better immune function, highlighting the importance of mindfulness in supporting restful sleep.

Promoting Healthy Lifestyle Choices

Mindfulness encourages a greater awareness of one's body and its needs, often leading to healthier lifestyle choices. This heightened awareness can result in better dietary habits, regular physical activity, and avoidance of harmful behaviors such as smoking and excessive alcohol consumption—all of which are critical for maintaining a strong immune system.

A study in *Appetite* found that mindfulness practices were associated with healthier eating behaviors, such as reduced binge eating and improved portion control. These healthier choices contribute to overall well-being and immune health, as proper nutrition and regular exercise are fundamental components of a robust immune system.

Enhancing Lymphatic Flow and Circulation

Mindfulness practices often include elements of gentle movement, such as mindful walking or yoga. These activities promote better circulation and lymphatic flow, which are crucial for immune function. The lymphatic system helps remove toxins and waste from the body, while proper circulation ensures that immune cells are efficiently transported to where they are needed.

Research in the *Journal of Physiological Anthropology* suggests that practices like yoga, which combine mindfulness with movement, can enhance lymphatic flow and improve overall circulation. This supports the immune system by facilitating the efficient removal of toxins and the delivery of immune cells throughout the body.

Building Resilience and Well-Being

Mindfulness practices also foster a sense of resilience and overall well-being. This psychological resilience can enhance immune function by providing a positive outlook and coping mechanisms in the face of stress and illness. A positive mental state is linked to better immune responses and a lower risk of chronic diseases.

A study in *Psychoneuroendocrinology* showed that individuals with higher levels of psychological resilience had stronger immune responses to vaccinations. This suggests that mindfulness practices, by building resilience, can enhance the body's ability to respond to immune challenges effectively.

Book 20: Mental and Emotional Health: The Barbara O'Neill Approach

Harmonizing Minds, Nurturing Hearts - Holistic Insights for Mental and Emotional Wellness

Chapter 1: Foundations of Mental and Emotional Wellbeing

1.1 Importance of Mental and Emotional Health

Mental and emotional health are integral to overall well-being, significantly impacting every aspect of our lives. Understanding and prioritizing mental and emotional health is not just essential, it's empowering. It affects our physical health, relationships, productivity, and quality of life. By grasping its importance, we can take control and achieve a balanced, fulfilling, and resilient life.

Physical Health and Well-being

Mental and emotional health are closely linked to physical health. Chronic stress, anxiety, and depression can lead to a variety of physical health issues. However, the good news is that good mental health promotes better physical health. It reduces stress levels, improves sleep quality, and enhances the body's ability to heal and recover. Regular mental health practices can significantly improve physical health outcomes, giving us hope and optimism for a healthier future.

Relationships and Social Connections

Our mental and emotional state dramatically influences how we interact with others. Positive mental health plays a crucial role in fostering healthy relationships. It enables effective communication, empathy, and emotional regulation. Individuals with good mental health are more likely to engage in supportive, fulfilling relationships, which provide emotional support and a sense of belonging. This understanding can make us feel more connected and understood in our relationships.

Productivity and Performance

Mental and emotional health is not just about personal well-being; it's also crucial for cognitive functions such as attention, memory, and decision-making. Good mental health can significantly enhance productivity and performance in both personal and professional settings. Individuals with positive mental health are better able to focus, solve problems, and manage time effectively. They are also more resilient to setbacks and challenges, maintaining motivation and perseverance. Conversely, mental health issues like anxiety, depression, and burnout can impair cognitive function, leading to decreased productivity, absenteeism, and lower overall performance. Investing in mental health can lead to improved job satisfaction, creativity, and career success.

Quality of Life and Fulfillment

Mental and emotional well-being are key determinants of overall quality of life. Good mental health allows individuals to experience joy, contentment, and fulfillment. It enables them to pursue their goals, hobbies, and passions with enthusiasm and purpose. Individuals with positive mental health are more likely to engage in healthy behaviors, such as regular exercise, balanced nutrition, and adequate sleep, further enhancing their quality of life. Poor mental health, on the other hand, can lead to a diminished sense of purpose, reduced interest in activities, and an overall lower quality of life. Prioritizing mental health is essential for achieving a balanced and fulfilling life.

<u>Resilience and Coping Skills</u>

Mental and emotional health are critical for building resilience and effective coping skills. Life is full of stressors, challenges, and uncertainties, and how we respond to these situations significantly impacts our well-being. Good mental health equips individuals with the tools to cope with stress, adapt to change, and recover from setbacks. Resilient individuals are better able to navigate life's ups and downs, maintaining a positive outlook and emotional stability. Developing coping skills through mental health practices, such as mindfulness, cognitive-behavioral techniques, and stress management, enhances resilience and overall mental well-being.

<u>Stigma and Access to Care</u>

Despite its importance, mental health is often stigmatized, leading to barriers in accessing care and support. Addressing the stigma surrounding mental health is crucial for encouraging individuals to seek help when needed. Promoting mental health awareness and education can help reduce stigma, fostering a more supportive and understanding environment. Access to mental health care, including therapy, counseling, and psychiatric services, is essential for addressing mental health issues and promoting emotional well-being. It is important to advocate for better access to mental health services and support systems to ensure that everyone has the opportunity to achieve optimal mental and emotional health.

Mental and emotional health are fundamental to overall well-being, influencing physical health, relationships, productivity, quality of life, and resilience. Prioritizing mental health through awareness, education, and access to care is essential for achieving a balanced and fulfilling life. By understanding the importance of mental and emotional health and taking proactive steps to maintain it, individuals can enhance their overall well-being, leading to a healthier, happier, and more resilient life.

1.2 Holistic Approach to Mental Wellness

A holistic approach to mental wellness considers the whole person—mind, body, and spirit—rather than focusing solely on the symptoms of mental health conditions. This comprehensive method emphasizes the interconnectedness of physical health, emotional well-being, and spiritual fulfillment, aiming to create a balanced and harmonious life. By integrating various therapies, lifestyle changes, and self-care practices, a holistic approach can significantly enhance mental wellness and overall quality of life.

<u>Understanding Holistic Mental Wellness</u>

The holistic approach to mental wellness is rooted in the belief that mental health cannot be isolated from other aspects of a person's life. It recognizes that physical ailments, emotional distress, and spiritual disconnect can all contribute to mental health issues. Therefore, treatment plans often include a combination of medical care, psychological support, lifestyle modifications, and alternative therapies. This multi-faceted approach aims to address the underlying causes of mental health conditions and promote long-term well-being.

<u>Physical Health and Mental Wellness</u>

Physical health is a fundamental component of mental wellness. The mind and body are intricately connected, and physical ailments can exacerbate mental health issues. A holistic approach emphasizes maintaining a healthy lifestyle through regular exercise, balanced nutrition, and adequate sleep. Exercise, for instance, has been shown to reduce symptoms of depression and anxiety by releasing endorphins and improving brain function. Nutrition also plays a critical role, as deficiencies in certain nutrients can lead to mood disturbances and cognitive impairments. Ensuring a diet rich in vitamins, minerals, and omega-3 fatty acids can support brain health and emotional stability.

Emotional Well-being and Self-care

Emotional well-being is central to holistic mental wellness. This involves recognizing and understanding one's emotions, developing healthy coping mechanisms, and fostering positive relationships. Mindfulness, meditation, and journaling can help individuals process their feelings and reduce stress. Mindfulness, in particular, encourages a present-focused awareness that can alleviate anxiety and depression by breaking the cycle of negative thought patterns. Additionally, engaging in hobbies, spending time with loved ones, and practicing gratitude can enhance emotional resilience and happiness.

Spiritual Fulfillment

Spiritual fulfillment, whether through religious practices, connection with nature, or personal introspection, is another crucial aspect of holistic mental wellness. Spirituality can provide a sense of purpose, meaning, and connection that transcends everyday stressors. Yoga, meditation, and prayer can help individuals connect with their inner selves and cultivate peace and contentment. For many, spirituality also involves community, which can offer support and a sense of belonging.

Alternative and Complementary Therapies

Holistic mental wellness often includes alternative and complementary therapies alongside conventional treatments. These therapies can provide additional support and address specific aspects of mental health. Examples include acupuncture, aromatherapy, and herbal medicine. Acupuncture, for instance, has been found to reduce symptoms of anxiety and depression by balancing the body's energy flow. Using essential oils like lavender and chamomile, aromatherapy can promote relaxation and alleviate stress. Herbal remedies, such as St. John's Wort and valerian root, have been used to manage symptoms of depression and anxiety.

Integrative Mental Health Care

Integrative mental health care combines conventional medical treatments with holistic practices to create a comprehensive treatment plan. This approach often involves collaboration between healthcare providers, including doctors, therapists, nutritionists, and alternative medicine practitioners. By addressing all aspects of a person's health, integrative care can provide more effective and personalized treatment. For example, a person with depression might receive medication and therapy while also incorporating yoga, dietary changes, and acupuncture into their routine.

Lifestyle Modifications

Lifestyle modifications are a key element of the holistic approach to mental wellness. This can include stress management techniques, such as time management, relaxation exercises, and boundary setting. It also involves creating a supportive environment, both at home and at work, that promotes mental health. Reducing exposure to toxic relationships, environments, and substances can have a profound impact on mental well-being.

Preventative Measures

A holistic approach to mental wellness also emphasizes prevention. By adopting healthy habits and practices, individuals can reduce their risk of developing mental health issues. This includes regular physical activity, a nutritious diet, sufficient sleep, and stress management techniques. Building a strong support network and seeking help early when issues arise are also important preventative measures.

A holistic approach to mental wellness provides a comprehensive framework for achieving and maintaining mental health. By considering the interconnectedness of physical health, emotional well-being, and spiritual fulfillment, this approach addresses the root causes of mental health issues and promotes long-term wellness. Integrating conventional treatments with alternative therapies, lifestyle modifications, and self-care practices can lead to a balanced and harmonious life. Adopting a holistic approach empowers individuals to take control of their mental health and live more fulfilling, resilient lives.

1.3 Relationship Between Mind, Body, and Emotions

The relationship between mind, body, and emotions is a complex, interwoven network that profoundly influences overall health and well-being. Understanding this intricate connection is not just fundamental, but also empowering, to achieving holistic wellness. The mind, body, and emotions do not operate in isolation; they are in constant interaction, each affecting the others in myriad ways. Recognizing and nurturing this relationship can lead to a more balanced and healthier life, putting you in control of your well-being.

1.3.1 The Mind-Body Connection

The mind-body connection is the bidirectional relationship between our mental processes and physical states. This connection is evident in how psychological stress can manifest as physical symptoms and vice versa. For example, anxiety and chronic stress are known to contribute to various physical health issues such as hypertension, gastrointestinal problems, and weakened immune function. Conversely, physical illnesses or pain can lead to psychological distress, including anxiety and depression.

One of the key mechanisms behind the mind-body connection is the role of the nervous system, particularly the autonomic nervous system, which regulates involuntary bodily functions such as heart rate, digestion, and respiratory rate. When a person experiences stress, the sympathetic nervous system triggers the "fight or flight" response, releasing stress hormones like cortisol and adrenaline. These hormones prepare the body to face a threat, but prolonged activation can lead to health problems such as insomnia, cardiovascular disease, and metabolic disorders.

1.3.2 The Role of Emotions

Emotions play a critical role in the interplay between the mind and body. They are not just psychological experiences, but they also involve physiological changes. For instance, feelings of fear or anger can increase the heart rate, cause muscles to tense, and lead to rapid breathing. Conversely, positive emotions, such as joy and love, can have calming effects, promoting relaxation and reducing stress.

Emotions are also closely linked to the endocrine system, which secretes hormones that influence nearly every cell, organ, and function of our bodies. Emotional states can alter hormonal balance, affecting energy levels and immune function. For example, chronic stress and negative emotions can lead to elevated levels of cortisol, which, over time, can suppress the immune system, increase inflammation, and even affect brain function, contributing to mood disorders.

1.3.3 Psychoneuroimmunology

The field of psychoneuroimmunology (PNI) explores the connections between psychological processes, the nervous system, and the immune system. It provides scientific evidence of how stress and emotions influence immune function and overall health. Research in PNI has shown that chronic stress can weaken the immune system, making the body more susceptible to infections and diseases. Positive emotional states, on the other hand, can enhance immune function and promote faster recovery from illness.

1.3.4 The Impact of Thoughts

Thoughts, both conscious and unconscious, significantly impact the mind-body-emotion relationship. Negative thought patterns, such as rumination, pessimism, and self-criticism, can contribute to mental health issues like depression and anxiety. These thoughts can also manifest physically, leading to tension, fatigue, and other stress-related symptoms.

Conversely, positive thinking and mindfulness practices can have beneficial effects on both mental and physical health. Mindfulness, which involves staying present and fully engaging with the current moment, has been shown to reduce stress, enhance emotional regulation, and improve physical health outcomes. Meditation, deep breathing, and progressive muscle relaxation can help calm the mind, reduce stress hormones, and promote well-being.

1.3.5 Emotional Intelligence

Emotional intelligence (EI) is recognizing, understanding, managing, and utilizing emotions effectively. High EI is not just associated with better mental health, healthier relationships, and improved physical health, but it is also a key to promoting holistic wellness. Individuals with high EI are better able to cope with stress, communicate effectively, and maintain emotional balance. Developing EI involves self-awareness, self-regulation, motivation, empathy, and social skills, all contributing to a healthier mind-body-emotion relationship and a more balanced life.

1.3.6 Holistic Approaches to Wellness

A holistic approach to wellness acknowledges the interdependence of mind, body, and emotions. This approach includes various practices and therapies designed to enhance the health of all three components. For instance, integrative medicine combines conventional medical treatments with complementary therapies such as acupuncture, yoga, and massage therapy. These practices address physical symptoms and promote mental and emotional well-being.

Regular physical activity is another essential component of holistic wellness. Exercise not only strengthens the body but also profoundly affects the mind and emotions. It releases endorphins, the body's natural painkillers and mood elevators, which can reduce stress, improve mood, and enhance overall mental health.

Nutrition also plays a crucial role. A balanced diet rich in nutrients supports brain function and emotional health. Certain foods, like those high in omega-3 fatty acids, antioxidants, and vitamins, can help reduce inflammation and support cognitive function, enhancing emotional well-being.

1.3.7 Practical Strategies

Implementing practical strategies to nurture the mind-body-emotion relationship can significantly improve overall health. Some strategies include:

1. Mindfulness Practices: Engage in daily mindfulness exercises such as meditation, deep breathing, or yoga to reduce stress and enhance emotional regulation.

2. Regular Physical Activity: Incorporate regular exercise into your routine to boost mood, reduce stress, and improve physical health.

3. Healthy Nutrition: Follow a balanced diet rich in whole foods, healthy fats, lean proteins, and plenty of fruits and vegetables to support brain and body health.

4. Emotional Intelligence Development: Work on improving your emotional intelligence through self-reflection, empathy-building exercises, and effective communication practices.

5. Stress Management Techniques: Practice stress management techniques such as time management, relaxation exercises, and setting healthy boundaries to maintain emotional balance and physical health.

Chapter 2: Nutrition and Mental Health

2.1 Nutritional Factors Affecting Mental Wellbeing

Nutrition plays a pivotal role in mental wellbeing, influencing cognitive function, mood, and overall mental health. The foods we consume provide the necessary nutrients that support brain function and emotional stability. Poor dietary choices can contribute to mental health issues, while a balanced diet rich in essential nutrients can enhance mental wellbeing. Understanding the nutritional factors affecting mental health is crucial for adopting dietary habits that promote psychological resilience and emotional balance.

The Brain-Gut Connection

The brain-gut connection underscores the significant impact of nutrition on mental wellbeing. The gut and brain communicate through the gut-brain axis, involving biochemical signaling between the gastrointestinal tract and the central nervous system. The gut microbiota, consisting of trillions of microorganisms, plays a vital role in this communication. A healthy gut microbiome supports the production of neurotransmitters such as serotonin, which regulates mood, anxiety, and happiness.

Dietary choices can influence the composition of the gut microbiome. Diets high in processed foods, sugar, and unhealthy fats can disrupt the balance of gut bacteria, leading to inflammation and negatively impacting mental health. Conversely, a diet rich in fiber, fruits, vegetables, and fermented foods promotes a healthy gut microbiome, enhancing mental wellbeing.

Essential Nutrients for Mental Health

Certain nutrients are particularly important for maintaining mental health. These include omega-3 fatty acids, vitamins, minerals, and amino acids.

1. Omega-3 Fatty Acids: Found in fatty fish, flaxseeds, chia seeds, and walnuts, omega-3 fatty acids are essential for brain health. They have anti-inflammatory properties and play a role in neurotransmitter function. Studies have shown that omega-3 supplementation can reduce symptoms of depression and anxiety.

2. B Vitamins: B vitamins, including B6, B12, and folate, are crucial for brain function and the synthesis of neurotransmitters. Deficiencies in these vitamins are linked to depression, fatigue, and cognitive decline. Leafy greens, legumes, nuts, and seeds are excellent sources of B vitamins.

3. Vitamin D: Known as the "sunshine vitamin," vitamin D is synthesized in the skin in response to sunlight. It is also found in fatty fish, fortified foods, and supplements. Low levels of vitamin D are associated with an increased risk of depression and mood disorders.

4. Magnesium: Magnesium is involved in over 300 biochemical reactions in the body, including those related to brain function. It helps regulate neurotransmitters and has a calming effect on the nervous system. Foods rich in magnesium include dark chocolate, avocados, nuts, and leafy greens.

5. Amino Acids: Amino acids, the building blocks of protein, are necessary for the production of neurotransmitters. Tryptophan, found in turkey, chicken, and eggs, is a precursor to serotonin. Tyrosine, found in dairy products, meat, and fish, is a precursor to dopamine. Adequate protein intake ensures the availability of these amino acids for neurotransmitter synthesis.

Impact of Processed Foods and Sugar

Processed foods and high sugar intake are detrimental to mental health. Diets high in refined sugars and unhealthy fats can lead to inflammation and oxidative stress, which are linked to mental health disorders. Sugar consumption can cause spikes and crashes in blood glucose levels, leading to mood swings, irritability, and fatigue.

Moreover, processed foods often lack essential nutrients and contain additives and preservatives that can negatively affect brain function. Studies have shown a correlation between the consumption of processed foods and an increased risk of depression and anxiety.

Hydration and Mental Health

Adequate hydration is essential for optimal brain function. Even mild dehydration can impair cognitive function, concentration, and mood. Water is vital for the delivery of nutrients to the brain and the removal of toxins. Drinking sufficient water throughout the day and consuming hydrating foods like fruits and vegetables supports mental clarity and emotional stability.

Balancing Blood Sugar Levels

Maintaining stable blood sugar levels is crucial for mental wellbeing. Fluctuations in blood glucose can affect energy levels, mood, and cognitive function. A diet that includes complex carbohydrates, protein, and healthy fats helps stabilize blood sugar levels. Whole grains, legumes, nuts, seeds, and lean proteins provide sustained energy and prevent mood swings.

Role of Antioxidants

Antioxidants protect the brain from oxidative stress and inflammation, both of which are linked to mental health disorders. Foods rich in antioxidants, such as berries, nuts, dark chocolate, and colorful vegetables, support brain health by reducing oxidative damage and promoting the production of neurotransmitters.

Probiotics and Fermented Foods

Probiotics, found in fermented foods like yogurt, kefir, sauerkraut, and kimchi, can positively influence mental health by improving gut health. Probiotics help maintain a healthy balance of gut bacteria, which is crucial for the production of neurotransmitters and the regulation of the immune response. A healthy gut microbiome is associated with reduced symptoms of anxiety and depression.

2.2 Supplements for Cognitive Function and Emotional Balance

Supplements can play a vital role in supporting cognitive function and emotional balance, particularly when dietary intake alone may not provide all the necessary nutrients. These supplements can help enhance brain health, improve mood, reduce stress, and support overall mental wellbeing. Understanding which supplements are beneficial and how they work can help individuals make informed decisions about their mental health regimen.

2.2.1 Omega-3 Fatty Acids

Omega-3 fatty acids, particularly eicosapentaenoic acid (EPA) and docosahexaenoic acid (DHA), are crucial for brain health. These essential fats, found in fish oil supplements, play a significant role in maintaining the structure and function of brain cells. They have anti-inflammatory properties that protect the brain from damage and support the production of neurotransmitters, which are critical for mood regulation. Studies have shown that omega-3 supplementation can help alleviate symptoms of depression and anxiety, improve memory, and enhance overall cognitive function.

2.2.2 B Vitamins

B vitamins, including B6, B12, and folate, are essential for brain health and emotional stability. They are involved in the production of neurotransmitters such as serotonin, dopamine, and norepinephrine, which regulate mood and cognitive function. Deficiencies in B vitamins are linked to mood disorders, cognitive decline, and mental fatigue. Supplementing with B-complex vitamins can support brain function, enhance energy levels, and improve emotional balance.

2.2.3 Vitamin D

Vitamin D, known as the "sunshine vitamin," is vital for brain health and mood regulation. It helps regulate the production of serotonin, a neurotransmitter that influences mood, sleep, and anxiety levels. Low levels of vitamin D are associated with an increased risk of depression and cognitive decline. Vitamin D supplements, especially in individuals with limited sun exposure or low dietary intake, can help improve mood and cognitive function.

2.2.4 Magnesium

Magnesium is a critical mineral for brain health and emotional balance. It plays a role in over 300 biochemical reactions in the body, including those involved in brain function and the regulation of neurotransmitters. Magnesium has a calming effect on the nervous system and can help reduce symptoms of anxiety and depression. Supplementing with magnesium can support relaxation, improve sleep quality, and enhance overall mental wellbeing.

2.2.5 Ginkgo Biloba

Ginkgo biloba is a herbal supplement known for its cognitive-enhancing properties. It improves blood flow to the brain, which supports cognitive function and memory. Ginkgo biloba also has antioxidant properties that protect the brain from oxidative stress and inflammation. Studies suggest that ginkgo biloba can improve cognitive performance, particularly in individuals with age-related cognitive decline, and may also help reduce symptoms of anxiety.

2.2.6 Rhodiola Rosea

Rhodiola rosea is an adaptogenic herb that helps the body cope with stress and improves mental resilience. It supports the production of neurotransmitters involved in mood regulation and cognitive function. Rhodiola rosea has been shown to reduce symptoms of fatigue, anxiety, and depression, and to enhance cognitive performance, particularly under stressful conditions. Supplementing with rhodiola rosea can help improve emotional balance and mental clarity.

2.2.7 L-Theanine

L-theanine is an amino acid found in tea leaves, particularly green tea. It promotes relaxation without causing drowsiness and can help reduce stress and anxiety. L-theanine enhances alpha brain wave activity, which is associated with a relaxed but alert mental state. It also supports the production of neurotransmitters such as serotonin and dopamine. Supplementing with L-theanine can improve focus, reduce stress, and enhance emotional balance.

2.2.8 Probiotics

Probiotics, beneficial bacteria found in the gut, play a significant role in brain health and emotional wellbeing. The gut-brain axis involves communication between the gut microbiota and the brain. A healthy gut microbiome supports the production of neurotransmitters and helps regulate the immune response, which can influence mood and cognitive function. Probiotic supplements can help maintain a healthy balance of gut bacteria, reduce symptoms of anxiety and depression, and support overall mental health.

Chapter 3: Herbal Remedies for Emotional Support

3.1 Herbs Known for Their Calming and Mood-Stabilizing Effects

Herbs have been used for centuries to promote mental and emotional well-being. Certain herbs are particularly renowned for their calming and mood-stabilizing effects. These herbs can help alleviate symptoms of anxiety, stress, and depression and support overall mental health. Here are some of the most effective herbs known for their calming and mood-stabilizing properties:

1. Ashwagandha

Ashwagandha (Withania somnifera) is an adaptogenic herb widely used in Ayurvedic medicine to combat stress and promote relaxation. It helps the body adapt to stress by regulating cortisol levels, which are often elevated during periods of stress. Ashwagandha also supports the nervous system, improves sleep quality, and enhances overall mood. Research indicates that ashwagandha can significantly reduce symptoms of anxiety and depression, making it a valuable herb for emotional balance.

2. Lavender

Lavender (Lavandula angustifolia) is well-known for its calming aroma and has been used for centuries to promote relaxation and reduce anxiety. Lavender essential oil can be inhaled or applied topically to induce a state of calm and improve sleep quality. Studies have shown that lavender can reduce symptoms of anxiety, depression, and insomnia. Its soothing properties make it popular for those seeking natural ways to enhance mood and relaxation.

3. Valerian Root

Valerian root (Valeriana officinalis) is commonly used to alleviate insomnia and anxiety. It works by increasing gamma-aminobutyric acid (GABA) levels in the brain, a neurotransmitter that promotes relaxation and reduces stress. Valerian root is often used as a natural remedy for sleep disorders and can help improve sleep quality without causing morning grogginess. Its calming effects extend to reducing anxiety and promoting a sense of tranquility.

4. Chamomile

Chamomile (Matricaria chamomilla) is a gentle herb known for its soothing properties. Chamomile tea is a popular bedtime beverage due to its mild sedative effects. It helps relax the nervous system, ease tension, and promote restful sleep. Chamomile has been shown to reduce symptoms of generalized anxiety disorder and depression. Its anti-inflammatory and antioxidant properties also contribute to its mood-stabilizing effects.

5. Passionflower

Passionflower (Passiflora incarnata) is traditionally used to treat anxiety and insomnia. It works by increasing GABA levels in the brain, promoting relaxation, and reducing nervous activity. Passionflower is effective in reducing symptoms of anxiety and can help improve sleep quality. Its calming effects make it a valuable herb for managing stress and enhancing emotional well-being.

6. St. John's Wort

St. John's Wort (Hypericum perforatum) is widely recognized for its antidepressant properties. It works by increasing serotonin, dopamine, and norepinephrine levels in the brain, which are neurotransmitters associated with mood regulation. St. John's Wort is commonly used to treat mild to moderate depression and anxiety. However, it can interact with various medications, so it should be used under the guidance of a healthcare professional.

7. Lemon Balm

Lemon balm (Melissa officinalis) is a calming herb that helps reduce stress and anxiety. It has mild sedative properties and is often used to promote relaxation and improve sleep. Lemon balm is effective in reducing symptoms of anxiety and enhancing mood. It can be consumed as a tea or a supplement to support emotional balance and mental clarity.

8. Rhodiola Rosea

Rhodiola rosea is an adaptogenic herb that helps the body cope with stress and fatigue. It supports the production of neurotransmitters that regulate mood and cognitive function. Rhodiola rosea has been shown to reduce symptoms of anxiety, depression, and mental fatigue. Its mood-stabilizing effects make it a valuable herb for enhancing mental resilience and emotional stability.

9. Holy Basil

Holy basil (Ocimum sanctum), or Tulsi, is an adaptogenic herb used in Ayurvedic medicine to reduce stress and promote mental clarity. It helps balance cortisol levels, support the nervous system, and enhance overall mood. Holy basil is effective in reducing symptoms of anxiety and depression, making it a powerful herb for emotional well-being.

10. Kava Kava

Kava kava (Piper methysticum) is a herb traditionally used in the South Pacific to promote relaxation and social harmony. It has anxiolytic properties that help reduce anxiety and induce a state of calm. Kava kava is effective in managing anxiety disorders and promoting relaxation without impairing cognitive function. However, it should be used with caution, as excessive use can affect liver health.

3.2 How to Use Herbal Remedies Safely for Emotional Health

Herbal remedies have been used for centuries to support emotional health, offering natural solutions for managing stress, anxiety, depression, and other mood disorders. While these remedies can be highly effective, it is crucial to use them safely to avoid potential side effects and interactions with other medications. Here are key considerations for safely using herbal remedies to support emotional health.

1. Understanding Herb Properties and Dosages

Different herbs have varying effects on the body and mind, so it is essential to understand the specific properties and appropriate dosages of each herb you intend to use. For instance, St. John's Wort is known for its antidepressant effects but can interact with many prescription medications, including antidepressants, birth control pills, and blood thinners. Valerian root is effective for anxiety and insomnia but can cause drowsiness and should not be used in combination with alcohol or sedatives.

Dosage Guidelines:

- St. John's Wort: Typically, 300 mg taken three times daily.

- Valerian Root: 400-900 mg taken 30 minutes to two hours before bedtime.

- Ashwagandha: 300-500 mg taken once or twice daily.

Always start with the lowest effective dose and gradually increase as needed, monitoring for any adverse effects.

2. Consulting Healthcare Professionals

Before starting any herbal regimen, especially if you have pre-existing conditions or are taking other medications, consult with a healthcare professional. This consultation helps prevent potential interactions and ensures the herbs you choose are appropriate for your specific health needs. A healthcare provider can also guide you on the proper dosages and duration of use.

3. Choosing Quality Products

The efficacy and safety of herbal remedies largely depend on the quality of the products. Select products from reputable brands that provide clear information on sourcing, processing, and standardization of active ingredients. Look for third-party testing and certifications to ensure purity and potency. Avoid products with additives, fillers, or artificial ingredients.

4. Monitoring for Side Effects

Even natural remedies can cause side effects, especially when used improperly or in high doses. Common side effects may include digestive issues, headaches, dizziness, and allergic reactions. If you experience any adverse effects, discontinue use immediately and consult a healthcare provider. Keep a journal to track your response to the herbs, noting any changes in symptoms or side effects.

5. Considering Long-Term Use and Cycling

While some herbs can be used long-term, others may be more appropriate for short-term use. For instance, adaptogens like ashwagandha and rhodiola are generally safe for extended use, but herbs like kava kava and valerian root should be cycled to prevent tolerance and dependency. A typical cycle might involve using the herb for six weeks followed by a two-week break.

6. Combining Herbs and Other Therapies

Herbal remedies can be used in conjunction with other natural therapies to enhance their effects. For example, combining herbal treatments with practices like meditation, yoga, and mindfulness can provide a more comprehensive approach to managing emotional health. However, be cautious when combining multiple herbs or therapies, as this can increase the risk of interactions and side effects.

7. Personalized Approaches

Each individual's response to herbal remedies can vary based on factors such as genetics, overall health, and the specific nature of their emotional health issues. Personalize your approach by starting with one herb at a time, allowing you to accurately assess its effects. Adjust dosages and combinations based on your body's response and consult with a healthcare provider for personalized recommendations.

8. Legal and Ethical Considerations

Be aware of the legal status of certain herbs in your region, as some herbs may be restricted or regulated. Additionally, consider the ethical sourcing of herbs, ensuring they are harvested sustainably and ethically to protect the environment and support fair trade practices.

3.3 Blending Essential Oils for Emotional Balance

Essential oils have long been revered for their therapeutic properties, particularly in promoting relaxation, relieving anxiety, and enhancing mood. These potent plant extracts can be a powerful tool in supporting mental and emotional well-being when used correctly. Here, we explore some of the most effective essential oils for these purposes and provide guidelines for their safe and effective use.

3.3.1 Lavender Essential Oil

Lavender is one of the most popular and versatile essential oils, widely known for its calming and soothing properties. It is particularly effective in reducing anxiety, promoting relaxation, and improving sleep quality. Studies have shown that inhaling lavender oil can reduce stress and anxiety levels, making it an excellent choice for those experiencing heightened emotional tension.

Usage:

- Diffusion: Add a few drops of lavender oil to a diffuser to fill your space with its calming aroma.

- Topical Application: Dilute with a carrier oil (such as jojoba or almond oil) and apply to the wrists, temples, or the soles of the feet.

3.3.2 Bergamot Essential Oil

Bergamot oil is known for its uplifting and mood-enhancing effects. It has a unique citrusy aroma that can help reduce feelings of anxiety and depression. Bergamot has been shown to lower cortisol levels, which are often elevated during stress, making it a valuable oil for emotional balance.

Usage:

- Inhalation: Add a few drops to a cotton ball or handkerchief and inhale deeply.

- Bath: Add 5-10 drops to a warm bath for a relaxing soak.

3.3.3 Ylang Ylang Essential Oil

Ylang ylang oil is often used to promote relaxation and reduce stress and anxiety. Its sweet, floral scent can create a sense of calm and well-being. This oil also has sedative properties that can help in reducing symptoms of depression.

Usage:

- Massage: Mix with a carrier oil and use in a calming massage.

- Diffusion: Use in an essential oil diffuser to create a tranquil environment.

3.3.4 Chamomile Essential Oil

Chamomile oil, particularly Roman chamomile, is renowned for its soothing effects. It can help alleviate anxiety and promote a sense of peace. Its gentle and calming aroma makes it an excellent choice for reducing stress and supporting relaxation.

Usage:

- Topical Application: Dilute with a carrier oil and apply to the skin, focusing on areas such as the neck and shoulders.

- Inhalation: Add a few drops to a bowl of hot water and inhale the steam.

3.3.5 Frankincense Essential Oil

Frankincense oil has a grounding and calming effect, making it ideal for reducing stress and promoting emotional balance. It has been used for centuries in meditation practices due to its ability to enhance mental clarity and focus.

Usage:

- Meditation: Diffuse during meditation sessions to deepen relaxation.

- Topical Application: Dilute and apply to pulse points for a grounding effect.

3.3.6 Clary Sage Essential Oil

Clary sage oil is known for its ability to reduce anxiety and promote a sense of well-being. It has a warm, herbal scent that can help calm the mind and improve mood.

Usage:

- Inhalation: Add to a diffuser or inhale directly from the bottle.

- Massage: Combine with a carrier oil and use in a relaxing massage.

While essential oils can offer significant benefits, it is important to use them safely to avoid potential side effects. Always dilute essential oils with a carrier oil before applying them to the skin to prevent irritation. Conduct a patch test before using a new oil to check for any allergic reactions. Use essential oils in moderation, as excessive use can lead to sensitization or adverse reactions. Pregnant women, children, and individuals with certain medical conditions should consult a healthcare professional before using essential oils.

Chapter 5: Mind-Body Techniques for Stress Reduction

5.1 Meditation and Its Benefits for Mental Health

Meditation is a practice that holds profound benefits for mental health, offering a pathway to inner peace, emotional resilience, and overall well-being. Rooted in ancient traditions across various cultures, meditation has evolved into diverse forms, each emphasizing mindfulness, concentration, or contemplation. One of the primary benefits of meditation lies in its ability to reduce stress and anxiety levels. By engaging in meditation, individuals can cultivate a state of deep relaxation, which counters the body's stress response by lowering cortisol levels and promoting a sense of calm.

Beyond stress reduction, meditation serves as a powerful tool for enhancing emotional regulation. Through regular practice, individuals develop heightened self-awareness, enabling them to observe their thoughts and emotions without judgment. This awareness fosters greater emotional resilience, allowing individuals to respond to challenging situations with clarity and composure rather than react impulsively. As a result, meditation can significantly improve one's ability to manage and mitigate symptoms of anxiety, depression, and other mood disorders.

Moreover, meditation has been shown to enhance cognitive function and promote mental clarity. By quieting the mind and improving concentration, meditation supports cognitive processes such as decision-making, problem-solving, and memory retention. Studies have demonstrated that regular meditation practice can lead to structural changes in the brain, including increased gray matter density in regions associated with learning and memory, which further underscores its potential to enhance cognitive abilities.

Another critical benefit of meditation is its role in promoting overall psychological well-being. It encourages a positive outlook on life by fostering a sense of inner peace, gratitude, and compassion. Meditation practices often include techniques aimed at cultivating loving-kindness and empathy, which not only strengthen interpersonal relationships but also contribute to a deeper sense of connection with oneself and others. This aspect of meditation is particularly valuable in combating feelings of loneliness and isolation, common contributors to poor mental health.

Furthermore, meditation can be tailored to meet specific mental health goals. For instance, mindfulness meditation emphasizes present-moment awareness, teaching individuals to focus on the here and now rather than dwelling on past regrets or worrying about the future. This aspect of mindfulness can be particularly beneficial for those struggling with anxiety disorders, helping them break free from cycles of rumination and catastrophizing thoughts.

Meditation offers a multifaceted approach to enhancing mental health by reducing stress, improving emotional regulation, enhancing cognitive function, and promoting overall psychological well-being. Its profound benefits extend beyond mere relaxation to encompass transformative effects on how individuals perceive and navigate life's challenges. As meditation continues to gain recognition in mainstream psychology and healthcare, its integration into daily routines represents a powerful strategy for cultivating resilience, fostering emotional balance, and nurturing mental health.

5.2 Mindfulness Practices for Emotional Resilience

Mindfulness practices are instrumental in cultivating emotional resilience, offering valuable tools to navigate life's challenges with greater equanimity and clarity. Rooted in Buddhist traditions and now widely studied in psychology and neuroscience, mindfulness involves paying attention to the present moment without judgment. This deliberate awareness allows individuals to observe thoughts, emotions, and bodily sensations as they arise, fostering a deeper understanding of oneself and the world.

One of the primary benefits of mindfulness for emotional resilience is its capacity to enhance self-awareness. Through mindfulness meditation and daily mindful living practices, individuals develop a keen sense of internal states, including emotions and triggers. This heightened self-awareness enables individuals to recognize and acknowledge their emotional responses without becoming overwhelmed by them. By embracing emotions with acceptance and curiosity rather than resistance, individuals can skillfully navigate challenging situations with greater clarity and emotional balance.

Moreover, mindfulness practices cultivate the ability to regulate emotions effectively. By becoming more attuned to the present moment, individuals can intentionally choose how to respond to stressful or triggering events. Mindfulness techniques such as mindful breathing or body scan exercises promote a sense of calm and relaxation, counteracting the body's stress response and reducing physiological symptoms of anxiety or agitation. This emotional regulation not only improves immediate well-being but also builds resilience over time, enhancing one's capacity to bounce back from adversity.

Furthermore, mindfulness fosters a non-reactive stance toward thoughts and emotions. Instead of automatically acting on impulse or getting caught up in negative thought patterns, individuals learn to observe thoughts as passing mental events. This perspective cultivates a sense of detachment from distressing thoughts and emotions, reducing their impact on overall emotional well-being. This aspect of mindfulness is particularly beneficial for individuals prone to rumination, worry, or anxiety disorders, offering a pathway to break free from cycles of negative thinking.

Another essential aspect of mindfulness practices is their role in promoting stress reduction and relaxation. By focusing on the present moment and grounding oneself in sensory experiences, individuals can alleviate mental tension and physical discomfort associated with stress. Mindfulness-based stress reduction (MBSR) programs, which integrate mindfulness meditation with yoga and cognitive-behavioral techniques, have been shown to reduce symptoms of anxiety, depression, and chronic pain while enhancing overall psychological resilience.

Additionally, mindfulness practices cultivate empathy and compassion toward oneself and others. Through practices such as loving-kindness meditation, individuals cultivate a sense of interconnectedness and goodwill, which strengthens social connections and supports emotional resilience. This compassionate attitude extends to self-care practices, encouraging individuals to prioritize their mental and emotional well-being through nurturing activities and positive self-talk.

Mindfulness practices are invaluable for enhancing emotional resilience by promoting self-awareness, emotional regulation, non-reactivity to thoughts and emotions, stress reduction, and cultivating empathy and compassion. These practices offer practical tools to manage stress, navigate challenging emotions, and foster a deeper connection with oneself and others. As mindfulness continues to gain recognition in therapeutic settings and everyday life, its integration represents a profound approach to cultivating emotional resilience and promoting overall well-being.

5.3 Yoga and Tai Chi for Stress Management and Emotional Balance

Yoga and Tai Chi are ancient practices renowned for their profound benefits in stress management and fostering emotional balance. Rooted in Eastern philosophies, both disciplines offer holistic approaches to harmonizing the mind, body, and spirit, promoting overall well-being through movement, breathwork, and mindfulness.

Yoga, originating from ancient India, encompasses a diverse range of practices that include physical postures (asanas), breath control (pranayama), meditation, and ethical principles. The integration of these elements in yoga practice contributes to stress reduction and emotional balance in various ways.

Firstly, the physical postures in yoga help release tension and promote relaxation by stretching and strengthening muscles, improving flexibility, and enhancing blood circulation. The deliberate focus on alignment and mindful movement encourages practitioners to be fully present in their bodies, reducing mental chatter and promoting a sense of calm.

Moreover, yoga emphasizes the connection between breath and movement through pranayama techniques. Controlled breathing patterns such as ujjayi (victorious breath) or deep belly breathing activate the parasympathetic nervous system, eliciting a relaxation response that counteracts the body's stress response. This practice not only calms the mind but also improves respiratory efficiency and oxygenation, enhancing overall physical and mental well-being.

Beyond the physical aspects, yoga incorporates meditation and mindfulness practices that cultivate present-moment awareness and emotional resilience. Mindfulness meditation, often integrated into yoga sessions or practiced independently, involves observing thoughts and sensations without judgment. This practice helps individuals develop a non-reactive stance toward stressors, promoting emotional regulation and reducing anxiety and depressive symptoms over time.

Tai Chi, originating from ancient China, is another mind-body practice renowned for its gentle, flowing movements and meditative qualities. Often referred to as "moving meditation," Tai Chi promotes stress reduction and emotional balance through slow, deliberate movements coordinated with deep breathing and focused attention.

The slow, fluid movements of Tai Chi promote relaxation and muscular relaxation, similar to yoga, facilitating the release of physical tension and enhancing flexibility and balance. The mindful attention to body posture and movement patterns encourages a deep sense of relaxation and presence, reducing mental stress and promoting mental clarity.

Additionally, Tai Chi incorporates principles of traditional Chinese medicine, including the concept of Qi (life force energy) and meridian pathways. The practice is believed to improve the flow of Qi throughout the body, harmonizing internal energy and promoting overall vitality and emotional balance.

Both yoga and Tai Chi offer profound psychological benefits by fostering a sense of inner peace, resilience, and emotional stability. Regular practice can lead to reduced levels of cortisol (the stress hormone), improved mood, and enhanced cognitive function. Moreover, these practices provide a supportive community environment and promote social connection, which are crucial factors in reducing feelings of isolation and loneliness that contribute to stress and emotional imbalance.

Yoga and Tai Chi are powerful practices for stress management and promoting emotional balance through their integration of physical postures, breathwork, meditation, and mindfulness. These ancient disciplines offer accessible and effective tools for individuals seeking to cultivate resilience, manage stress more effectively, and enhance overall well-being. As research continues to demonstrate their therapeutic benefits, integrating yoga or Tai Chi into one's routine represents a proactive approach to nurturing mental and emotional health in the modern world.

Chapter 6: Physical Activity and Its Impact on Mental Health

6.1 Exercise as a Tool for Stress Relief and Mood Elevation

Exercise is a powerful tool for stress relief and mood elevation, offering numerous physical and psychological benefits to overall well-being. Whether engaging in aerobic activities, strength training, yoga, or other forms of bodily movement, exercise profoundly impacts the body's stress response systems and emotional state.

Physical activity triggers the release of endorphins, often called "feel-good" hormones, in the brain. Endorphins are neurotransmitters that act as natural painkillers and mood elevators, promoting feelings of euphoria and reducing perceptions of pain and stress. This neurochemical response, commonly known as the "runner's high, " can be experienced during and after exercise sessions.

Moreover, regular exercise helps regulate the body's stress hormones, such as cortisol and adrenaline. Cortisol, released in response to stress, can accumulate in the body if not adequately managed, contributing to feelings of anxiety, irritability, and physical tension. Exercise helps lower cortisol levels, improving stress resilience and a more balanced emotional state.

Beyond its immediate effects on neurotransmitters and hormones, exercise offers long-term mental health and well-being benefits. Regular physical activity has been shown to reduce symptoms of depression and anxiety, with research indicating that exercise can be as effective as traditional therapies in alleviating mild to moderate depression. The rhythmic movements and focused attention required in activities like yoga or tai chi promote relaxation and mindfulness, contributing to stress reduction and emotional balance.

In addition to directly impacting mood, exercise enhances overall physical health, supporting mental well-being. Physical fitness contributes to cardiovascular health, strengthens the immune system, improves sleep quality, and enhances cognitive function. These physiological benefits create a foundation for resilience against stressors and contribute to a positive outlook on life.

Furthermore, exercise is a natural outlet for pent-up energy and emotions, providing a healthy way to cope with stress and emotional challenges. Engaging in physical activity allows individuals to channel their frustration or anxiety into productive movements, promoting a sense of empowerment and control over one's emotions.

The type and intensity of exercise can vary based on individual preferences and fitness levels. From the exhilaration of aerobic exercises like running, swimming, or cycling to the strength-building benefits of weight training, there's a wide range of options to explore. Each type of exercise offers unique benefits, promoting both physical and emotional well-being.

Mind-body exercises like yoga, tai chi, or Pilates integrate physical movement with breath awareness and mindfulness practices. These disciplines promote relaxation, improve flexibility and balance, and cultivate inner peace and emotional stability.

Incorporating exercise into daily routines can be a proactive strategy for managing stress and promoting mental health. Whether scheduling regular gym sessions, taking brisk walks during breaks, or participating in group fitness classes, finding enjoyable physical activity is key to sustaining long-term engagement and reaping the benefits.

It's important to note that while exercise is a powerful tool for stress relief and mood elevation, it should be approached mindfully and balanced with adequate rest and recovery. Overtraining or excessive exercise can lead to physical strain, fatigue, and increased stress levels. Listening to the body's signals and incorporating variety into fitness routines can help prevent burnout and support overall well-being.

Exercise is a multifaceted approach to stress management and emotional balance, offering immediate and long-term mental health benefits. By engaging in regular physical activity, individuals can enhance mood, reduce stress levels, and cultivate resilience against life's challenges. Incorporating exercise into daily life promotes holistic well-being and supports a positive mental and emotional health outlook.

6.2 Incorporating Movement into Daily Routine for Emotional Health

Incorporating movement into daily routines is beneficial for physical fitness and plays a crucial role in enhancing emotional health and overall well-being. The connection between physical activity and emotional well-being is well-established, with research consistently showing that regular exercise and movement can profoundly affect mood, stress levels, and mental clarity.

One primary way movement benefits emotional health is through the release of endorphins, neurotransmitters in the brain known for their ability to reduce pain and produce feelings of euphoria and well-being. Our bodies naturally produce endorphins when we engage in physical activity, whether it's a brisk walk, yoga session, or dance class. This "exercise high" can help alleviate symptoms of anxiety and depression, improve mood, and increase feelings of happiness and relaxation.

Moreover, regular movement helps regulate stress hormones such as cortisol and adrenaline. These hormones are released in response to stressors, triggering the body's "fight or flight" response. Prolonged or chronic stress can lead to elevated cortisol levels, which may contribute to anxiety, irritability, and difficulty concentrating. Exercise helps reduce these stress hormones, promoting a more balanced emotional state and enhancing resilience to stress.

Incorporating movement into daily routines also provides an opportunity for mindfulness and stress reduction. Mindfulness practices, such as yoga and tai chi, emphasize present-moment awareness and conscious breathing techniques. These activities promote physical flexibility, strength, and balance and cultivate mental clarity, focus, and relaxation. By connecting mind and body, mindfulness-based movement practices can help individuals manage stress more effectively and improve emotional resilience.

Furthermore, regular physical activity supports better sleep quality, essential for emotional well-being. Sleep is critical in regulating mood, cognitive function, and emotional processing. Exercise has been shown to promote deeper and more restorative sleep, reducing the likelihood of sleep disturbances and insomnia. Adequate sleep enhances emotional regulation and supports overall mental health.

Another important aspect of incorporating movement into daily routines for emotional health is its role in self-care and stress management. Engaging in physical activity provides a healthy outlet for pent-up energy and emotions, allowing individuals to release tension, frustration, and anxiety constructively. Whether going for a run, practicing yoga, or participating in a group fitness class, movement can be a form of self-expression and empowerment, boosting self-esteem and confidence.

Moreover, physical activity can foster social connections and community support, vital for emotional well-being. Joining exercise classes, sports teams, or outdoor activities can create opportunities to meet new people, build friendships, and strengthen existing relationships. Social interaction and support networks contribute to a sense of belonging and emotional resilience, buffering against stress and promoting overall life satisfaction.

Incorporating movement into daily routines doesn't necessarily require a gym membership or structured exercise regimen. Simple activities such as taking the stairs instead of the elevator, walking or biking to work, gardening, or playing with pets can all contribute to increased physical activity levels and improved emotional health. The key is to find enjoyable, sustainable activities that fit into daily schedules.

For those with sedentary jobs or lifestyles, incorporating movement breaks throughout the day can be particularly beneficial. Stretching exercises, short walks, or desk yoga poses can help alleviate muscle tension, improve circulation, and boost energy levels. These micro-breaks enhance physical health and support mental clarity and productivity.

Chapter 7: Sleep and Its Role in Emotional Resilience

7.1 Importance of Quality Sleep for Mental Health

Quality sleep is not merely a rest period but a vital pillar of mental health and overall well-being. The significance of sleep transcends its therapeutic effects on the body; it plays a crucial role in maintaining cognitive function, emotional regulation, and psychological resilience. Scientifically, sleep is considered a dynamic process during which the brain consolidates memories, processes information, and clears out toxins accumulated during wakefulness. This nightly restoration is pivotal for optimal brain function and mental clarity throughout the day.

One of the primary benefits of quality sleep lies in its profound impact on cognitive abilities. Studies consistently show that adequate sleep enhances attention, concentration, problem-solving, and decision-making abilities. Conversely, sleep deprivation or poor sleep quality can impair these cognitive functions, leading to difficulties in learning, memory retention, and overall cognitive performance.

Furthermore, sleep is intricately linked to emotional regulation and mental health. Sleep deficiency has been associated with increased susceptibility to stress, anxiety, and depression. Sleep plays a crucial role in regulating emotions and processing emotional experiences. During sleep, the brain processes and integrates emotions, helping individuals maintain emotional stability and resilience in the face of daily challenges.

Beyond cognitive and emotional benefits, quality sleep is also essential for physical health. It supports the immune system, promotes tissue healing and repair, regulates hormone levels, and supports cardiovascular health. Chronic sleep deprivation, on the other hand, is linked to a higher risk of various health conditions, including obesity, diabetes, and cardiovascular disease.

Creating a consistent sleep routine and prioritizing sleep hygiene are essential strategies for improving sleep patterns. This includes establishing a regular sleep schedule, creating a conducive sleep environment (e.g., dark, cool, and quiet), limiting exposure to screens before bedtime, and practicing relaxation techniques such as meditation or deep breathing exercises.

Quality sleep is a cornerstone of mental health and well-being, influencing cognitive function, emotional resilience, and overall physical health. Incorporating habits that promote restorative sleep can significantly enhance one's ability to cope with stress, maintain optimal mental functioning, and achieve overall wellness.

7.2 Strategies for Improving Sleep Patterns

Improving sleep patterns is crucial for overall health and well-being, as quality sleep plays a vital role in maintaining physical, mental, and emotional balance. Here are several strategies that can help enhance sleep patterns and promote restful sleep:

1. Establishing a Consistent Sleep Schedule: Setting a regular sleep-wake cycle helps regulate the body's internal clock, making it easier to fall asleep and wake up naturally. Aim to go to bed and wake up at the same time every day, even on weekends, to reinforce the body's sleep-wake rhythm.

2. Creating a Relaxing Bedtime Routine: Engaging in relaxing activities before bed signals to the body that it's time to wind down. Activities such as reading a book, taking a warm bath, practicing gentle yoga or meditation, or listening to calming music can help transition from wakefulness to sleepiness.

3. Optimizing Sleep Environment: Make your bedroom conducive to sleep by creating a comfortable and relaxing environment. Ensure the room is cool, dark, and quiet, and consider using blackout curtains, earplugs, or a white noise machine to minimize disruptions. Invest in a comfortable mattress and pillows that support your sleeping posture.

4. Limiting Exposure to Screens: The blue light emitted by smartphones, tablets, computers, and TVs can interfere with the production of melatonin, a hormone that regulates sleep-wake cycles. To improve sleep quality, avoid using screens at least an hour before bedtime. Instead, engage in low-light activities that promote relaxation.

5. Managing Stress and Anxiety: Stress and anxiety can significantly impact sleep quality. Practice stress-reducing techniques such as deep breathing exercises, progressive muscle relaxation, or mindfulness meditation to calm the mind and body before bedtime. Journaling or writing down worries can also help clear the mind.

6. Regular Physical Activity: Engaging in regular exercise can promote better sleep, but timing is key. Aim for moderate aerobic exercise earlier in the day or at least a few hours before bedtime. Avoid vigorous exercise close to bedtime, as it may stimulate the body and make it harder to fall asleep.

7. Mindful Eating Habits: Avoid heavy meals, caffeine, and alcohol close to bedtime, as they can interfere with sleep. Instead, opt for light snacks if needed and consider herbal teas such as chamomile or valerian root, which are known for their calming properties and can support relaxation before sleep.

8. Cognitive Behavioral Therapy for Insomnia (CBT-I): CBT-I is a structured program designed to address the underlying causes of insomnia through cognitive restructuring and behavioral changes. It focuses on improving sleep habits, changing negative thoughts about sleep, and promoting relaxation techniques.

9. Natural Supplements and Herbs: Some individuals find relief from sleep disturbances with natural supplements such as melatonin, magnesium, or herbal remedies like valerian root or passionflower. However, it's essential to consult with a healthcare provider before starting any new supplement regimen.

10. Seeking Professional Help if Needed: If sleep problems persist despite trying these strategies, it may be beneficial to consult with a healthcare professional or sleep specialist. They can help identify underlying sleep disorders or medical conditions contributing to sleep disturbances and recommend appropriate treatment options.

By incorporating these strategies into your daily routine and making sleep a priority, you can improve sleep patterns and promote better overall health and well-being. Consistency and patience are key as you work to establish healthy sleep habits that support restful and rejuvenating sleep each night.

Book 21: Holistic Living and Preventive Care with Barbara O'Neill

Holistic Living and Preventive Care with Comprehensive Health and Wellness Strategies

Chapter 1: Foundations of Holistic Living

1.1 What is Holistic Living?

Holistic living is a philosophy and lifestyle approach emphasizing mind, body, spirit, and environment interconnectedness. It encompasses various aspects of life, promoting balance, harmony, and well-being through integrated practices and mindful choices. At its core, holistic living acknowledges that each individual is a complex system influenced by internal and external factors. It seeks to cultivate optimal health and vitality by addressing these dimensions comprehensively.

1.1.1 Core Principles of Holistic Living

Holistic living is guided by several core principles that shape its approach to health and wellness:

Whole-Person Perspective: Holistic living recognizes that individuals are more than their physical bodies. It acknowledges health's mental, emotional, spiritual, and social dimensions, viewing these aspects as interconnected and equally important in achieving overall well-being.

Prevention and Wellness: Rather than focusing solely on treating symptoms or diseases, holistic living emphasizes prevention through lifestyle choices that support health and vitality. It promotes proactive measures such as healthy eating (e.g., a balanced diet rich in fruits and vegetables), regular exercise (e.g., yoga, walking, or swimming), stress management (e.g., meditation or deep breathing exercises), and adequate sleep to maintain wellness and prevent illness.

Balance and Harmony: Achieving balance in all aspects of life—physical, emotional, mental, and spiritual—is not just a goal of holistic living, but a way of life. This balance fosters harmony within oneself and with the surrounding environment, promoting a sense of wholeness and integration that brings a profound sense of peace.

Individualized Care: Holistic living is not a one-size-fits-all approach. It recognizes that each person has unique needs, preferences, and circumstances that influence their health. It encourages personalized approaches to health care and lifestyle choices, considering genetics, lifestyle, beliefs, and goals, making each individual feel understood and catered to.

Mind-Body-Spirit Connection: Holistic living emphasizes the interconnectedness of the mind, body, and spirit. It recognizes that mental and emotional well-being can impact physical health and vice versa. Meditation, yoga, and mindfulness are often integrated to nurture this connection.

Environmental Awareness: Holistic living extends beyond personal health to include environmental stewardship. It encourages sustainable practices that promote the planet's health, such as reducing waste, conserving resources, and supporting eco-friendly products and practices.

1.1.2 Practices and Components of Holistic Living

Holistic living encompasses a wide range of practices and components that contribute to overall well-being.

Nutrition: A cornerstone of holistic living is nourishing the body with whole, nutrient-dense foods that support optimal health. Emphasis is placed on fresh fruits and vegetables, whole grains, lean proteins, and healthy fats while minimizing processed foods, sugars, and artificial additives.

Physical Activity: Regular exercise is essential for physical health and mental well-being. Holistic living encourages a balanced approach to fitness, incorporating activities that promote cardiovascular health, strength, flexibility, and overall vitality.

Stress Management: Effective stress management techniques are integral to holistic living. Meditation, deep breathing exercises, yoga, and tai chi help reduce stress levels, promote relaxation, and support emotional resilience.

Mindfulness and Meditation: These practices cultivate present-moment awareness and promote mental clarity, emotional stability, and spiritual connection. Mindfulness techniques can be integrated into daily life to enhance well-being and reduce stress.

Emotional and Spiritual Growth: Holistic living encourages self-reflection, personal growth, and spiritual exploration. Practices such as journaling, therapy, and participation in community or spiritual groups support emotional healing and inner peace.

Complementary Therapies: Holistic living often incorporates complementary therapies such as acupuncture, chiropractic care, massage therapy, and herbal medicine to support health and healing. These therapies are used in conjunction with conventional medical treatments to address underlying causes and promote holistic well-being.

Environmental Consciousness: Awareness of environmental impact and sustainable living practices are integral to holistic living. This includes reducing exposure to toxins, supporting eco-friendly products and practices, and fostering a connection to nature.

1.2 Benefits of Holistic Living

Adopting a holistic approach to life can lead to numerous benefits:

1. Enhanced Overall Health: Holistic living promotes physical, mental, emotional, and spiritual health, leading to improved quality of life and increased vitality.

2. Improved Resilience: By addressing multiple aspects of health, holistic living enhances resilience to stress, illness, and life challenges.

3. Personal Empowerment: Holistic practices empower individuals to take an active role in their health and well-being, fostering a sense of control and autonomy.

4. Greater Life Satisfaction: Achieving balance and harmony in life through holistic practices can enhance life satisfaction and fulfillment.

5. Reduced Healthcare Costs: Prevention-focused approaches and lifestyle modifications may lead to fewer medical interventions and lower healthcare costs over time.

In essence, holistic living offers a comprehensive framework for nurturing health, fostering resilience, and promoting overall well-being by addressing the interconnected aspects of mind, body, spirit, and environment. By embracing holistic principles and practices, individuals can cultivate a balanced and harmonious life that supports health, vitality, and fulfillment.

1.3 Principles of Holistic Health and Wellness

Holistic health and wellness encompass a multifaceted approach to well-being that integrates various aspects of an individual's life, emphasizing the interconnectedness of mind, body, spirit, and environment. This holistic approach operates on several core principles that guide its philosophy and practices, aiming to optimize health, vitality, and overall quality of life.

One of the fundamental principles of holistic health and wellness is the recognition of individuals as complex beings with interconnected dimensions. This perspective views health not just as the absence of disease but as a state of optimal well-being that encompasses physical, mental, emotional, and spiritual aspects. Holistic practitioners believe that these dimensions are interdependent and influence each other profoundly. For instance, emotional stress can manifest physically through symptoms like headaches or digestive issues, highlighting the importance of addressing the root causes holistically.

Holistic health emphasizes the importance of proactive measures and preventive care to maintain health and wellness. Rather than focusing solely on treating symptoms, holistic practices advocate for lifestyle choices that promote long-term well-being. This includes adopting a balanced diet rich in nutrients, engaging in regular physical activity, managing stress effectively, getting adequate sleep, and minimizing exposure to toxins. By nurturing overall health and resilience, individuals can potentially reduce the risk of developing chronic illnesses and enhance their quality of life.

Achieving balance and harmony is central to holistic health and wellness. This principle acknowledges the dynamic interplay between various aspects of life—physical, emotional, mental, and spiritual—and emphasizes the importance of equilibrium among these dimensions. For instance, maintaining a balanced diet, managing stress levels, fostering positive relationships, and engaging in activities that promote relaxation and inner peace contribute to overall harmony. When these elements are in balance, individuals are more likely to experience a sense of wholeness and well-being.

Holistic health recognizes that each person is unique, with distinct needs, preferences, and circumstances that influence their health journey. Therefore, personalized care and treatment plans are essential in holistic practices. This approach considers factors such as genetics, lifestyle, environmental influences, and personal beliefs to tailor interventions and recommendations accordingly. By acknowledging individual differences and preferences, holistic practitioners empower individuals to take an active role in their health and make informed decisions that align with their values and goals.

The interconnectedness of the mind, body, and spirit is a core principle of holistic health. This principle underscores the notion that mental and emotional well-being significantly impact physical health and vice versa. Practices such as meditation, yoga, mindfulness, and spiritual exploration are integral to nurturing this connection. These practices promote self-awareness, emotional resilience, and spiritual growth, fostering a deeper understanding of oneself and one's place in the world.

Holistic health embraces integrative approaches that combine conventional and complementary therapies to address health concerns comprehensively. Integrative medicine integrates evidence-based practices from both conventional medicine and alternative therapies, such as acupuncture, chiropractic care, herbal medicine, and massage therapy. This collaborative approach allows for a more holistic assessment and treatment of health conditions, considering the whole person rather than just the symptoms.

Holistic health extends beyond individual well-being to include the health of the environment. Environmental factors play a crucial role in overall health, and holistic practices emphasize sustainability and environmental stewardship. This includes supporting eco-friendly practices, reducing exposure to environmental toxins, and fostering a connection to nature. By promoting a healthy environment, holistic health advocates contribute to the well-being of communities and future generations.

1.4 Benefits of Holistic Health and Wellness

Embracing holistic health and wellness principles offers numerous benefits that contribute to a balanced and fulfilling life:

1. Enhanced Overall Health: By addressing multiple dimensions of health, holistic practices support physical vitality, mental clarity, emotional resilience, and spiritual well-being.

2. Empowerment and Self-Care: Holistic health empowers individuals to take an active role in their health through informed decision-making, self-care practices, and lifestyle modifications that promote well-being.

3. Prevention of Illness: Proactive measures and preventive care in holistic health may reduce the risk of developing chronic conditions and enhance longevity.

4. Improved Quality of Life: Achieving balance and harmony through holistic practices can lead to greater life satisfaction, increased energy levels, and enhanced personal fulfillment.

5. Comprehensive Approach: Holistic health addresses the root causes of health issues rather than just managing symptoms, promoting long-term health benefits and sustainable wellness.

Holistic health and wellness principles offer a comprehensive framework for nurturing health, vitality, and overall well-being by addressing the interconnected aspects of mind, body, spirit, and environment. By embracing these principles, individuals can cultivate a balanced and harmonious life that supports optimal health, resilience, and quality of life.

1.5 Benefits of Adopting a Holistic Lifestyle

Adopting a holistic lifestyle encompasses embracing practices that prioritize overall well-being by considering the interconnectedness of various aspects of life—physical, mental, emotional, and spiritual. This approach offers many benefits that contribute to enhanced health, vitality, and quality of life.

One of the primary benefits of adopting a holistic lifestyle is its focus on comprehensive health improvement. Unlike conventional approaches that often treat symptoms in isolation, holistic practices aim to address the underlying causes of health issues. By integrating physical health with mental, emotional, and spiritual well-being, individuals experience a more balanced approach to health management. This can lead to enhanced vitality, reduced incidence of chronic illnesses, and improved overall health outcomes over time.

Holistic living is not just about practices, it's about empowerment. It empowers individuals to actively participate in their health and well-being. Through mindful eating, regular physical activity, stress management techniques, and self-care rituals, individuals become more attuned to their bodies' needs and preferences. This empowerment fosters a sense of control over one's health journey, promoting self-confidence, resilience, and a proactive approach to maintaining wellness.

Holistic practices emphasize stress reduction techniques such as meditation, yoga, deep breathing exercises, and mindfulness practices. For instance, meditation can be as simple as taking a few minutes each day to sit quietly and focus on your breath, while yoga can involve a series of gentle stretches and poses. These techniques help individuals manage daily stressors more effectively and enhance emotional resilience. By cultivating a calm and centered mind, individuals experience reduced anxiety levels, improved mood stability, and a greater capacity to cope with life's challenges. This holistic approach to emotional well-being promotes mental clarity, inner peace, and overall emotional balance.

Nutrition plays a crucial role in holistic living, focusing on consuming whole, nutrient-dense foods that nourish the body and support optimal function. A holistic diet emphasizes fresh fruits and vegetables, lean proteins, healthy fats, and complex carbohydrates while minimizing processed foods, sugars, and artificial additives. By prioritizing nutrition, individuals experience improved digestive health, enhanced nutrient absorption, increased energy levels, and a strengthened immune system. This holistic approach to nutrition not only supports long-term health, vitality, and resilience but also brings a sense of balance and harmony to one's life.

Holistic living emphasizes the profound connection between the mind and body, recognizing that mental and emotional states significantly impact physical health. Meditation, biofeedback, yoga, and tai chi promote mind-body awareness and integration. By fostering a harmonious mind-body connection, individuals become more aware and in tune with their bodies, leading to improved sleep quality, reduced inflammation, enhanced immune function, and accelerated healing processes. This holistic approach supports overall well-being by promoting physical health, mental clarity, and emotional stability.

For many individuals, holistic living includes nurturing spiritual well-being and personal growth. Spiritual health is not necessarily tied to a specific religion, but rather to a sense of connection to something greater than oneself. This may involve prayer, meditation, mindfulness, journaling, or engaging in meaningful community activities. Cultivating spiritual health provides a sense of purpose, inner peace, and fulfillment, contributing to overall life satisfaction and happiness. By aligning personal values with daily actions, individuals experience greater authenticity, resilience, and a deeper connection to themselves and others.

Holistic living extends beyond personal well-being to include environmental stewardship and sustainability. This may involve adopting eco-friendly practices such as recycling, reducing waste, conserving energy, supporting local agriculture, and minimizing exposure to environmental toxins.

Chapter 2: Nutrition as Preventive Medicine

2.1 Role of Nutrition in Preventing Illness and Promoting Health

Nutrition plays a fundamental role in preventing illness and promoting overall health by providing essential nutrients that support various bodily functions, enhance immune response, and reduce the risk of chronic diseases. A balanced and nutrient-rich diet is crucial not only for maintaining optimal physical health but also for supporting mental and emotional well-being.

<u>Essential Nutrients and Their Functions</u>

Nutrition provides the body with essential nutrients such as vitamins, minerals, protein, carbohydrates, fats, and water. Each nutrient plays a unique role in maintaining health:

- Vitamins and minerals are vital for immune function, energy production, bone health, and maintaining the nervous system.

- Proteins are necessary for muscle repair and growth, enzyme production, and hormone regulation.

- Carbohydrates serve as the body's primary source of energy.

- Healthy fats support brain function, hormone production, and the absorption of fat-soluble vitamins.

- Water is essential for hydration, digestion, nutrient transport, and temperature regulation.

<u>Immune Support and Disease Prevention</u>

A well-balanced diet rich in vitamins, minerals, antioxidants, and phytonutrients supports a robust immune system, helping the body defend against infections and diseases. Nutrients like vitamin C, vitamin D, zinc, and antioxidants found in fruits, vegetables, nuts, and seeds strengthen immune response and reduce the severity of illnesses. Studies show that deficiencies in key nutrients can impair immune function, making individuals more susceptible to infections and chronic diseases.

<u>Role in Chronic Disease Prevention</u>

Chronic diseases such as cardiovascular diseases, diabetes, obesity, and certain cancers are often influenced by dietary habits. A diet high in processed foods, saturated fats, sugars, and low in fiber can increase the risk of developing these conditions. Conversely, a diet rich in whole grains, lean proteins, healthy fats, fruits, and vegetables can reduce the risk of chronic diseases. For example, diets high in fiber promote digestive health and reduce the risk of colorectal cancer, while omega-3 fatty acids found in fish support heart health and reduce inflammation.

<u>Mental and Emotional Well-being</u>

Nutrition also plays a significant role in mental and emotional well-being. Research indicates that deficiencies in certain nutrients, such as omega-3 fatty acids, B vitamins, and minerals like magnesium and zinc, may contribute to mood disorders such as depression and anxiety. Conversely, consuming a nutrient-dense diet that includes whole foods and adequate hydration can support brain function, stabilize mood, and improve cognitive performance.

Gut Health and Immune Function

The gut microbiome, composed of trillions of bacteria and other microorganisms, plays a crucial role in immune function and overall health. A diet rich in fiber, prebiotics (found in foods like garlic, onions, and bananas), and probiotics (found in fermented foods like yogurt, kefir, and sauerkraut) promotes a diverse and healthy gut microbiota. This, in turn, enhances immune function, reduces inflammation, and supports digestion and nutrient absorption.

Personalized Nutrition Approaches

Individual nutritional needs vary based on factors such as age, sex, genetics, lifestyle, and health status. Personalized nutrition approaches take these factors into account to optimize health outcomes. Registered dietitians and nutritionists can help individuals develop personalized nutrition plans tailored to their specific needs and goals. This may include addressing nutrient deficiencies, managing chronic conditions through diet, supporting athletic performance, or promoting healthy aging.

Sustainable Food Choices

In addition to promoting personal health, nutrition also influences environmental sustainability. Sustainable food choices, such as consuming locally grown produce, reducing food waste, and choosing plant-based proteins over animal products, can have positive effects on both human health and the environment. By supporting sustainable agriculture practices, individuals contribute to preserving natural resources, reducing greenhouse gas emissions, and promoting biodiversity.

Education and Empowerment

Education about nutrition empowers individuals to make informed food choices that support their health and well-being. Nutrition education can encompass understanding food labels, meal planning, cooking skills, and recognizing the importance of balanced nutrition across the lifespan. By promoting nutrition literacy and encouraging healthy eating habits from an early age, communities can foster a culture of wellness and disease prevention.

Nutrition plays a pivotal role in preventing illness and promoting health by providing essential nutrients that support immune function, disease prevention, mental and emotional well-being, gut health, and personalized nutrition approaches. A balanced and nutrient-rich diet not only supports physical health but also contributes to environmental sustainability and empowers individuals to make informed food choices. By prioritizing nutrition as a cornerstone of health, individuals can enhance their quality of life, reduce the risk of chronic diseases, and support overall well-being throughout the lifespan.

2.2 Foods and Nutrients for Long-Term Health and Vitality

To promote long-term health and vitality, a balanced and nutrient-rich diet is essential. Incorporating a variety of foods that provide essential nutrients can significantly contribute to overall well-being. One of the foundational principles of a healthy diet is ensuring a diverse intake of fruits and vegetables. These foods are rich in vitamins, minerals, antioxidants, and dietary fiber, which are crucial for maintaining optimal health.

Fruits and vegetables provide an array of vitamins such as vitamin C, vitamin A, and various B vitamins, all of which play critical roles in supporting immune function, vision health, energy metabolism, and more. Antioxidants found in these foods, such as beta-carotene, lycopene, and flavonoids, help protect cells from oxidative stress and inflammation, thereby reducing the risk of chronic diseases like heart disease and cancer.

Whole grains are another essential component of a nutritious diet, offering complex carbohydrates, fiber, B vitamins, and minerals like iron and magnesium. They provide sustained energy levels and support digestive health. Including a variety of whole grains such as oats, quinoa, brown rice, and whole wheat in meals can help regulate blood sugar levels, improve satiety, and reduce the risk of type 2 diabetes.

Healthy fats, such as those found in avocados, nuts, seeds, and fatty fish like salmon and mackerel, are crucial for brain health, hormone production, and the absorption of fat-soluble vitamins like vitamin D. These fats also contain omega-3 fatty acids, which have anti-inflammatory properties and contribute to heart health.

Protein is essential for building and repairing tissues, supporting immune function, and maintaining muscle mass. Lean sources of protein such as poultry, fish, beans, lentils, tofu, and Greek yogurt provide necessary amino acids without the excess saturated fat found in some animal products.

In addition to macronutrients, micronutrients like calcium, potassium, and magnesium are critical for bone health, nerve function, and muscle contraction. Dairy products, leafy greens, nuts, seeds, and fortified foods are excellent sources of these minerals.

Hydration is often overlooked but is fundamental to maintaining health. Water plays a crucial role in regulating body temperature, aiding digestion, transporting nutrients, and eliminating waste products. Herbal teas and fresh fruits and vegetables with high water content also contribute to overall hydration.

Adopting a diet rich in fruits, vegetables, whole grains, lean proteins, healthy fats, and adequate hydration provides the body with essential nutrients needed for optimal health and vitality. By prioritizing nutrient-dense foods and maintaining a balanced diet, individuals can support their long-term well-being and reduce the risk of chronic diseases. Regular physical activity and mindful eating habits complement a nutritious diet, enhancing overall health and quality of life.

Chapter 3: Herbal Remedies for Preventive Care

3.1 Using Herbs to Maintain Health and Prevent Illness

Using herbs to maintain health and prevent illness is rooted in centuries-old practices that harness the natural healing properties of plants. Herbs offer a holistic approach to health, supporting various bodily systems and promoting overall well-being through their diverse array of medicinal compounds.

One of the primary benefits of using herbs is their rich content of vitamins, minerals, antioxidants, and phytochemicals. These bioactive compounds contribute to the herbs' therapeutic effects, helping to strengthen the immune system, combat inflammation, and protect against oxidative stress. For example, herbs like echinacea, elderberry, and garlic are known for their immune-boosting properties, helping to ward off infections and support immune function.

Herbs also play a significant role in promoting digestive health. Plants such as ginger, peppermint, and chamomile possess carminative properties that aid digestion, alleviate indigestion, and soothe gastrointestinal discomfort. They can also be natural remedies for bloating, gas, and nausea.

Furthermore, herbs are commonly used to support cardiovascular health. Hawthorn, garlic, and turmeric may help lower blood pressure, reduce cholesterol levels, and improve circulation. These herbs contain compounds that support heart muscle function, regulate blood vessel tone, and provide antioxidant protection to blood vessels.

In addition to physical health, herbs benefit mental and emotional well-being. Adaptogenic herbs like ashwagandha, Rhodiola, and holy basil help the body adapt to stress, support adrenal function and promote a sense of calm and balance. Herbs such as lavender, lemon balm, and passionflower are known for their calming effects, helping to reduce anxiety, improve sleep quality, and enhance overall mood.

Using herbs as a preventive health strategy involves incorporating them into daily routines. This can be achieved through herbal teas, culinary herbs in cooking, herbal supplements, or topical applications like herbal salves and essential oils. Herbal teas are a convenient way to enjoy herbs' benefits, providing hydration and therapeutic effects. Culinary herbs not only enhance the flavor of dishes but also impart their medicinal properties when consumed regularly.

When using herbs for preventive health, it's essential to consider quality and sourcing. Organic, sustainably harvested herbs ensure purity and potency, minimizing exposure to pesticides and contaminants. Understanding the appropriate dosage and potential interactions with medications is crucial, and consulting with a qualified herbalist or healthcare provider can provide personalized guidance.

Herbs offer a natural and holistic approach to maintaining health and preventing illness by supporting immune function, promoting digestive health, enhancing cardiovascular health, and supporting mental well-being. Incorporating a variety of herbs into daily routines can provide a wide range of health benefits, contributing to overall vitality and resilience. By harnessing the therapeutic potential of herbs, individuals can empower themselves to take proactive steps toward optimal health and well-being.

3.2 Key Herbs for Preventive Care

Key herbs for preventive care encompass a diverse array of plants traditionally used for their health-promoting properties across different cultures and traditions. These herbs are valued for their nutritional content and their bioactive compounds that contribute to their therapeutic effects. Here, we explore some key herbs known for their preventive care benefits.

Echinacea (Echinacea purpurea, Echinacea angustifolia): Echinacea is perhaps one of the most well-known herbs for immune support. It is widely used to prevent and reduce the severity of common colds and upper respiratory infections. Echinacea enhances immune function by stimulating the production of white blood cells and promoting the activity of other immune cells. Regular use of echinacea during cold and flu season may help reduce the risk of infections and shorten the duration of illness.

Garlic (Allium sativum): Garlic has been revered for centuries for its medicinal properties. It contains sulfur compounds such as allicin, which have potent antimicrobial and immune-stimulating effects. Garlic is known for supporting cardiovascular health by helping lower blood pressure and cholesterol levels. It also possesses antioxidant properties that protect cells from oxidative damage, thus contributing to overall health and longevity.

Ginger (Zingiber officinale): Ginger is a versatile herb known for its anti-inflammatory and digestive benefits. It contains bioactive compounds like gingerol and shogaol, which have potent antioxidant and anti-inflammatory properties. Ginger is often used to alleviate nausea, improve digestion, and reduce inflammation in conditions such as arthritis. Regularly consuming ginger tea or incorporating fresh ginger into meals can support digestive health and overall well-being.

Turmeric (Curcuma longa): Turmeric, with its active compound curcumin, is renowned for its powerful anti-inflammatory and antioxidant properties. It supports joint health, reduces inflammation, and helps protect against chronic diseases such as heart disease and cancer. Turmeric is commonly used in traditional Ayurvedic and Chinese medicine for its broad health benefits, including immune support and cognitive function.

Holy Basil (Ocimum sanctum, Ocimum tenuiflorum): Holy basil, also known as tulsi, is considered a sacred herb in Ayurvedic medicine. It is revered for its adaptogenic properties, which help the body adapt to stress and support adrenal function. Holy basil also has antioxidant, antimicrobial, and anti-inflammatory properties, making it beneficial for immune health and overall vitality. It is often consumed as a tea to promote relaxation, enhance mood, and support respiratory health.

Ashwagandha (Withania somnifera): Ashwagandha is an adaptogenic herb that helps the body cope with stress and maintain balance. It supports adrenal health, improves resilience to stress, and promotes overall energy levels. Ashwagandha also has immune-modulating effects, helping to enhance immune function and protect against infections. It is commonly used in Ayurvedic medicine to promote longevity, vitality, and cognitive function.

Elderberry (Sambucus nigra): Elderberry is rich in antioxidants and flavonoids, which have immune-enhancing properties. It is traditionally used to prevent and shorten the duration of colds and flu. Elderberry syrup or tea is a popular remedy for respiratory infections and seasonal allergies. The berries also contain vitamins A and C, which support immune function and protect against oxidative stress.

Chamomile (Matricaria chamomilla): Chamomile is a gentle herb known for its calming and soothing effects on the nervous system. It promotes relaxation, reduces anxiety, and improves sleep quality. Chamomile tea is often consumed to relieve digestive discomfort, promote restful sleep, and support overall well-being. Its anti-inflammatory and antioxidant properties contribute to its preventive care benefits.

Incorporating these key herbs into daily routines can provide various preventive health benefits, supporting immune function, promoting cardiovascular health, reducing inflammation, and enhancing overall well-being.

Whether consumed as teas, added to culinary dishes, or taken in supplement form, these herbs offer natural and effective ways to maintain health and vitality. As with any herbal therapy, consulting with a healthcare provider or qualified herbalist is essential to ensure safety, appropriate dosage, and potential interactions with medications. By harnessing the power of these herbs, individuals can take proactive steps toward preventive care and holistic wellness.

Chapter 4: Essential Oils for Holistic Health

4.1 Aromatherapy Techniques for Wellbeing and Prevention

Aromatherapy encompasses a variety of techniques that promote overall wellbeing and preventive health benefits through the use of essential oils derived from plants. These techniques leverage the aromatic and therapeutic properties of essential oils to support physical, emotional, and mental health. Here are some key aromatherapy techniques that are widely used for wellbeing and prevention:

Inhalation is one of the most common and effective methods of aromatherapy. It involves breathing in the aroma of essential oils, which stimulates the olfactory system and promotes various physiological and psychological responses. Inhalation can be done through:

- Direct Inhalation: This involves inhaling essential oils directly from the bottle or a few drops on a tissue. It is convenient and provides immediate benefits, such as uplifting mood, reducing stress, and enhancing mental clarity.

- Steam Inhalation: Adding a few drops of essential oils to hot water and inhaling the steam can help clear nasal passages, relieve respiratory congestion, and support respiratory health. It is beneficial during cold and flu seasons or for sinusitis relief.

Topical application involves applying diluted essential oils directly to the skin. This method allows for absorption through the skin, where the oils can exert their therapeutic effects locally and systemically. Popular methods include:

- Massage: Diluted essential oils are combined with carrier oils and massaged into the skin. This technique promotes relaxation, relieves muscle tension, improves circulation, and supports overall wellbeing. Massaging essential oils on specific areas can target pain relief or promote relaxation, depending on the blend used.

- Compresses: Adding a few drops of essential oils to warm or cold water and soaking a cloth in the mixture to apply to a specific area of the body can provide relief from inflammation, pain, or muscle soreness. This method is soothing and effective for localized issues.

Adding essential oils to bathwater allows for a relaxing and therapeutic experience. Essential oils are mixed with a dispersant (like a carrier oil or bath salt) before adding to warm water. The oils disperse through the water, and their aroma fills the air, providing benefits such as relaxation, stress relief, and skin nourishment. Aromatherapy baths are ideal for promoting relaxation, easing muscle tension, and improving sleep quality.

Diffusing essential oils into the air creates a calming and inviting atmosphere while dispersing the oils' therapeutic properties throughout the room. Diffusers disperse microscopic oil droplets into the air, allowing inhalation and absorption through the respiratory system. This method is effective for enhancing mood, purifying the air, and supporting respiratory health. Different types of diffusers, such as ultrasonic, nebulizing, and heat-based diffusers, offer various ways to disperse essential oils into the environment.

Regular use of aromatherapy techniques can contribute to overall wellbeing and prevent various health issues. Essential oils like tea tree, eucalyptus, and lavender have antimicrobial properties that can help purify the air and reduce airborne pathogens. Diffusing these oils in living spaces or using them in cleaning products can support a healthier environment and prevent the spread of germs. Additionally, inhaling uplifting essential oils like citrus oils can enhance mood, reduce stress levels, and promote a positive outlook, contributing to overall emotional and mental health.

Aromatherapy techniques offer versatile and effective methods for promoting wellbeing and preventive health. Whether through inhalation, topical application, aromatherapy baths, diffusion, or using essential oils for prevention, integrating these practices into daily routines can support physical, emotional, and mental balance. By harnessing the natural benefits of essential oils, individuals can enhance their overall health, strengthen immunity, reduce stress, and cultivate a sense of wellbeing in their lives.

4.2 Essential Oils for Supporting Physical, Emotional, and Mental Health

Essential oils have gained popularity for their diverse therapeutic benefits in supporting physical, emotional, and mental health. Derived from aromatic plants, these oils contain concentrated compounds that interact with the body through inhalation, topical application, and sometimes ingestion, providing holistic wellness support. Here's how essential oils can benefit different aspects of health:

Physical Health

Essential oils are known for their potent properties that can support physical health in various ways:

- Pain Relief: Oils like peppermint, eucalyptus, and lavender are popular choices for their analgesic properties. They can help alleviate muscle aches, joint pain, headaches, and even chronic pain conditions like arthritis.

- Respiratory Support: Eucalyptus, tea tree, and peppermint oils are effective in promoting respiratory health. Inhalation of these oils can help clear nasal congestion, reduce inflammation in the airways, and provide relief from symptoms of allergies, colds, and sinus infections.

- Immune Boosting: Many essential oils, including lemon, tea tree, and frankincense, have antimicrobial properties that can support the immune system. They can help fend off infections, purify the air, and enhance overall immunity.

- Digestive Aid: Peppermint and ginger oils are commonly used to support digestive health. They can help alleviate symptoms of indigestion, bloating, and nausea, promoting better digestive function.

Emotional Health

Essential oils are powerful tools for emotional wellbeing and can positively influence mood and emotions:

- Stress Relief: Lavender, chamomile, and bergamot oils are renowned for their calming and stress-relieving properties. Diffusing these oils or using them in a relaxing bath can help reduce feelings of anxiety, promote relaxation, and improve overall mood.

- Mood Enhancement: Citrus oils like orange, lemon, and grapefruit are uplifting and can help uplift mood, increase energy levels, and promote a positive outlook.

- Sleep Support: Essential oils such as lavender, cedarwood, and roman chamomile are beneficial for promoting relaxation and improving sleep quality. Using these oils in a diffuser before bedtime or adding them to a bedtime routine can enhance relaxation and support restful sleep.

Mental Health

Essential oils can also support cognitive function and mental clarity:

- Focus and Concentration: Rosemary and peppermint oils are known for their stimulating properties, which can enhance focus, concentration, and cognitive performance. Diffusing these oils in a workspace or using them during study or work sessions can improve mental alertness.

- Memory Support: Oils like lemon, basil, and rosemary have been studied for their potential to support memory retention and cognitive function. Incorporating these oils into a daily routine may help improve memory recall and mental clarity.

- Emotional Balance: Frankincense and sandalwood oils are often used in aromatherapy practices to promote emotional stability, reduce feelings of anxiety, and support overall emotional balance.

Incorporating essential oils into daily routines through aromatherapy practices can provide multifaceted support for physical, emotional, and mental health. However, it's essential to use essential oils safely and according to recommended guidelines. Diluting oils with a carrier oil before topical application, using a diffuser for inhalation, and consulting with a qualified aromatherapist or healthcare professional for personalized recommendations are advisable steps. With their diverse therapeutic properties, essential oils offer a natural and holistic approach to enhancing overall health and wellbeing.

4.3 Creating Personalized Essential Oil Blends for Preventive Care

Creating personalized essential oil blends for preventive care involves understanding the therapeutic properties of different oils and tailoring them to support specific health goals. Here's how you can create effective blends for preventive care.

Understanding Essential Oil Properties

To create effective blends, it's crucial to understand the properties of various essential oils:

- Antimicrobial: Oils like tea tree, eucalyptus, and lavender have antimicrobial properties that can help ward off infections and support immune health.

- Anti-inflammatory: Oils such as chamomile, frankincense, and rosemary can reduce inflammation, which is beneficial for preventing chronic diseases and supporting overall wellness.

- Calming and Relaxing: Lavender, chamomile, and bergamot oils are known for their calming effects, which can reduce stress and promote emotional balance.

- Energizing: Citrus oils like lemon, orange, and grapefruit are uplifting and energizing, promoting vitality and mental clarity.

Tailoring Blends to Specific Needs

Depending on your health concerns and goals, you can tailor essential oil blends accordingly:

- Immune Support Blend: Create a blend using tea tree, eucalyptus, and lemon oils to support immune function and protect against seasonal illnesses. Diffuse these oils at home or use them in a roller bottle diluted with a carrier oil for topical application.

- Stress Relief Blend: Combine lavender, chamomile, and frankincense oils to create a calming blend that promotes relaxation and reduces stress levels. Use this blend in a diffuser or add a few drops to a warm bath for a soothing experience.

- Digestive Support Blend: Use peppermint, ginger, and fennel oils to create a blend that aids digestion and relieves symptoms of indigestion or bloating. Dilute this blend in a carrier oil and apply it topically to the abdomen or inhale it directly from the bottle.

Methods of Application

There are several ways to use essential oil blends for preventive care:

- Aromatherapy: Diffuse essential oils using a diffuser to purify the air and promote respiratory health. This method also helps to create a pleasant and therapeutic atmosphere in your home or workspace.

- Topical Application: Dilute essential oils with a carrier oil like coconut or jojoba oil before applying them to the skin. This method is effective for targeted relief and can be used in massage or as part of a skincare routine.

- Inhalation: Add a few drops of essential oil blend to a bowl of hot water and inhale the steam to support respiratory health and clear nasal passages.

Safety Considerations

It's essential to use essential oils safely to prevent adverse reactions:

- Always dilute essential oils before applying them to the skin to avoid irritation or sensitization.

- Conduct a patch test before using a new essential oil to check for any allergic reactions.

- Consult with a qualified aromatherapist or healthcare professional, especially if you have existing health conditions, are pregnant, or are taking medications.

Chapter 5: Mind-Body Techniques for Stress Prevention

5.1 Stress Reduction and Its Role in Preventive Health

Stress reduction plays a pivotal role in preventive health by mitigating the detrimental impact of chronic stress on the body and mind. Chronic stress is linked to a wide range of health issues, including cardiovascular disease, immune system suppression, digestive disorders, and mental health conditions such as anxiety and depression. Therefore, adopting effective stress reduction techniques is crucial for maintaining overall well-being and preventing the onset of these conditions.

One of the primary benefits of stress reduction in preventive health is its positive impact on the immune system. Prolonged stress can weaken immune function, making individuals more susceptible to infections and illnesses. By implementing stress reduction techniques such as mindfulness meditation, yoga, deep breathing exercises like the 4-7-8 technique, or regular physical activity such as brisk walking or swimming, individuals can bolster their immune response and enhance their ability to fight pathogens.

Moreover, stress reduction techniques contribute to cardiovascular health by lowering blood pressure, reducing heart rate, and decreasing the production of stress hormones like cortisol and adrenaline. High levels of these hormones over an extended period can lead to hypertension and increase the risk of heart disease. Engaging in activities that promote relaxation and calmness, such as tai chi or progressive muscle relaxation, can help maintain a healthy cardiovascular system.

Another significant aspect of stress reduction in preventive health is its role in promoting mental and emotional well-being. Chronic stress is a known contributor to anxiety, depression, and other mood disorders. By incorporating stress reduction practices into daily routines, individuals can manage and alleviate symptoms of these conditions. Art therapy, journaling, or time in nature can provide emotional support and enhance resilience against life's challenges.

Furthermore, stress reduction techniques improve sleep quality, which is essential for overall health and immune function. The value of a good night's rest cannot be overstated. Poor sleep from stress can disrupt the body's natural circadian rhythms and impair cognitive function, mood regulation, and metabolic processes. Practicing relaxation techniques before bedtime, such as calming music or a warm bath, can promote restful sleep and support optimal health, highlighting the importance of sleep in our stress management journey.

Incorporating stress reduction into preventive health strategies also extends to lifestyle modifications, including dietary choices and social interactions. A balanced diet rich in whole foods, antioxidants, and omega-3 fatty acids can provide nutritional support for stress management. But equally important are the social connections we maintain. Seeking support from friends, family, or support groups can help buffer the effects of stress and enhance overall resilience, underscoring the importance of these relationships in our health journey.

Ultimately, stress reduction techniques empower individuals to actively maintain their health and prevent the onset of chronic diseases. By cultivating mindfulness, resilience, and emotional balance through various practices, individuals can mitigate the adverse effects of stress on their physical, emotional, and mental well-being. This sense of empowerment puts individuals in control of their health, enhancing their quality of life and promoting longevity and vitality for years to come

5.2 Meditation, Mindfulness, and Relaxation Techniques

Meditation, mindfulness, and relaxation techniques are invaluable practices that promote mental clarity, emotional stability, and overall well-being. Each approach offers unique benefits while collectively contributing to reducing stress, enhancing focus, and fostering inner peace.

Meditation is a centuries-old practice rooted in various cultural and spiritual traditions. It involves focusing the mind on a particular object, thought, or activity to achieve a state of mental clarity and emotional calmness. There are several types of meditation, including mindfulness, transcendental, loving-kindness, and guided meditation. These practices differ in techniques but share the goal of cultivating awareness and presence in the moment.

On the other hand, mindfulness is a state of being fully present and engaged in the current moment, without judgment or distraction.

Mindfulness techniques can be practiced formally through meditation or informally throughout daily activities. The core principle of mindfulness involves paying attention to thoughts, sensations, and emotions as they arise, fostering a deeper understanding of oneself and one's surroundings. Mindfulness-based stress reduction (MBSR) programs have gained popularity in clinical settings for their efficacy in managing stress, anxiety, chronic pain, and improving overall mental health.

Relaxation techniques encompass a range of practices designed to induce relaxation and reduce physiological and psychological arousal. Techniques such as progressive muscle relaxation, deep breathing exercises (diaphragmatic breathing), guided imagery, and autogenic training help activate the body's relaxation response. These methods promote physical relaxation by lowering heart rate, reducing muscle tension, and calming the nervous system. By incorporating relaxation techniques into daily routines, individuals can alleviate stress, improve sleep quality, and enhance overall emotional resilience.

The benefits of meditation, mindfulness, and relaxation techniques extend beyond immediate stress relief to encompass long-term improvements in mental and physical health. Scientific research supports their effectiveness in various areas:

Stress Reduction: These practices are renowned for reducing the production of stress hormones like cortisol and adrenaline, promoting a more balanced physiological response to stressors. Regular practice can lower overall stress levels and increase resilience to future stressors.

Emotional Regulation: Meditation and mindfulness cultivate emotional awareness and regulation by fostering a non-reactive attitude towards emotions. This allows individuals to respond to challenging situations with more excellent stability and clarity.

Improved Cognitive Function: Studies have shown that meditation can enhance cognitive abilities such as attention, memory, and decision-making. Mindfulness practices encourage present-moment awareness, which can sharpen focus and concentration.

Enhanced Emotional Wellbeing: Regular practitioners often report reduced symptoms of anxiety, depression, and mood disturbances. These techniques promote positive emotions such as gratitude, compassion, and joy.

Physical Health Benefits: Beyond mental health, meditation and relaxation techniques have been associated with improved cardiovascular health, immune function, and pain management. By reducing inflammation and promoting relaxation, these practices support overall physical wellbeing.

Incorporating meditation, mindfulness, and relaxation techniques into daily life can be transformative, but consistency and commitment are key to reaping their full benefits. Beginners may start with short sessions and gradually increase duration as they become more comfortable. Integrating these practices into morning or evening routines can set a positive tone for the day or facilitate relaxation before bedtime.

Meditation, mindfulness, and relaxation techniques ultimately empower individuals to cultivate a deeper connection with themselves, manage stress more effectively, and enhance their overall quality of life. As evidence of their effectiveness grows, these practices are increasingly recognized as essential tools for promoting mental clarity, emotional resilience, and holistic wellbeing in today's fast-paced world.

5.3 Yoga and Tai Chi for Stress Management and Wellbeing

Yoga and Tai Chi are ancient practices that have gained widespread recognition for their profound benefits in promoting stress management, overall wellbeing, and holistic health. Rooted in different cultural traditions, these practices share common principles of mindfulness, breath awareness, and gentle movement, making them accessible to people of all ages and fitness levels.

Yoga, originating from ancient India, encompasses a variety of practices that unite the mind, body, and spirit. The word "yoga" itself means union, emphasizing the integration of physical postures (asanas), breath control (pranayama), and meditation to achieve a harmonious balance within oneself. There are numerous styles of yoga, ranging from vigorous and dynamic forms like Vinyasa and Power Yoga to more gentle and restorative practices such as Yin Yoga and Hatha Yoga.

Central to yoga's effectiveness in stress management is its emphasis on mindful movement and breath awareness. Practicing yoga postures not only improves flexibility, strength, and posture but also encourages present-moment awareness and relaxation. The synchronization of movement with breath helps calm the nervous system, reduce cortisol levels (the stress hormone), and promote a sense of inner peace and tranquility.

Tai Chi, also known as Tai Chi Chuan, originated in ancient China as a martial art and has evolved into a graceful form of exercise characterized by slow, flowing movements. Often described as "meditation in motion," Tai Chi integrates gentle physical movements, breath control, and mindfulness. The practice emphasizes relaxation, balance, and the smooth flow of energy (Qi or Chi) through the body's energy channels.

Both yoga and Tai Chi offer a multitude of benefits for stress management and overall wellbeing:

1. Stress Reduction: Regular practice of yoga and Tai Chi has been shown to lower stress levels by promoting relaxation responses, reducing the impact of stress hormones on the body, and enhancing resilience to stressors. The mindful, meditative aspects of these practices cultivate a sense of calm and mental clarity.

2. Physical Health: Yoga and Tai Chi improve physical fitness by increasing strength, flexibility, and balance. They support cardiovascular health, joint mobility, and muscle tone, which contribute to overall physical wellbeing and vitality.

3. Emotional Balance: These practices promote emotional resilience and wellbeing by fostering self-awareness, emotional regulation, and a positive outlook. The mindfulness cultivated through yoga and Tai Chi helps individuals manage emotions more effectively and develop a deeper sense of inner peace.

4. Mind-Body Connection: Both yoga and Tai Chi emphasize the connection between body and mind. By practicing mindful movement and breath awareness, individuals develop greater body awareness, enhance proprioception (the sense of body position), and improve coordination.

5. Cognitive Benefits: Research suggests that yoga and Tai Chi can enhance cognitive function, including memory, concentration, and decision-making abilities. These practices stimulate neuroplasticity, the brain's ability to form new connections and adapt to changes.

6. Community and Social Support: Participating in yoga classes or Tai Chi sessions provides opportunities for social interaction and community support, which are important factors in maintaining mental and emotional wellbeing.

Incorporating yoga or Tai Chi into one's daily routine can be transformative, whether practiced alone or in a group setting. Beginners can start with gentle, beginner-friendly classes and gradually progress to more advanced levels as their confidence and familiarity with the practice grow.

Ultimately, yoga and Tai Chi offer holistic approaches to stress management and overall wellbeing by integrating physical, mental, and emotional aspects of health. These ancient practices continue to be valued in modern society for their profound benefits in promoting relaxation, enhancing vitality, and fostering a balanced, harmonious lifestyle. Whether seeking stress relief, physical fitness, or inner peace, yoga and Tai Chi provide powerful tools for cultivating a healthier, more resilient mind and body.

Chapter 6: Physical Activity and Preventive Health

6.1 Benefits of Regular Exercise for Preventing Illness

Regular exercise is widely recognized as a cornerstone of preventive health. It offers a myriad of benefits that extend beyond physical fitness to encompass mental and emotional well-being. Consistent physical activity plays a crucial role in reducing the risk of chronic illnesses and promoting overall longevity.

Firstly, regular exercise contributes significantly to maintaining a healthy body weight. By burning calories and increasing metabolism, exercise helps to prevent obesity, which is a known risk factor for numerous health conditions such as type 2 diabetes, cardiovascular disease, and certain cancers. Moreover, physical activity helps build and maintain lean muscle mass, which supports metabolic health and insulin sensitivity.

Exercise also plays a pivotal role in cardiovascular health. Aerobic activities such as brisk walking, running, swimming, and cycling strengthen the heart and lungs, improving circulation and lowering blood pressure. This reduces the risk of developing heart disease, stroke, and other cardiovascular conditions. Additionally, regular exercise helps to manage cholesterol levels, increasing high-density lipoprotein (HDL) cholesterol often referred to as "good" cholesterol, and decreasing low-density lipoprotein (LDL) cholesterol, known as "bad" cholesterol.

Furthermore, physical activity is essential for enhancing immune function. Moderate exercise has been shown to boost the immune system by promoting the circulation of immune cells throughout the body, thus improving the body's ability to fight off infections and illnesses. Regular exercise also reduces inflammation, which is associated with many chronic diseases.

Beyond physical health, exercise has profound effects on mental and emotional well-being. It is a natural mood enhancer, stimulating the production of endorphins—neurotransmitters that promote happiness and relaxation. Exercise also reduces levels of stress hormones such as cortisol and adrenaline, alleviating symptoms of anxiety and depression. Regular physical activity is associated with improved sleep quality, cognitive function, and overall mental resilience.

Moreover, exercise plays a crucial role in bone health and joint function. Weight-bearing exercises such as walking, jogging, dancing, and resistance training help strengthen bones and prevent osteoporosis, a condition characterized by weak and brittle bones. Additionally, regular physical activity supports joint flexibility, reducing the risk of joint pain and stiffness associated with arthritis and other musculoskeletal disorders.

Regular exercise is essential for maintaining overall health and preventing a wide range of chronic illnesses. The American College of Sports Medicine and other health organizations recommend at least 150 minutes of moderate-intensity aerobic exercise per week and muscle-strengthening activities on two or more days per week. This can be achieved through activities such as brisk walking, jogging, swimming, cycling, dancing, or participating in sports.

Ultimately, the benefits of regular exercise extend far beyond physical fitness, encompassing mental, emotional, and overall wellbeing. By adopting a consistent exercise regimen, individuals can significantly reduce their risk of chronic diseases, enhance immune function, improve cardiovascular health, and promote longevity. Regular physical activity is a powerful preventive measure that empowers individuals to lead healthier, more vibrant lives.

6.2 Types of Physical Activities Promoting Longevity and Vitality

Physical activities promoting longevity and vitality are not just a necessity, but also a source of joy and pleasure. These exercises, which contribute to overall health and well-being, are enjoyable and essential for maintaining physical fitness, mental acuity, and emotional balance throughout life.

Aerobic exercises, such as brisk walking, jogging, swimming, cycling, and dancing, are excellent choices for promoting longevity. These activities elevate the heart rate and improve cardiovascular health by strengthening the heart and lungs. Aerobic exercises also enhance circulation, supporting the delivery of oxygen and nutrients throughout the body while removing metabolic waste products.

Strength training exercises, including weightlifting, resistance band workouts, and bodyweight exercises like push-ups, squats, and planks, are crucial for maintaining muscle mass and bone density as we age. By challenging muscles against resistance, strength training helps to preserve lean muscle tissue, which naturally declines with age. Strong muscles support joint stability, balance, and overall functional movement, reducing the risk of falls and injuries.

Flexibility and stretching exercises, such as yoga and Pilates, contribute to longevity by improving joint mobility and muscle flexibility. These activities promote better posture, range of motion, and overall body alignment, which can alleviate stiffness and discomfort associated with aging. Enhanced flexibility also supports ease of movement and reduces the likelihood of muscle strains or injuries.

Balance exercises, such as tai chi and specific yoga poses, promote longevity by enhancing stability and coordination. These activities help to improve proprioception—the body's sense of its position in space—and reduce the risk of falls, especially among older adults. Balance exercises also engage core muscles, which support posture and overall spinal health.

Incorporating various physical activities into a weekly routine is a significant achievement that promotes overall vitality and longevity. Meeting the recommended 150 minutes of moderate-intensity aerobic activity or 75 minutes of vigorous-intensity aerobic activity per week, combined with muscle-strengthening exercises on two or more days, is a source of pride. Additionally, incorporating flexibility and balance exercises two to three times per week enhances overall physical fitness and reduces the risk of injury, further adding to the sense of accomplishment.

Regular physical activity contributes to physical health and plays a significant role in mental and emotional well-being. Exercise stimulates the release of endorphins—natural mood elevators—and reduces levels of stress hormones such as cortisol and adrenaline. This can lead to improved mood, reduced anxiety and depression symptoms, and enhanced cognitive function.

Overall, maintaining an active lifestyle that includes various physical activities is a powerful tool for promoting longevity and vitality. It supports cardiovascular health, muscle strength, flexibility, balance, and mental well-being, empowering individuals to enhance their quality of life and enjoy the benefits of a healthier, more active lifestyle well into old age.

Chapter 7: Sleep and Its Importance in Preventive Health

7.1 Understanding the Role of Sleep in Overall Wellbeing

Sleep's role in overall well-being is fundamental to maintaining a healthy lifestyle and optimizing physical, mental, and emotional health. Sleep is a complex physiological process essential for the body to rest, repair, and rejuvenate. It plays a crucial role in various bodily functions, including metabolism, immune function, cognitive performance, mood regulation, and overall quality of life.

One of sleep's primary functions is to facilitate physical restoration and repair. During sleep, the body undergoes processes that repair tissues, muscles, and cells. This includes the production of growth hormone, which is essential for muscle growth and repair. Adequate sleep also supports immune function by allowing the body to produce cytokines, a protein that helps fight infections and inflammation.

Sleep is equally vital for cognitive function and mental clarity. It is critical in memory consolidation, learning, and problem-solving skills. During sleep, the brain processes information gathered throughout the day, strengthening neural connections and forming memories. Lack of sleep can impair cognitive function, leading to difficulties in concentration, decision-making, and emotional regulation.

Furthermore, sleep has a profound impact on mood and emotional well-being. Adequate sleep helps regulate mood by influencing neurotransmitter levels and emotional processing in the brain. Chronic sleep deprivation is associated with increased irritability, anxiety, and feelings of stress. Sleep also plays a role in regulating emotions, with studies showing that insufficient sleep can make it challenging to manage emotions effectively.

Regarding physical health, sleep plays a crucial role in maintaining a healthy weight and metabolism. Sleep deprivation disrupts the balance of hunger hormones, ghrelin, and leptin, leading to increased appetite and cravings for high-calorie foods. This can contribute to weight gain and metabolic disorders over time. Adequate sleep supports hormone regulation, including insulin sensitivity, crucial for maintaining blood sugar levels and reducing the risk of type 2 diabetes.

Moreover, sleep is essential for cardiovascular health. Research has shown that poor sleep quality and insufficient sleep duration are associated with an increased risk of hypertension, heart disease, and stroke. During sleep, the cardiovascular system undergoes critical vital processes, including lowering blood pressure and inflammation. Chronic sleep deprivation can disrupt these processes and contribute to cardiovascular dysfunction.

Creating a conducive sleep environment and practicing good sleep hygiene are essential for optimizing sleep quality and duration. This includes maintaining a consistent sleep schedule, establishing a relaxing bedtime routine, and ensuring a comfortable sleep environment free of disruptions. Limiting exposure to electronic devices and stimulating activities before bedtime can promote better sleep quality.

Overall, understanding the role of sleep in overall well-being underscores its importance for physical health, cognitive function, emotional regulation, and quality of life. Prioritizing adequate and restful sleep is essential for maintaining optimal well-being and supporting long-term health outcomes.

7.2 Strategies for Improving Sleep Quality

Improving sleep quality is essential for overall health and well-being, influencing everything from cognitive function to immune response and emotional stability. Here are several strategies that can help enhance sleep quality:

Firstly, establishing a consistent sleep schedule is crucial. Going to bed and waking up simultaneously every day, even on weekends, helps regulate your body's internal clock, promoting better sleep quality over time. This consistency reinforces the natural sleep-wake cycle, known as the circadian rhythm, which governs when you feel sleepy and awake.

Creating a relaxing bedtime routine can signal your body that it's time to wind down. Activities such as reading a book, taking a warm bath, or practicing relaxation techniques like deep breathing or meditation can help prepare your mind and body for sleep. Avoiding stimulating activities or electronic devices close to bedtime can promote relaxation and reduce sleep disturbances.

Ensuring a comfortable sleep environment is another critical factor. Your bedroom should be calm, quiet, and dark, as these conditions are conducive to quality sleep. Investing in a comfortable mattress and pillows that support your sleeping position can also improve sleep quality by reducing discomfort and promoting better alignment.

Limiting exposure to light, incredibly blue light emitted by screens, in the hours leading up to bedtime is crucial. Blue light suppresses melatonin production, a hormone that regulates sleep-wake cycles. Dimming the lights and using amber-colored or blue light-blocking glasses in the evening can help signal your body that it's time to prepare for sleep.

Managing stress and anxiety is essential for improving sleep quality. Stress can interfere with the ability to fall asleep and stay asleep. Stress-reducing techniques such as mindfulness meditation, progressive muscle relaxation, or journaling can help calm the mind and promote relaxation before bedtime.

Monitoring and moderating your caffeine intake is essential, as caffeine is a stimulant that can disrupt sleep patterns. Limiting caffeine consumption, especially in the afternoon and evening hours, ensures that its effects do not interfere with your ability to fall or stay asleep.

Regular physical activity has been shown to improve sleep quality by promoting relaxation and reducing insomnia symptoms. However, it's essential to time exercise appropriately. Exercising earlier in the day or at least a few hours before bedtime allows your body temperature to return to normal, promoting better sleep.

Finally, practicing good sleep hygiene involves adopting habits that support healthy sleep patterns. This includes avoiding large meals, nicotine, and alcohol close to bedtime, as these can interfere with sleep quality. Creating a sleep-friendly routine and environment that prioritizes relaxation and comfort can significantly improve sleep quality and overall well-being.

By incorporating these strategies into your daily routine and addressing any underlying sleep disorders or conditions with professional guidance, you can enhance sleep quality and reap the benefits of restorative and rejuvenating sleep for optimal health and well-being.

7.3 Creating Healthy Sleep Habits for Preventive Care

Creating healthy sleep habits is fundamental for preventive care and overall well-being. Sleep plays a crucial role in maintaining physical health, cognitive function, and emotional balance. Establishing consistent routines and optimizing your sleep environment can significantly enhance the quality and duration of your sleep, which is crucial for these aspects of your health.

Firstly, let's delve into the benefits of maintaining a regular sleep schedule. This is not just a routine, it's a commitment to your well-being. Going to bed and waking up at the same time each day, even on weekends, helps regulate your body's internal clock, known as the circadian rhythm. This consistency supports the natural sleep-wake cycle, making it easier to fall asleep and wake up refreshed. Irregular sleep patterns can disrupt this cycle, leading to sleep deprivation and potential health consequences. So, let's make a commitment to our bodies and our health by sticking to a regular sleep schedule.

Creating a bedtime routine can signal your body that it's time to wind down. Engaging in calming activities such as reading a book, taking a warm bath, or practicing relaxation techniques like deep breathing or meditation can promote relaxation and reduce stress, making it easier to transition into sleep. Avoiding stimulating activities such as intense exercise, and electronics like smartphones, tablets, and computers before bedtime is essential, as the blue light emitted by screens can suppress the production of melatonin, a hormone that regulates sleep.

Optimizing your sleep environment is essential for promoting restful sleep. Your bedroom should be relaxed, with a comfortable mattress and pillows supporting your preferred sleeping position. Ensure that the room is calm, quiet, and dark, as these conditions can enhance sleep quality. Consider using blackout curtains, earplugs, or white noise machines to minimize external noise and light disruptions.

Practicing good sleep hygiene involves adopting habits that support healthy sleep patterns. Sleep hygiene refers to a variety of different practices and habits that are necessary to have good nighttime sleep quality and full daytime alertness. Avoid consuming large meals, caffeine, nicotine, and alcohol close to bedtime, as these substances can interfere with your ability to fall asleep and stay asleep. Limiting daytime naps and establishing a relaxing pre-sleep routine can also improve sleep quality.

Managing stress and anxiety is not just a suggestion, it's a powerful tool in your arsenal for improving sleep habits and overall well-being. Chronic stress can disrupt sleep patterns and lead to insomnia. But you have the power to change that. Stress-reducing activities such as mindfulness meditation, progressive muscle relaxation, or journaling can help calm the mind and promote relaxation before bedtime. Addressing underlying stressors and developing effective coping strategies are essential in creating a supportive sleep environment. So, let's take control of our stress and take back our sleep.

Regular physical activity is not just good for your body, it's great for your sleep. It can promote better sleep by reducing anxiety and promoting relaxation. However, it's essential to time exercise appropriately. Exercising earlier in the day or at least a few hours before bedtime allows your body temperature to return to normal, which can facilitate falling asleep. So, let's lace up our shoes and get moving for a better night's sleep.

Book 22: Integrating Herbal Remedies into Daily Life

Practical Strategies for Enhancing Health and Well-Being Through Nature

Chapter 1: Tips for Incorporating herbs into your daily routine

Incorporating herbs into your daily routine can be a simple and rewarding way to enhance your overall health and well-being. Herbs offer a natural, holistic approach to managing various health concerns and promoting a balanced lifestyle. Here are some practical tips to help you seamlessly integrate herbs into your everyday life:

1) Start with a Morning Routine

One of the easiest ways to include herbs in your daily routine is by starting your morning with herbal teas or infusions. Herbal teas such as green tea, peppermint, or chamomile can offer a gentle boost of energy or calmness to kickstart your day. Here's how you can do it:

Select an herb that aligns with your morning needs. For energy and focus, consider green tea or ginseng. For a calm and centered start, try chamomile or lemon balm.

Boil water and pour it over the selected herb in teabag or loose-leaf form. Let it steep for 5-10 minutes.

Sip your herbal tea while planning your day or during your morning meditation.

2) Incorporate Herbs into Meals

Adding herbs to your meals is an excellent way to reap their health benefits without altering your routine significantly. Fresh and dried herbs can enhance your dishes' flavor and nutritional value. Here are some ideas:

Cooking with Fresh Herbs. Add herbs like basil, oregano, thyme, or rosemary to your soups, stews, and salads. You can also blend fresh herbs into sauces and dressings.

Herbal Spices. When cooking, use powdered herbs such as turmeric, ginger, and cinnamon. These spices not only add flavor but also provide various health benefits.

Herbal Oils and Vinegars. Infuse olive oil or vinegar with herbs like garlic, rosemary, or thyme. Use these infused oils and vinegars as dressings for salads or marinades for meats.

3) Use Herbal Supplements

Herbal supplements are a convenient way to incorporate herbs into your daily routine, especially if you have a busy lifestyle. These supplements are available in various forms, including capsules, tinctures, and powders.

Capsules: Herbal capsules are easy to take and can be included in your daily vitamin regimen. For example, consider taking a daily ashwagandha capsule for stress management or a turmeric capsule for anti-inflammatory benefits.

<u>Tinctures</u>: Herbal tinctures are concentrated extracts of herbs. They can be taken directly or added to water or juice. For instance, a few drops of echinacea tincture can support your immune system.

<u>Powders</u>: Herbal powders can be mixed into smoothies, yogurt, or oatmeal. Spirulina, chlorella, and maca powders are popular for boosting energy and nutrition.

4) Herbal Baths and Skin Care

Incorporating herbs into your skincare and self-care routines can enhance relaxation and promote healthy skin. Herbal baths and homemade skincare products are excellent ways to enjoy the benefits of herbs.

Add dried herbs or essential oils to your bathwater. Lavender, chamomile, and rose petals are perfect for a relaxing bath. Place the herbs in a muslin bag or add a few drops of essential oil.

Create DIY skincare products using herbs. For example, make a soothing face mask with honey and turmeric, or use aloe vera gel for its moisturizing properties. Herbal-infused oils, like calendula oil, can be used as natural moisturizers.

5) Stay Consistent

Consistency is key when it comes to reaping the benefits of herbal remedies. Make a habit of incorporating herbs into your routine, and give your body time to adjust and respond. Here are some tips for staying consistent:

Use a journal or an app to remind you to take herbal supplements or prepare herbal tea. Add herbs to activities you already do daily. For instance, you can add herbal tinctures to your morning smoothie or take a relaxing herbal bath as part of your evening wind-down routine. Not all herbs will work the same way for everyone. Feel free to experiment with different herbs and methods until you find what works best.

6) Educate Yourself

Understanding the properties and uses of different herbs can help you make informed choices about which herbs to incorporate into your routine. Here are some ways to educate yourself:

Numerous resources are available on herbal medicine. Invest in a few good books or follow reputable websites and blogs. Enroll in online or local courses on herbal medicine to gain a deeper understanding. Don't hesitate to seek advice from herbalists or healthcare providers who are knowledgeable about herbal medicine.

Following these tips, you can seamlessly incorporate herbs into your daily routine and enjoy their numerous health benefits. Herbs offer a natural and effective solution to boost your energy, manage stress, or enhance your overall well-being. Always consult a healthcare professional before starting any new herbal regimen to ensure it is safe and appropriate for your specific health needs.

Chapter 2: Additional tips for your daily routine

Incorporating herbs into your daily routine can significantly enhance your health and well-being. Beyond the foundational tips, numerous creative and practical ways to make herbs a regular part of your life exist. Here are additional tips to help you seamlessly integrate herbs into your everyday activities.

1) Herbal Smoothies and Juices

Incorporate herbs into your smoothies and juices for an easy and delicious way to enjoy their benefits.

Green Smoothies: Add herbs like parsley, cilantro, or mint to your green smoothies. These herbs not only provide a nutritional boost but also add fresh flavor.

Herbal Juices: Mix fresh herbs such as basil, mint, or dandelion greens into your vegetable juices. Spinach, cucumber, and mint make a refreshing and healthful drink.

2) Herbal Snacks

Herbs can be added to snacks for an extra health kick.

Herbal Dips: Make dips using herbs like dill, chives, or parsley. For example, a yogurt-based dip with garlic and dill is tasty and beneficial for digestion.

Herb-Infused Snacks: Prepare herbal popcorn by tossing freshly popped corn with olive oil and dried herbs such as rosemary or thyme. You can also bake kale chips seasoned with sea salt and herbs.

3) Incorporating Herbs into Desserts

Herbs can enhance the flavor and health benefits of your desserts.

For a unique and refreshing dessert, infuse your homemade ice cream with herbs like lavender, mint, or basil.

Infuse honey with herbs such as lavender, thyme, or chamomile. Drizzle this herbal honey over desserts like yogurt, fruit, or pancakes.

4) Herbal Oils and Vinegars

Infusing oils and vinegars with herbs can make meal preparation more flavorful and healthful.

Herbal Olive Oil: Create your own herbal-infused olive oil using rosemary, basil, or garlic. Use this oil for cooking or as a salad dressing.

Herbal Vinegar: Infuse vinegar with herbs like tarragon, thyme, or oregano. These vinegars can be used in dressings, marinades, or as a tangy addition to cooked vegetables.

5) Herbal Ice Cubes

Make herbal ice cubes to add flavor and health benefits to your drinks. Freeze herbs like mint, basil, or lemon balm in ice cube trays with water. Add these cubes to your water, iced tea, or cocktails for a refreshing twist.

6) Using Herbs in Baking

Herbs can add unique flavors to your baked goods.

Add rosemary, thyme, or sage to bread dough before baking. Herbal breads are delicious and pair well with soups and salads.

Incorporate herbs into baked goods like cookies, cakes, and muffins. Lavender cookies or rosemary shortbread are delightful examples.

7) Herbal Baths and Skincare

Enhance your self-care routine with herbs for relaxation and skin health.

Create bath salts with dried herbs like lavender, chamomile, or calendula. Mix these with Epsom salts and a few essential oils for a relaxing bath. Prepare a facial steam with herbs like chamomile, rosemary, and mint. Boil water, add the herbs, and lean over the bowl with a towel over your head to capture the steam.

8) Growing Your Herbs

Growing herbs home ensures a fresh supply and enhances your connection to natural remedies.

Start a small herb garden in your backyard or pots on your windowsill. Herbs like basil, mint, and rosemary are easy to grow and maintain. If outdoor space is limited, consider indoor planters for herbs. Grow lights can help provide the necessary conditions for year-round growth.

9) Herbal Supplements for Pets

Incorporate herbs into your pet care routine for their health and well-being. Make homemade pet treats using pet-safe herbs like parsley or chamomile. These treats can help with digestion and anxiety. Consult a veterinarian about adding herbal supplements like milk thistle or turmeric to your pet's diet for liver health and anti-inflammatory benefits.

10) Herbal Wellness Rituals

Establishing wellness rituals can make herbs a meaningful part of your day.

Develop an evening routine with a calming herbal tea like chamomile or valerian root to promote restful sleep.

Take a break during the day with a refreshing herbal tea such as peppermint or ginseng to boost energy and focus.

11) Staying Educated and Engaged

Continuously learning about herbs can keep you motivated and informed.

Participate in online forums, local herbal groups, or social media communities dedicated to herbal medicine. Sharing experiences and tips can enhance your knowledge and keep you engaged.

Look for workshops, webinars, and classes on herbal medicine. Learning from experts can provide deeper insights and practical skills.

12) Creating Herbal Routines for Family

Incorporate herbs into your family's daily routines for collective health benefits.

Create a family tradition of drinking herbal tea together. Choose kid-friendly herbs like lemon balm or chamomile for a safe and enjoyable experience.

Teach children about the benefits of herbs through fun activities like planting a small herb garden or making herbal crafts.

By following these additional tips, you can more effectively integrate herbs into your daily routine and enjoy their numerous health benefits. Whether through your diet, skincare, self-care rituals, or even pet care, herbs offer a versatile and natural approach to enhancing your well-being. Always consult with a healthcare professional before starting any new herbal regimen to ensure it is appropriate for your specific needs and health conditions.

Chapter 3: Lifestyle changes and dietary advice

Embracing lifestyle changes and making informed dietary choices can significantly enhance your health and well-being. These changes are fundamental to supporting the body's natural healing processes and maintaining long-term vitality. Here are some practical and effective lifestyle changes and dietary advice to incorporate into your daily routine.

3.1 Balanced Diet

A balanced diet provides your body with the essential nutrients to function optimally.

Whole Foods: Focus on consuming whole, unprocessed foods such as fruits, vegetables, whole grains, lean proteins, and healthy fats. These foods are rich in vitamins, minerals, and antioxidants that support overall health.

Variety: Include a variety of colors and types of foods in your diet. Different foods provide different nutrients, so eating a wide range ensures a comprehensive nutritional profile.

Portion Control: Be mindful of portion sizes to avoid overeating. Eating smaller, more frequent meals can help maintain steady energy levels throughout the day.

Hydration: Drink plenty of water to stay hydrated. Proper hydration is essential for digestion, nutrient absorption, and overall bodily functions.

3.2 Incorporating Herbs into Your Diet

Herbs can be a valuable addition to your diet, providing flavor and health benefits.

1) Herbal Teas

Replace sugary drinks with herbal teas such as green tea, chamomile, or peppermint. These teas are not only refreshing but also offer various health benefits.

2) Cooking with Herbs

Use fresh and dried herbs like basil, oregano, thyme, and rosemary in your cooking. They can enhance the flavor of your meals and provide additional nutrients.

3) Herbal Supplements

Consider taking herbal supplements to support specific health goals. Always consult with a healthcare provider before starting any new supplement.

3.3 Regular Physical Activity

Regular physical activity is essential for maintaining a healthy weight, improving cardiovascular health, and boosting overall well-being.

Exercise Routine: Aim for at least 150 minutes of moderate-intensity weekly exercise. This can include activities like brisk walking, cycling, or swimming.

Strength Training: Include strength training exercises at least twice weekly to build and maintain muscle mass.

Flexibility and Balance: Incorporate exercises that enhance flexibility and balance, such as yoga or tai chi. These activities can improve posture, reduce the risk of injury, and promote relaxation.

3.4 Stress Management

Effective stress management is vital for maintaining mental and emotional health.

1) Mindfulness and Meditation

Practice mindfulness and meditation techniques to reduce stress and enhance mental clarity. Even a few minutes a day can make a significant difference.

2) Deep Breathing

Engage in deep breathing exercises to calm the mind and reduce anxiety. Techniques such as diaphragmatic breathing can be very effective.

3) Hobbies and Interests

Make time for hobbies and activities that you enjoy. Engaging in creative or recreational activities can be a great way to relieve stress.

3.5 Adequate Sleep

Getting enough sleep is essential for overall health and well-being.

Maintain a consistent sleep schedule by going to bed and waking up at the same time every day, even on weekends.

Create a conducive sleep environment by keeping your bedroom cool, dark, and quiet. Invest in a comfortable mattress and pillows.

Develop a wind-down routine to signal your body that it's time to sleep. This could include reading, taking a warm bath, or practicing gentle stretching exercises.

3.6 Limiting Unhealthy Habits

Reducing or eliminating unhealthy habits is crucial for long-term health.

1) Avoid Smoking

If you smoke, seek help to quit. Smoking is linked to numerous health problems, and quitting can significantly improve your health.

2) Limit Alcohol

Limit alcohol consumption to moderate levels. For most adults, this means up to one drink per day for women and two for men.

3) Reduce Sugar and Processed Foods

Minimize your intake of added sugars and highly processed foods, which can contribute to weight gain and chronic health conditions.

3.7 Regular Health Check-Ups

Regular health check-ups and screenings are essential for early detection and prevention of health issues.

Schedule regular check-ups with your healthcare provider to monitor your health and address concerns early.

Based on your age and risk factors, participate in recommended preventive screenings, such as blood pressure checks, cholesterol tests, and cancer screenings.

Stay informed about your health conditions and treatment options. Being proactive and knowledgeable can help you make better health decisions.

You can significantly improve your overall health and well-being by making these lifestyle changes and following this dietary advice. These changes are not only beneficial for your physical health but also for your mental and emotional well-being. Consistency is key, and minor, incremental changes can lead to significant long-term benefits. Always consult with healthcare professionals when making substantial changes to your diet or lifestyle to ensure they are appropriate for your health needs.

Chapter 4: How to improve preventive health measures

Improving preventive health measures is essential for safeguarding long-term well-being and reducing the likelihood of developing chronic illnesses. Individuals can effectively enhance their overall quality of life by integrating a holistic approach to health management. Here are comprehensive strategies and tips to elevate your preventive health efforts:

1) Maintain a Nutrient-Rich Diet

Embrace a balanced diet emphasizing whole foods such as fruits, vegetables, whole grains, lean proteins, and healthy fats. This diet, by minimizing processed foods, sugars, and excessive salt intake, fortifies your body with essential vitamins, minerals, and antioxidants crucial for immune function and overall vitality, thereby playing a key role in preventive health.

2) Regular Physical Activity

Incorporate regular exercise into your routine to support cardiovascular health, muscular strength, and flexibility. By committing to at least 150 minutes of moderate-intensity aerobic activity per week, supplemented with strength training exercises, you can take control of your fitness levels and promote longevity, a key goal of preventive health. This empowerment over your health can instill a sense of confidence and well-being.

3) Optimize Sleep Patterns

Establish consistent sleep patterns by creating a conducive sleep environment and adhering to a regular sleep schedule. Strive for 7-9 hours of quality sleep per night to facilitate optimal cognitive function, mood regulation, and physical recovery, all of which are crucial for preventive health.

4) Stress Management Techniques

Implement stress-reduction strategies such as mindfulness meditation, deep breathing exercises, yoga, or tai chi to mitigate the adverse effects of chronic stress. Cultivating relaxation techniques fosters emotional resilience, improves mental clarity, and supports overall mental health.

5) Avoid Harmful Substances

Limit alcohol consumption and refrain from smoking or using recreational drugs, as these habits significantly increase the risk of cardiovascular diseases, respiratory ailments, and various cancers. Adopting a smoke-free lifestyle and practicing moderation with alcohol promotes long-term health and well-being.

6) Hydration and Hygiene Practices

Drink plenty of water throughout the day to maintain adequate hydration. Proper hydration supports optimal bodily functions, aids digestion, and enhances skin health. Additionally, practice good hygiene by washing hands frequently with soap and water to prevent the spread of infections and maintain overall cleanliness.

7) Social Engagement

Cultivate a strong support network and foster meaningful connections with family, friends, and community members. Social interaction promotes mental well-being, reduces feelings of isolation, and enhances overall life satisfaction. It also contributes to emotional resilience and improves overall quality of life. This sense of connection and support can make your health journey more enjoyable and rewarding, making you feel more connected and less isolated.

8) Educate and Empower Yourself

Stay informed about current health guidelines, preventive screenings, and vaccination recommendations relevant to your age, gender, and medical history. Regularly consult healthcare professionals for personalized health assessments, preventive screenings, and tailored advice to optimize your preventive health efforts. This knowledge and control over your health can empower you to make informed decisions about your well-being.

By embracing and incorporating these comprehensive strategies into your daily routine, you can proactively manage your health and reduce the risk of developing chronic diseases. Adopting a proactive approach to preventive health empowers individuals to cultivate resilience, vitality, and longevity, promoting a higher quality of life both now and in the future. Remember, small, consistent steps toward better health yield significant long-term benefits.

Book 23: Advanced Techniques and Formulations

Elevating Your Herbal Practice with Expert Methods and Innovations

Chapter 1: Creating complex herbal blends

Creating complex herbal blends involves combining various herbs thoughtfully to achieve synergistic health benefits and balanced flavors. Understanding each herb's properties and interactions is critical to creating effective and enjoyable blends, whether you're crafting teas, tinctures, salves, or culinary mixes. Here's a detailed exploration of how to create complex herbal blends:

Before blending herbs, it's essential to grasp their properties, including taste, aroma, medicinal qualities, and potential interactions. Herbs can be categorized based on their primary effects:

Adaptogens: Herbs like ashwagandha, rhodiola, and holy basil help the body adapt to stress and support overall resilience.

Nervines: Herbs such as chamomile, lemon balm, and passionflower have calming effects on the nervous system, promoting relaxation and reducing anxiety.

Digestives: Herbs like peppermint, ginger, and fennel aid digestion, relieve bloating, and support gastrointestinal health.

Anti-inflammatories: Herbs such as turmeric, ginger, and boswellia reduce inflammation in the body, easing conditions like arthritis and promoting joint health.

Antimicrobials: Herbs like garlic, oregano, and thyme have antimicrobial properties that help fight infections and support immune function.

Circulatory Tonics: Herbs such as hawthorn, ginkgo, and cayenne improve circulation and cardiovascular health.

1.1 Principles of Herbal Blending

Establishing a Purpose

Define the goal of your blend. Are you creating a tea for relaxation, a tincture for immune support, or a salve for skin healing? Clarifying your intention guides herb selection and proportions.

Selecting Complementary Herbs

Choose herbs that complement each other in flavor and function. Consider their medicinal properties and potential interactions to create a balanced blend. For example:

Blend bitter herbs like dandelion with sweeter herbs like licorice to improve palatability.

Combine calming nervines like chamomile with digestive herbs like peppermint for a soothing digestive tea.

Mix herbs with different medicinal actions, such as anti-inflammatory turmeric with adaptogenic ashwagandha, for a multi-purpose blend.

Understanding Dosages and Potencies

Ensure you understand each herb's recommended dosages and potencies to avoid adverse effects and optimize therapeutic benefits. Start with small quantities and adjust ratios based on personal preferences and desired effects.

Considering Synergy and Interaction

Some herbs work synergistically, enhancing each other's effects when combined. For instance:

Turmeric and Black Pepper: Black pepper enhances the absorption of curcumin, the active compound in turmeric, maximizing its anti-inflammatory benefits.

Chamomile and Lemon Balm: Combining these calming nervines amplifies their relaxing effects on the nervous system.

1.2 Methods for Blending Herbs

Tea Blends

Teas are a popular way to blend herbs for medicinal and culinary purposes. To create herbal tea blends:

Combine herbs in varying ratios based on their desired effects (e.g., 1 part chamomile, 1 part lemon balm, 1/2-part lavender).

Steep the blend in hot water for 5-10 minutes, adjusting steeping times based on herb potency.

Taste test to adjust flavors and potency before straining and serving.

Tinctures and Extracts

Tinctures are concentrated herbal extracts made by soaking herbs in alcohol or glycerin. To create tincture blends:

Calculate herb ratios based on desired potency (e.g., 1:2 herb-to-alcohol ratio for fresh herbs, 1:5 for dried). Allow herbs to macerate in alcohol or glycerin for 4-6 weeks, shaking daily to extract medicinal compounds.

Strain and Store: Strain the liquid in dark glass bottles in a cool, dark place for long-term preservation.

Salves and Ointments

Salves and ointments blend herbs with oils or beeswax for topical applications. To create herbal salves:

Infuse dried herbs in carrier oils like olive or coconut over low heat for several hours.

Strain the oil and mix with beeswax to create a solid salve or ointment consistency.

Pour into containers and allow to cool and solidify before sealing and storing in a cool, dark place.

1.3 Safety and Considerations

Be mindful of potential allergens and sensitivities when blending herbs, especially if individuals have known allergies.

Consult with an herbalist or healthcare provider, especially when blending for specific health conditions or taking medications.

Label blends with ingredients, proportions, and instructions to ensure safe and effective use.

Creating complex herbal blends is both an art and a science, requiring knowledge of herbal properties, careful selection, and thoughtful formulation. Whether crafting teas, tinctures, or salves, mastering these principles allows for creating effective and enjoyable herbal remedies tailored to individual health needs and preferences.

Chapter 2: Use herbs in combination with other natural therapies

Using herbs in combination with other natural therapies can enhance their effectiveness and provide comprehensive support for various health concerns. Integrating herbs with complementary therapies such as aromatherapy, acupuncture, dietary adjustments, and lifestyle modifications offers a holistic approach to health and wellness. Here's an exploration of how herbs can synergize with other natural therapies:

Aromatherapy

Aromatherapy involves using essential oils extracted from plants to promote physical, emotional, and mental well-being. When combined with herbal remedies, aromatherapy can amplify therapeutic benefits and enhance overall treatment outcomes. For example:

- Essential Oil Blends: Creating synergistic blends of essential oils and herbal extracts can target specific health issues, such as lavender and chamomile for relaxation or eucalyptus and peppermint for respiratory support.

- Application Methods: Inhalation of essential oils through diffusers or topical application in diluted forms can complement herbal treatments, providing both aromatic and medicinal benefits.

Acupuncture

Acupuncture is a traditional Chinese medicine practice that involves inserting thin needles into specific points on the body to stimulate energy flow and promote healing. When combined with herbal therapy:

- Enhanced Energy Flow: Herbs such as ginger or ginseng can be used in conjunction with acupuncture to strengthen the body's energy (qi) and enhance treatment outcomes for conditions like chronic pain or digestive disorders.

- Holistic Treatment: Acupuncture and herbal remedies together provide a holistic approach to addressing underlying imbalances and promoting overall health and well-being.

Dietary Adjustments

Diet plays a crucial role in overall health and can significantly impact the effectiveness of herbal therapies. Integrating herbs into a balanced diet:

- Nutritional Support: Incorporating herbs like turmeric, garlic, and ginger into daily meals can provide additional nutritional support and enhance immune function, digestion, and overall vitality.

- Herbal Supplements: Herbal supplements, such as capsules or powders, can complement dietary adjustments by providing concentrated doses of beneficial herbs for specific health goals.

Lifestyle Modifications

Lifestyle factors, including stress management, sleep hygiene, and physical activity, greatly influence health outcomes. Combining herbal therapies with lifestyle modifications:

- Stress Reduction: Herbs like ashwagandha or holy basil can be used alongside relaxation techniques such as yoga or meditation to support stress management and promote emotional well-being.

- Sleep Support: Herbal teas such as chamomile or valerian root can aid in improving sleep quality when combined with bedtime routines that promote relaxation and restfulness.

Integrative Wellness Plans

Developing personalized integrative wellness plans that incorporate multiple natural therapies:

- Individualized Approach: Herbalists, naturopathic doctors, or integrative healthcare providers can create customized treatment plans that integrate herbs with other natural therapies based on individual health needs, preferences, and goals.

- Collaborative Care: Working collaboratively with healthcare professionals ensures comprehensive support and holistic management of health conditions, fostering optimal outcomes and patient satisfaction.

Safety and Consultation

- Professional Guidance: It's essential to consult with qualified healthcare providers or herbalists when combining herbs with other natural therapies, especially if managing chronic conditions or taking medications.

- Potential Interactions: Be aware of potential interactions between herbs and other therapies, ensuring safe and effective integration into treatment protocols.

- Monitoring and Adjustments: Regular monitoring and adjustments to treatment plans may be necessary to optimize therapeutic benefits and address individual responses to combined therapies.

By incorporating herbs into comprehensive wellness strategies that include aromatherapy, acupuncture, dietary adjustments, and lifestyle modifications, individuals can harness the synergistic benefits of natural therapies for enhanced health and well-being. This integrative approach supports holistic healing and empowers individuals to take proactive steps towards achieving and maintaining optimal health naturally.

Chapter 3: Troubleshooting of common problems in herbal preparations

Troubleshooting common issues in herbal preparations is essential for ensuring the effectiveness, safety, and quality of herbal remedies. Whether you're creating herbal teas, tinctures, salves, or other preparations, encountering challenges is common but manageable with the right knowledge and approach. Here's a comprehensive guide to troubleshooting common issues in herbal preparations:

3.1 Insufficient Potency or Effectiveness

- Herb Quality: Ensure you're using high-quality herbs from reputable sources. Low-quality or old herbs may lack potency due to degradation of active compounds.

- Dosage: Review the dosage and proportion of herbs used in your preparation. Adjust the quantity of herbs to achieve the desired therapeutic effect.

- Extraction Time: Extend the steeping or maceration time for teas or tinctures to maximize extraction of medicinal compounds.

- Herb Freshness: Use fresh herbs whenever possible, as dried herbs lose potency over time. Consider growing your own herbs for optimal freshness.

3.2 Bitter or Unpleasant Taste

- Herb Selection: Choose herbs with milder flavors or balance bitter herbs with sweeter ones in blends. For example, mix dandelion with licorice root in teas to improve palatability.

- Steeping Time: Shorten the steeping time for teas or dilute tinctures with water or juice to reduce bitterness.

- Flavor Masking: Incorporate natural sweeteners like honey or stevia, or add citrus fruits or spices to mask bitter flavors.

- Cold Infusion: For sensitive herbs, use cold infusion methods that extract fewer bitter compounds.

3.3 Herb Sediment or Residue

- Straining Methods: Use fine mesh strainers or cheesecloth to remove sediment from herbal infusions or tinctures.

- Clarification: Allow herbal preparations to settle, then decant or carefully pour off the clear liquid while leaving sediment behind.

- Filtering Techniques: Consider using coffee filters or muslin bags for finer filtration of herbal extracts.

- Shaking Before Use: Shake tinctures well before use to redistribute any settled particles and ensure even distribution of active compounds.

3.4 Mold or Spoilage

- Proper Storage: Store herbal preparations in airtight containers in cool, dark places to prevent exposure to moisture and light.

- Alcohol Content: Ensure tinctures have sufficient alcohol content (at least 25-30% or higher) to preserve the preparation and inhibit mold growth.

- Quality Control: Inspect herbs for signs of mold or decay before preparation. Discard any herbs that appear moldy or have an off smell.

- Sanitization: Use clean utensils, containers, and hands during preparation to minimize contamination risks.

3.5 Allergic Reactions or Side Effects

- Individual Sensitivities: Be aware of potential allergens or sensitivities to specific herbs. Conduct patch tests or start with small doses to assess tolerance.

- Consultation: Consult with a healthcare professional or herbalist before starting herbal treatments, especially if you have underlying health conditions or are taking medications.

- Herb Interactions: Research potential interactions between herbs and medications. Adjust formulations or avoid herbs that may interfere with prescribed treatments.

- Discontinue Use: Discontinue use and seek medical advice if allergic reactions or adverse effects occur. Keep a record of herbs used and symptoms experienced for future reference.

3.6 Weak Color or Aroma

- Herb Quality: Use fresh, vibrant herbs with strong color and aroma for optimal sensory appeal and potency.

- Storage Conditions: Store dried herbs in airtight containers away from light and moisture to preserve color and aroma.

- Extraction Methods: Ensure proper extraction methods are used, such as heat infusion for teas or longer maceration times for tinctures, to enhance color and aroma.

- Blending Techniques: Blend herbs with complementary colors and aromas to create balanced and visually appealing preparations.

3.7 Clumping or Separation

- Emulsification: Use emulsifiers like vegetable glycerin or lecithin when combining herbs with oils or water-based solvents to prevent clumping.

- Agitation: Stir or shake herbal mixtures thoroughly during preparation to ensure even distribution of ingredients and prevent separation.

- Temperature Control: Maintain consistent temperatures during preparation and storage to prevent ingredients from separating.

- Quality Ingredients: Use high-quality, compatible ingredients in formulations to minimize clumping or separation issues.

3.8 General Tips for Successful Herbal Preparations

- Documentation: Keep detailed records of herbal recipes, including ingredients, proportions, and preparation methods, to replicate successful formulations.

- Quality Assurance: Source herbs from reputable suppliers and conduct quality checks to ensure purity and potency.

- Labeling: Clearly label herbal preparations with ingredients, dosage instructions, and expiration dates for safe and effective use.

- Continuous Learning: Stay informed about herbal medicine practices and techniques through reputable sources, workshops, or professional associations.

Chapter 4: Testimonials about the application of advanced techniques

Integrating advanced herbal techniques into daily health routines has proven transformative for many individuals seeking natural solutions to various health challenges. However, it's important to consult a healthcare professional before making any significant changes to your health regimen. Here are detailed testimonials from individuals who have experienced significant benefits from incorporating these herbal practices into their lifestyles.

Sarah B.: *"For years, I struggled with irritable bowel syndrome (IBS) that affected my daily life. Traditional medications provided only temporary relief and came with side effects. Seeking a natural approach, I consulted with an herbalist who crafted personalized herbal tinctures tailored to my digestive needs. Combining herbs like peppermint, chamomile, and marshmallow root, these tinctures have remarkably reduced my IBS symptoms. I no longer experience frequent bloating or abdominal discomfort, and my digestion feels more balanced. Integrating these herbal blends into my routine has been transformative, allowing me to regain control over my gut health without the drawbacks of conventional treatments."*

Michael S.: *"As someone who struggled with insomnia for years, finding effective remedies was a priority. Herbal teas suggested by my holistic practitioner, infused with herbs like valerian, passionflower, and lemon balm, have become my nightly ritual. The calming effects of these blends have significantly improved my sleep quality. I now fall asleep faster and wake up feeling refreshed, without the grogginess I experienced with prescription sleep aids. Incorporating these herbal teas into my bedtime routine has improved my sleep and enhanced my overall well-being, allowing me to approach each day with more energy and clarity."*

Emily R.: *"Athletic pursuits have always been a passion, but muscle soreness and joint stiffness often hindered my progress. Discovering herbal salves enriched with arnica, ginger, and cayenne through my herbalist's guidance has been a game-changer. These natural remedies provide immediate relief and promote faster recovery after intense workouts. The anti-inflammatory properties of these herbs soothe sore muscles and reduce joint pain, allowing me to maintain peak performance without relying on over-the-counter pain relievers. Incorporating these herbal salves into my fitness regimen has eased my physical discomfort and supported my long-term athletic goals."*

John K.: *"Managing stress in a demanding job has constantly challenged me. Seeking alternatives to traditional stress management techniques, I turned to adaptogenic herbs recommended by a wellness coach. Incorporating ashwagandha, Rhodiola, and holy basil into my daily routine has been transformative. These herbs help my body adapt to stress, enhance resilience, and promote well-being. Since integrating these adaptogens, I've noticed a significant reduction in anxiety levels and a more balanced mood throughout the day. These herbal blends have become vital to my self-care regimen, providing sustainable support in navigating life's pressures."*

Anna L.: *"Seasonal allergies have plagued me for years, challenging springtime activities due to sinus congestion and itchy eyes. Dissatisfied with the side effects of allergy medications, I explored herbal remedies like nettle leaf and elderflower under the guidance of an herbalist. Incorporating these herbs into my daily routine through teas and nasal rinses has been incredibly effective. I now experience milder allergy symptoms and improved respiratory health without the drowsiness caused by antihistamines. These natural solutions have allowed me to enjoy outdoor activities more comfortably, free from the usual allergy-related discomforts."*

Book 24: Herbal Remedies for Special Categories of people

Tailoring Natural Solutions for Unique Needs and Conditions

Chapter 1: Considerations for children

Considerations for children when using herbal remedies are crucial to ensure safety, efficacy, and appropriateness for their developing bodies. While herbs can offer gentle and practical support for children's health, it's essential to approach their use with careful consideration and informed guidance. Here's a comprehensive look at factors to consider when considering herbal remedies for children.

1.1 Safety and Dosage

The safety of herbal remedies for children hinges on several critical factors, including dosage, formulation, and age-appropriate considerations.

Unlike adults, children require smaller doses of herbs due to their smaller body size and different metabolic rates. Herbalists and healthcare providers, with their expertise, typically adjust dosages based on a child's age, weight, and health condition to minimize the risk of adverse effects, providing you with the reassurance and confidence you need.

It's important to note that while herbal remedies can be beneficial, they also carry potential risks and side effects. For instance, some herbs may cause allergic reactions or interact with medications. Therefore, it's crucial to research each herb thoroughly and consult with a healthcare professional or qualified herbalist before use. This will help ensure the safety and effectiveness of the herbal remedy for your child.

Different herbs are suitable for children at different stages of development. Gentle herbs like chamomile or catnip may be used for soothing digestive discomfort or promoting relaxation in infants and toddlers. As children grow older, herbs such as elderberry or echinacea may be introduced to support immune function during cold and flu seasons.

1.2 Choosing Suitable Herbs

Appropriate herbs for children involves considering their safety profile, efficacy, and potential interactions.

Some herbs are generally considered safe (GRAS) for children when used appropriately, such as chamomile for calming or ginger for digestive support. However, it's crucial to research each herb thoroughly and consult with a healthcare professional or qualified herbalist before use.

Herbs chosen for children should align with their specific health needs and conditions. For example, herbs like lemon balm may be beneficial for anxiety or restlessness, while calendula can soothe minor skin irritations.

Consider any potential interactions between herbs and medications your child may be taking. It's essential to inform healthcare providers about all herbal supplements to avoid adverse effects or interactions.

1.3 Administration and Compliance

Administering herbal remedies to children requires patience and careful attention to their preferences and reactions.

Many herbal preparations for children are formulated to be palatable, such as flavored syrups or herbal teas mixed with honey. Ensuring a pleasant taste can enhance compliance and effectiveness.

Depending on the child's age and preferences, herbal remedies can be administered in various ways, including mixing with food or drinks, using droppers for precise dosing, or applying topically in the case of salves or ointments.

Monitor your child's response to herbal remedies regularly and adjust dosages or formulations as needed. This adaptability empowers you to be in control of your child's health, paying attention to any changes in symptoms or adverse reactions, and consulting with healthcare providers if concerns arise.

1.4 Common Uses for Children

Herbal remedies can support various aspects of children's health and well-being:

Herbs like ginger, fennel, or peppermint can help relieve gas, bloating, or nausea in children and promote comfortable digestion.

Herbs such as elderberry, echinacea, or astragalus may help strengthen the immune system and reduce the frequency of colds or flu.

Calendula, chamomile, or lavender can be used topically to soothe minor skin irritations, diaper rash, or insect bites.

Herbs like lemon balm or passionflower may help calm anxiety, promote relaxation, or support healthy sleep patterns in children.

1.5 Considerations for Special Categories of People

Certain populations of children may require additional considerations when using herbal remedies:

Herbal remedies for infants should be used with caution and under the guidance of a healthcare provider due to their sensitive systems and limited ability to metabolize certain substances.

Children with chronic health conditions or long-term medications may require specialized herbal formulations or closer monitoring to ensure safety and effectiveness.

Be mindful of allergies or sensitivities to herbs, especially if children have known allergies to specific plants or foods.

Incorporating herbal remedies into children's healthcare requires careful consideration of safety, dosage, suitable herbs, administration methods, and collaboration with healthcare providers. By following these guidelines and working collaboratively with qualified professionals, parents can harness the benefits of herbal medicine to support children's health naturally and effectively, feeling supported and part of a team.

Chapter 2. Considerations for seniors

Considerations for the elderly when using herbal remedies are crucial to ensure safety, efficacy, and appropriateness, given their unique health needs and potential interactions with medications. As individuals age, physiological changes can affect how their bodies metabolize and respond to herbs, so careful consideration and informed guidance are essential. Here's a comprehensive exploration of considerations for using herbal remedies in the elderly.

2.1 Physiological Changes and Safety

Physiological changes associated with aging can impact the safety and efficacy of herbal remedies:

Aging often slows metabolism and alters how the body absorbs and processes substances, including herbs. This can affect how quickly herbs take effect and how long they remain active in the body.

Age-related changes in liver and kidney function may affect the clearance of herbal compounds from the body. Monitoring liver and kidney function is crucial when using herbs that could impact these organs.

Many elderly individuals take multiple prescription medications to manage chronic conditions. Herbal remedies can potentially interact with medications, affecting their efficacy or causing adverse effects. Considering these interactions and consult healthcare providers to avoid potential complications is essential.

2.2 Choosing Suitable Herbs

Selecting appropriate herbs for elderly individuals involves considering their health conditions, medication regimen, and potential sensitivities:

Herbs chosen for elderly individuals should address specific health concerns prevalent in this age group, such as joint stiffness, cognitive decline, cardiovascular health, or sleep disturbances.

Opt for herbs with a well-established safety profile for elderly use, such as ginger for digestive support or ginkgo biloba for cognitive function. Avoid herbs with known safety concerns or interactions with medications commonly prescribed to older adults.

Consult with healthcare providers, including geriatricians or herbalists specializing in elder care, to tailor herbal regimens to individual health needs and ensure compatibility with existing treatments.

2.3 Administration and Compliance

Administering herbal remedies to elderly individuals requires considerations for ease of use and compliance:

Choose herbal preparations that are easy to administer and digest, such as capsules, tinctures, or teas. Ensure formulations are palatable and well-tolerated to enhance compliance.

Adjust herbal dosages based on the individual's age, health status, and tolerance levels. Start with lower doses and gradually increase as needed while monitoring for adverse reactions.

Monitor the elderly individual's response to herbal remedies regularly, noting any changes in symptoms or unexpected side effects. Adjustments may be necessary to optimize efficacy and safety.

2.4 Common Uses for the Elderly

Herbal remedies can support various aspects of elderly health and well-being:

Herbs like turmeric, boswellia, or devil's claw may help reduce inflammation and alleviate joint pain associated with arthritis or stiffness.

Ginkgo biloba, bacopa, or rosemary are herbs known for their potential to support cognitive function and memory in elderly individuals.

Hawthorn berries, garlic, or hibiscus can support heart health and maintain healthy blood pressure levels.

Peppermint, fennel, or licorice root can aid in digestive comfort, reducing symptoms like bloating, gas, or indigestion.

2.5 Considerations for Specific Conditions

Certain health conditions common in the elderly may require tailored herbal approaches:

Herbs such as horsetail or nettle leaf may support bone health and mineral absorption, complementing conventional treatments.

Valerian root, passionflower, or chamomile are herbs known for their calming properties and may promote better sleep quality without the risks associated with sedative medications.

Calendula, comfrey, or aloe vera can be used topically to soothe dry skin, minor irritations, or wounds common in elderly skin.

2.6 Consulting Healthcare Providers

Collaboration with healthcare providers is essential when integrating herbal remedies into elderly care:

Discuss potential herb-drug interactions to avoid adverse effects and ensure herbal remedies complement prescribed medications.

To develop personalized herbal protocols, conduct a thorough assessment of the elderly individual's health history, current medications, and overall health goals.

Monitor the elderly individual's health status and response to herbal treatments regularly, adjusting protocols as needed based on changes in health or medication regimens.

2.7 Education and Empowerment

Educating elderly individuals and caregivers about herbal remedies promotes informed decision-making and enhances therapeutic outcomes:

Provide clear instructions on how to use herbal remedies safely and effectively, including dosage, administration methods, and potential side effects to watch for.

Encourage elderly individuals to actively participate in their health care decisions, including incorporating herbal remedies as part of a holistic approach to wellness.

Integrating herbal remedies into elderly care requires carefully considering physiological changes, health conditions, medication interactions, and individual preferences. By collaborating with healthcare providers and tailoring herbal regimens to specific needs, herbal medicine can effectively support elderly health and well-being, promoting quality of life and longevity.

Chapter 3: Considerations for people with chronic conditions

Considerations for individuals with chronic conditions when using herbal remedies are crucial for ensuring safety, efficacy, and compatibility with ongoing treatments. Chronic conditions such as diabetes, hypertension, autoimmune disorders, and others require careful management, and herbal remedies can play a supportive role when integrated thoughtfully into a comprehensive healthcare plan. Here's an in-depth exploration of considerations for using herbal remedies in individuals with chronic conditions.

Chronic conditions are persistent health issues that require ongoing management and care.

Diverse Health Needs. Individuals with chronic conditions often have diverse health needs that may include symptom management, disease progression control, and overall quality of life improvement.

Complex Treatment Regimens. Managing chronic conditions typically involves multiple medications, lifestyle modifications, and regular medical monitoring to optimize health outcomes.

Individual Variability. It's crucial to recognize that responses to herbal remedies can vary widely among individuals with chronic conditions. Factors such as disease severity, medication interactions, and underlying health status all contribute to this variability, underscoring the need for personalized care.

3.1 Safety and Compatibility

Safety is paramount when considering herbal remedies for individuals with chronic conditions:

Potential Interactions: Herbal remedies can interact with prescription medications, affecting efficacy or causing adverse effects. It is crucial to identify potential interactions and consult healthcare providers to minimize risks.

Herb-Drug Interactions: Certain herbs, such as St. John's wort, may interfere with the metabolism of medications used to treat chronic conditions like depression or heart disease. Understanding these interactions is essential for safe integration.

Allergies and Sensitivities: Individuals with chronic conditions may have heightened sensitivities or allergies to certain herbs. Careful selection and monitoring are necessary to prevent allergic reactions or worsening of symptoms.

3.2 Choosing Suitable Herbs

Selecting appropriate herbs involves considering their safety, efficacy, and potential benefits for specific chronic conditions:

Choose herbs with documented efficacy and safety profiles for managing symptoms associated with chronic conditions. For example, curcumin is used for its anti-inflammatory properties in arthritis, and garlic is used for cardiovascular support.

Consult with healthcare providers, including herbalists or integrative medicine practitioners, to select herbs that complement existing treatments and address individual health needs.

Consider herbs that not only manage symptoms but also support overall well-being and quality of life. These herbs can address symptoms beyond conventional treatment approaches, offering a ray of hope and enhancing the quality of life for individuals with chronic conditions.

3.3 Administration and Monitoring

Administering herbal remedies to individuals with chronic conditions requires careful monitoring and adjustments:

Dosage Considerations

Tailor herbal dosages based on individual health status, disease progression, and treatment goals. Start with lower doses and gradually increase as tolerated, monitoring for any adverse effects or improvements in symptoms.

Consistency and Compliance

Encourage consistent use of herbal remedies as part of a daily routine, ensuring compliance with prescribed dosages and administration methods.

Monitoring Effects

Assess the effects of herbal remedies on symptoms and overall health regularly. Document changes in health status, side effects, or improvements to guide ongoing management.

3.4 Common Uses for Chronic Conditions

Herbal remedies can offer support for various chronic conditions, including:

Pain Management: Herbs like turmeric, ginger, or white willow bark may help alleviate pain associated with arthritis or fibromyalgia.

Mood and Mental Health: St. John's wort, lavender, or passionflower can support mood stability and mental well-being in individuals with chronic depression or anxiety.

Digestive Health: Peppermint, ginger, or marshmallow root may aid in soothing digestive discomfort, such as irritable bowel syndrome (IBS) symptoms.

Immune Support: Echinacea, astragalus, or elderberry can strengthen immune function, reducing the frequency and severity of infections in individuals with chronic immune disorders.

3.5 Integrative Care Approach

Integrating herbal remedies into comprehensive care for chronic conditions requires collaboration and communication among healthcare providers:

Patient-Centered Care: It's essential to engage individuals in shared decision-making regarding herbal treatment options. This approach, emphasizing informed consent and realistic expectations, ensures that patients feel valued and respected in their healthcare journey.

Interdisciplinary Collaboration: To ensure the best possible care for individuals with chronic conditions, it's essential to collaborate with conventional healthcare providers and herbalists or integrative medicine specialists. This teamwork can help coordinate care and optimize treatment outcomes.

Education and Empowerment: By educating individuals about the benefits, risks, and proper use of herbal remedies, we can empower them to make informed choices and actively participate in their healthcare management. This patient involvement is a key aspect of the integrative care approach.

3.6 Monitoring and Adjustments

Regular monitoring and adjustments are essential for optimizing herbal therapy in individuals with chronic conditions:

Long-Term Management: Implement long-term monitoring plans to evaluate the efficacy and safety of herbal remedies, making adjustments as necessary based on changes in health status or treatment goals.

Adverse Effects Management: Promptly address any adverse effects or complications related to herbal use, ensuring timely intervention and adjustment of herbal protocols as needed.

Documentation and Reporting: Maintain comprehensive records of herbal therapy, including dosages, administration methods, and health outcomes. Share this information with all healthcare providers involved in the individual's care for informed decision-making.

Integrating herbal remedies into managing chronic conditions requires a nuanced approach considering safety, efficacy, compatibility with existing treatments, and individual health needs. By collaborating with healthcare providers and adopting a patient-centered approach, herbal medicine can complement conventional therapies, offering holistic support and enhancing the quality of life for individuals managing chronic health challenges.

Chapter 4: Adapting remedies for different needs

Adapting herbal remedies to meet different needs involves tailoring treatments to specific health conditions, preferences, and circumstances. This flexible approach allows herbalists and healthcare providers to address a wide range of health concerns while accommodating varying sensitivity levels, efficacy requirements, and personal preferences. Here's an exploration of how herbal remedies can be adapted to meet diverse needs:

Personalized Health Goals

Adapting herbal remedies begins with understanding an individual's unique health goals and preferences.

Herbalists assess specific health conditions, such as digestive issues, respiratory ailments, or emotional well-being, to determine the most appropriate herbs and formulations.

Tailoring herbal remedies focuses on effectively managing symptoms, whether they involve pain relief, immune support, stress reduction, or enhancing overall vitality.

Herbal treatments can also be adapted for preventive health measures, supporting immune function, cardiovascular health, and overall well-being to maintain optimal health.

Customized Herbal Formulations

Customizing herbal formulations ensures they meet the specific needs and preferences of individuals.

Choosing herbs based on their therapeutic properties and compatibility with an individual's health profile. For instance, adaptogens like ashwagandha or Rhodiola may be selected to support resilience to stress and promote overall vitality.

Herbalists may prepare remedies in various forms, including teas, tinctures, capsules, or topical applications, depending on the preferred method of administration and the targeted health benefit.

Adapting dosage levels according to age, health status, and sensitivity to ensure safety and optimize therapeutic effectiveness.

Herbal Synergy and Combinations

Combining herbs strategically enhances their synergistic effects and addresses multiple health concerns simultaneously.

Herbalists formulate blends that combine complementary herbs to amplify therapeutic benefits. For example, combining ginger for digestive support with peppermint for soothing effects may enhance overall gastrointestinal health.

Developing formulas tailored to specific health conditions, such as herbal blends for respiratory health, joint support, or sleep enhancement, allows for targeted treatment approaches.

Considering individual responses to herbs and adjusting combinations as needed to achieve optimal health outcomes and minimize adverse effects.

Cultural and Personal Preferences

Adapting herbal remedies respects cultural traditions and personal preferences.

Integrating herbs traditionally used in different cultural practices ensures relevance and respect for cultural beliefs and practices related to health and healing.

Adjusting herbal formulations to improve taste and enhance palatability encourages consistent use and compliance, which is particularly important for individuals sensitive to solid flavors or textures.

Choosing herbs sourced sustainably and ethically aligns with personal values and environmental stewardship, ensuring the integrity and purity of herbal preparations.

Age-Specific Adaptations

Adapting herbal remedies for different age groups considers developmental stages and specific health needs.

Use gentle herbs and age-appropriate formulations that are safe and effective for young individuals, such as soothing herbal teas for digestive comfort or herbal salves for skin irritations.

Tailoring herbal treatments to address common adult health concerns, such as stress management, hormonal balance, or cardiovascular health, with appropriate dosages and formulations.

Adjusting herbal therapies to accommodate age-related changes in metabolism, organ function, and potential interactions with medications, ensuring safety and efficacy in promoting healthy aging.

Integrative Approach to Conventional Medicine

Integrating herbal remedies with conventional medical treatments promotes comprehensive health care.

Consulting with healthcare professionals to coordinate herbal therapies with existing medical treatments, ensuring compatibility and safety.

Monitor health outcomes regularly and communicate changes in herbal use with healthcare providers, allowing for adjustments based on evolving health needs or treatment plans.

Providing education on herbal therapies' benefits and potential risks empowers individuals to make informed decisions and actively participate in their health care.

Evidence-Based Practice

Adapting herbal remedies based on scientific research and clinical evidence enhances efficacy and safety:

Incorporating herbs with proven therapeutic benefits supported by scientific studies and clinical trials ensures evidence-based practice in herbal medicine.

Selecting high-quality herbs from reputable sources and adhering to stringent manufacturing standards to guarantee potency, purity, and safety in herbal formulations.

Staying updated on the latest research and developments in herbal medicine to refine treatment approaches and optimize individual health outcomes.

Adapting herbal remedies involves a personalized approach considering individual health goals, preferences, cultural influences, and age-specific needs. By customizing herbal formulations, strategically combining herbs, respecting cultural traditions, and integrating with conventional medicine, herbalists and healthcare providers can effectively support diverse health concerns and promote holistic well-being across different populations.

Book 25: Ethical Harvesting and Sustainability

A Guide to Responsible Practices for Preserving Herbal Resources

Chapter 1: Sustainable practices in growing and harvesting herbs

Sustainable practices in growing and harvesting herbs are essential to ensure the health of the environment, the quality of the herbs, and the well-being of future generations. Adopting eco-friendly methods in herbal cultivation and collection helps maintain biodiversity, prevent soil degradation, and reduce the impact on natural resources. Here's an exploration of sustainable practices for growing and harvesting herbs:

1.1 Organic Cultivation

Organic cultivation of herbs is a reassuring choice, as it avoids synthetic chemicals and promotes a healthier ecosystem, ensuring the highest quality herbs for your use.

Compost, manure, and other organic matter enrich the soil naturally, providing essential nutrients without the adverse effects of chemical fertilizers.

Natural pest control methods, such as introducing beneficial insects, using neem oil, or companion planting, help manage pests without harming the environment.

Rotating crops and planting diverse herbs prevents soil depletion, reduces pest and disease cycles, and enhances soil health.

1.2 Water Conservation

Efficient water use is crucial in sustainable herb farming. Implementing drip irrigation systems minimizes water waste by delivering water directly to the plant roots, reducing evaporation and runoff.

Applying mulch around plants helps retain soil moisture, suppress weeds, and improve soil structure, reducing the need for frequent watering.

Collecting and storing rainwater provides an additional water source for irrigation, lessening the dependency on municipal water supplies and conserving natural resources.

1.3 Soil Health

Maintaining healthy soil is fundamental to sustainable herb cultivation.

Planting cover crops, such as clover or legumes, improves soil fertility, prevents erosion, and promotes beneficial microbial activity. Reducing tillage preserves soil structure, maintains organic matter, and supports a thriving ecosystem of soil organisms contributing to plant health.

Regular soil testing allows for precise nutrient management, ensuring the soil has the right balance of minerals to support healthy herb growth.

1.4 Ethical Wildcrafting

As herbalists and growers, your role in sustainable harvesting of wild herbs, or wildcrafting, is crucial. Your careful attention can help preserve natural populations for future generations.

Gathering herbs respecting the plant population ensures that sufficient plants continue reproducing. This may involve only taking a small portion of the plant or harvesting in a way that allows the plant to regenerate.

Your knowledge and skill in harvesting herbs during peak season ensures optimal potency and minimizes impact on plant communities. This understanding can also prevent overharvesting during vulnerable periods, showcasing your expertise in sustainable herb cultivation.

Avoiding the collection of rare or endangered herbs protects these species from extinction and helps maintain biodiversity.

1.5 Local and Community-Based Practices

Supporting local and community-based herb growing fosters sustainability and reduces environmental impact.

Sourcing herbs locally reduces transportation emissions and supports local economies. It also ensures fresher, higher-quality herbs. Participating in or supporting community herb gardens encourages local food production, reduces food miles, and provides educational opportunities about sustainable agriculture.

Saving seeds from healthy plants ensures a continuous supply of adapted, resilient plant varieties and reduces the need to purchase new seeds annually.

1.6 Renewable Energy Use

Integrating renewable energy sources in herb farming operations minimizes the carbon footprint:

Utilizing solar panels for energy needs in greenhouses, irrigation systems, and processing facilities reduces reliance on fossil fuels and promotes clean energy use.

Harnessing wind energy where feasible can power various farm operations, decreasing the environmental impact.

Implementing energy-efficient practices, such as using energy-saving lighting and equipment, conserves resources and reduces operational costs.

1.7 Education and Advocacy

Promoting sustainable herb growing and harvesting practices involves educating the community and advocating for environmental stewardship:

Offering workshops and training programs on sustainable agriculture practices empowers individuals to adopt eco-friendly methods in their herb cultivation efforts. Raising awareness about the importance of sustainability in herbal practices encourages consumers to support environmentally responsible products and practices.

Partnering with environmental organizations and advocacy groups strengthens efforts to promote and implement sustainable practices in the herbal industry.

Sustainable practices in growing and harvesting herbs are essential for maintaining ecological balance, ensuring the environment's health, and providing high-quality herbal products. By adopting organic cultivation methods, conserving water, preserving soil health, practicing ethical wildcrafting, supporting local initiatives, utilizing renewable energy, and educating the community, herbalists and growers can contribute to a more sustainable and resilient future.

Chapter 2: Ethical considerations in herbal medicine

Ethical considerations in herbal medicine are essential to ensure the responsible use, sourcing, and distribution of herbs. Ethical practices safeguard the well-being of individuals using herbal remedies, protect the environment, and respect cultural traditions and knowledge. This holistic approach to herbal medicine emphasizes integrity, accountability, and respect for nature and human communities. Here's an exploration of critical ethical considerations in herbal medicine:

Respect for Traditional Knowledge

Respecting traditional knowledge involves acknowledging and honoring the cultural heritage and wisdom of indigenous and local communities who have used herbs for centuries.

Herbalists should approach traditional herbal knowledge with respect and sensitivity, recognizing the deep cultural significance of these practices.

When using traditional herbal knowledge, providing fair compensation and recognition to the communities that have preserved and shared this knowledge is important.

Engaging in collaborative partnerships with indigenous and local communities ensures their voices are heard and their contributions are valued in herbal medicine.

Sustainable Sourcing and Environmental Stewardship

Ethical herbal medicine practices emphasize sustainable sourcing to protect natural habitats and ensure the long-term availability of medicinal plants.

Harvesting herbs that allow plant populations to regenerate ensures that they remain available for future generations. This involves techniques such as selective harvesting and rotating harvest locations.

Organic farming methods and minimizing synthetic chemicals protect the environment and ensure that herbs are free from harmful residues. Supporting conservation initiatives and organizations that protect endangered plant species and their habitats is crucial for preserving biodiversity.

Transparency and Honesty in Product Labeling

Transparency in product labeling ensures that consumers are fully informed about the herbal products they use.

Listing all ingredients, including the botanical names of herbs, allows consumers to make informed choices and avoid potential allergens or unwanted substances.

Information about herbs' source and origin helps consumers understand the product's journey and environmental impact.

Adhering to high quality standards and providing accurate information about herbal products' potency, purity, and safety builds trust with consumers.

Ensuring Safety and Efficacy

Ethical herbal medicine prioritizes the safety and efficacy of herbal treatments to protect public health.

Utilizing herbs with well-documented therapeutic benefits and scientific backing ensures effective and safe treatments.

Providing clear guidelines on the proper dosage and administration of herbal remedies minimizes the risk of adverse effects and maximizes therapeutic benefits.

Encouraging users to monitor their health and report adverse effects ensures that herbal treatments are used safely and effectively. This information can also contribute to ongoing research and improvements in herbal medicine.

Fair Trade and Economic Justice

Supporting fair trade practices in the herbal industry promotes economic justice and ethical business practices.

Ensuring that farmers and workers involved in cultivating and harvesting herbs receive fair wages and work in safe conditions is fundamental to ethical herbal medicine.

Investing in community development projects in regions where herbs are sourced supports local economies and improves the quality of life for residents.

Building transparent and ethical supply chains ensures that all parties involved in producing and distributing herbal products are treated fairly and ethically.

Respect for Individual Autonomy

Respecting individual autonomy involves empowering consumers to make informed decisions about their health and herbal treatments.

Providing comprehensive information about herbal treatments' benefits, risks, and alternatives ensures that individuals can make informed choices.

Tailoring herbal treatments to individual needs and preferences respects each person's unique health journey and promotes holistic well-being.

Educating consumers about herbal medicine and encouraging self-care practices empowers them to actively participate in their health.

Ethical Research Practices

Ethical research practices in herbal medicine ensure the integrity and credibility of scientific studies.

Obtaining informed consent from participants in herbal research studies ensures they are fully aware of the study's purpose, procedures, and potential risks.

Publishing research findings openly and honestly, regardless of the outcomes, contributes to the body of knowledge and promotes trust in herbal medicine research.

Conducting research ethically, without exploiting vulnerable populations or communities, ensures that research benefits are shared equitably.

Ethical considerations in herbal medicine encompass a wide range of practices prioritizing the well-being of individuals, the environment, and communities. Practitioners and companies can build a responsible and trustworthy herbal medicine industry by respecting traditional knowledge, ensuring sustainable sourcing, promoting transparency, prioritizing safety and efficacy, supporting fair trade, respecting individual autonomy, and adhering to ethical research. These ethical principles guide the responsible use and distribution of herbs, fostering a holistic approach that benefits both people and the planet.

Chapter 3: Supporting biodiversity and ecological health

Supporting biodiversity and ecological health is fundamental to sustainable herbal medicine practices. Ensuring the preservation and enhancement of biodiversity within ecosystems protects the environment and maintains the availability and potency of medicinal herbs. Here's an exploration of how supporting biodiversity and ecological health intersects with herbal medicine:

3.1 Preservation of Native Plant Species

Prioritizing the cultivation of native herbs supports local ecosystems by maintaining plant diversity and providing habitats for native wildlife. Native plants are well-adapted to the local environment, often requiring less water and fewer resources.

Preventing the spread of invasive species that can outcompete native plants is vital. Invasive species disrupt local ecosystems and reduce biodiversity, threatening the survival of native herbs.

Establishing seed banks and conservation gardens dedicated to preserving native and endangered plant species ensures these herbs are protected for future generations. These initiatives play a crucial role in safeguarding genetic diversity.

3.2 Sustainable Harvesting Practices

Harvesting only a portion of a plant or specific parts, such as leaves or flowers, allows the plant to continue growing and reproducing. This practice helps maintain healthy populations of wild herbs.

Collecting herbs during appropriate seasons ensures that plants have the opportunity to complete their reproductive cycles. This timing also ensures the harvested herbs reach their peak potency and nutritional value.

Using minimal-impact techniques, such as hand harvesting, reduces soil disruption and minimizes harm to surrounding plant and animal life. These methods help maintain the integrity of natural habitats.

3.3 Habitat Conservation

Participating in or supporting habitat restoration projects rehabilitating degraded ecosystems ensures they can support diverse plant and animal life. This might include reforestation efforts or wetland restoration.

Supporting the creation and maintenance of protected areas, such as nature reserves and national parks, ensures that ecosystems remain intact and free from destructive activities like logging, mining, or overharvesting.

Promoting the development of urban green spaces, such as community gardens and green roofs, enhances urban biodiversity and provides essential habitats for pollinators and other wildlife.

3.4 Pollinator Support

Planting various flowering plants that bloom at different times throughout the year provides continuous food sources for pollinators like bees, butterflies, and hummingbirds.

Reducing or eliminating the use of pesticides that harm pollinators helps maintain healthy pollinator populations. Organic and natural pest control methods are safer alternatives.

Providing habitats for pollinators, such as bee hotels and butterfly gardens, supports their life cycles and contributes to the pollination of herbs and other plants.

3.5 Soil Health and Microbial Diversity

Organic farming practices, such as composting and crop rotation, enriches the soil and promotes a diverse microbial community. Healthy soil supports robust plant growth and resilience to pests and diseases.

Encouraging mycorrhizal relationships between fungi and plant roots enhances nutrient uptake and soil structure. These symbiotic relationships are crucial for the health of many medicinal herbs.

Implementing erosion control measures, such as planting cover crops and mulches, prevents soil degradation and loss of valuable topsoil. This helps maintain soil fertility and plant diversity.

3.6 Community and Education

Involving local communities in conservation efforts and sustainable herb cultivation projects empowers them to preserve their natural heritage actively.

Educational programs and workshops about biodiversity, sustainable agriculture, and herbal medicine raise awareness and encourage sustainable practices.

Promoting public awareness campaigns highlighting the importance of biodiversity and ecological health can drive collective action and support conservation initiatives.

Supporting biodiversity and ecological health is integral to herbal medicine. By preserving native plant species, adopting sustainable harvesting practices, conserving habitats, supporting pollinators, maintaining soil health, and engaging communities, herbalists and growers can contribute to a sustainable and thriving environment. These efforts ensure that medicinal herbs remain available and effective for future generations while promoting ecosystems' overall health and resilience.

Chapter 4: Connecting with other herbalists and enthusiasts

Connecting with other herbalists and enthusiasts is vital for expanding knowledge, sharing experiences, and fostering a sense of community within the field of herbal medicine. Networking can lead to new opportunities, collaborations, and a deeper understanding of herbal practices. Here's an exploration of how to connect with others in the herbal community:

4.1 Attending Conferences and Workshops

Conferences and workshops offer excellent opportunities to meet fellow herbalists, learn from experts, and stay updated on the latest trends and research in herbal medicine.

National and International Conferences

Participating in national and international conferences dedicated to herbal medicine can provide exposure to various topics and practices. These events often feature keynote speakers, panel discussions, and hands-on workshops led by leading experts in the field. Attendees can learn about new research, innovative techniques, and emerging trends while networking with like-minded individuals.

Local Workshops and Seminars

Local workshops and seminars are more accessible and provide a platform for learning and networking within the local herbal community. These events can focus on specific topics, such as herb identification, cultivation techniques, or herbal remedy preparation. Engaging in these smaller, more intimate settings can facilitate deeper connections and foster ongoing collaborations with local herbalists and enthusiasts.

Online Webinars and Virtual Conferences

With the rise of digital technology, online webinars and virtual conferences have become increasingly popular. To make the most of these virtual events, consider preparing questions in advance, participating in the interactive sessions, and actively engaging in the networking opportunities through chat rooms and social media groups. These events often include live presentations, interactive Q&A sessions, and networking opportunities through chat rooms and social media groups.

4.2 Joining Herbal Associations and Groups

Herbal associations and groups provide a structured environment for ongoing education, support, and networking among herbalists and enthusiasts. Joining these groups can give you a sense of belonging and being part of a larger community.

Professional Herbal Associations

Joining professional herbal associations, such as the American Herbalists Guild (AHG) or the National Institute of Medical Herbalists (NIMH), offers access to a wealth of resources. These may include journals with the latest research, newsletters with updates on industry trends, and continuing education opportunities to further your knowledge. Membership in these organizations can also enhance credibility and provide a platform for professional development and advocacy.

Local Herbal Clubs and Groups

Local herbal clubs and groups offer a more grassroots approach to networking and education. To find and join these groups, consider searching online, asking at local herb shops, or attending community events. These groups often organize regular meetings, herb walks, and study groups where members can share knowledge, discuss challenges, and collaborate on projects. Being part of a local group fosters a sense of community and provides valuable support from peers who share a passion for herbal medicine.

Online Forums and Social Media Groups

Online forums and social media groups, such as those on Facebook, Reddit, or specialized herbalist websites, provide a platform for herbalists and enthusiasts to connect, share experiences, and seek advice. These virtual communities offer a convenient way to stay connected with others in the field, participate in discussions, and access vast information and resources.

4.3 Collaborative Projects and Research

Collaborative projects and research initiatives can lead to significant advancements in herbal medicine and foster strong connections among participants. Participating in these can empower you to make a real difference in the field.

Community Gardens and Herb Farms

Participating in or establishing community gardens and herb farms provides a hands-on opportunity to work with others in growing and harvesting medicinal herbs. These collaborative efforts enhance practical skills, strengthen bonds within the community, and promote the sustainable cultivation of herbs.

Research Partnerships

Collaborating on research projects with other herbalists, universities, or research institutions can contribute to the scientific validation of herbal practices and the discovery of new therapeutic uses for herbs. Joint research often involves sharing knowledge, resources, and expertise, producing more robust and impactful findings.

Educational Workshops and Retreats

Organizing or participating in educational workshops and retreats focused on herbal medicine allows for in-depth learning and collaboration. These events can provide a sense of achievement as you gain new knowledge and build lasting professional relationships.

Connecting with other herbalists and enthusiasts is essential for personal and professional growth in herbal medicine. By attending conferences and workshops, joining herbal associations and groups, and engaging in collaborative projects and research, individuals can expand their knowledge, share experiences, and build a supportive community. These connections enhance the practice of herbal medicine and contribute to the broader goals of sustainability, education, and the advancement of natural health practices. Embracing these opportunities for networking and collaboration ensures a vibrant and dynamic future for the herbal community.

Chapter 5: Online resources, forums, and groups

In the digital age, online resources, forums, and groups have become invaluable tools for herbalists and enthusiasts to connect, learn, and share knowledge. These platforms offer a wealth of information and provide opportunities for networking and collaboration that transcend geographical boundaries. Here's a look at how to effectively utilize these online resources to enhance your practice and knowledge in herbal medicine:

Online Educational Resources

The internet is rich with educational resources that cater to both novice and experienced herbalists. Websites, e-books, and online courses provide comprehensive information on various aspects of herbal medicine:

- *Websites and Blogs*: Reputable websites such as the American Herbalists Guild (AHG) and Herbal Academy offer articles, research papers, and guides on a wide range of topics. Many herbalists also run personal blogs where they share their insights, experiences, and recipes, providing a more personalized learning experience.

- *E-Books and Online Libraries*: Digital books and online libraries provide in-depth knowledge on specific herbs, their uses, and preparation methods. These resources are often written by experts and cover both traditional knowledge and modern scientific findings.

- *Online Courses and Webinars*: Many institutions and herbalists offer online courses and webinars that cover everything from the basics of herbal medicine to advanced topics. These structured learning experiences often include video lectures, reading materials, and interactive components, allowing for a comprehensive understanding of the subject matter.

Forums and Discussion Boards

Online forums and discussion boards are excellent places to ask questions, share experiences, and learn from others. These platforms create a sense of community and provide peer support:

- *Specialized Herbal Forums*: Websites like HerbMentor and Reddit have dedicated forums where herbalists can discuss specific topics, share advice, and troubleshoot common issues. These forums are moderated by experienced herbalists who ensure that the information shared is accurate and helpful.

- *General Health and Wellness Forums*: Broader health and wellness forums often have sections dedicated to herbal medicine. Participating in these discussions can provide insights into how herbal practices integrate with other health modalities and offer a wider perspective on wellness.

Online resources, forums, and groups are indispensable for anyone involved in herbal medicine. They offer a platform for continuous learning, community support, and professional networking. By actively engaging with these digital tools, herbalists can enhance their knowledge, share their expertise, and build a supportive community that promotes the responsible and effective use of herbal medicine.

Chapter 6: Continuing education and certification programs

Continuing education and certification programs are essential for herbalists who seek to deepen their knowledge, stay updated with the latest developments, and enhance their credibility in herbal medicine. These programs provide structured learning opportunities that cover various aspects of herbal practice, from foundational knowledge to advanced techniques. Here's a closer look at the importance and benefits of these educational pathways.

6.1 Importance of Continuing Education

The field of herbal medicine is continuously evolving with new research findings and scientific advancements. Continuing education helps herbalists stay informed about the latest studies, emerging trends, and innovative practices, ensuring that their knowledge remains current and relevant.

Advanced courses and workshops allow herbalists to refine their skills and expand their expertise. Whether it's learning new methods of herb preparation, understanding complex phytochemistry, or exploring integrative health approaches, continuing education provides the tools needed to grow professionally.

Many professional herbal organizations require members to participate in continuing education to maintain their certification. This ensures that practitioners uphold high standards of practice and stay committed to lifelong learning.

6.2 Certification Programs

Certification programs formalize an herbalist's skills and knowledge, which can enhance professional credibility and open up new career opportunities.

Programs like those offered by the American Herbalists Guild (AHG) provide rigorous training and assessment to certify practitioners as Registered Herbalists (RH). This certification demonstrates a high level of competency and commitment to ethical practice.

Herbalists can also pursue specialized certifications in clinical herbalism, ethnobotany, or aromatherapy. These programs often include focused coursework and practical experience, allowing practitioners to develop expertise in specific fields of interest. With the rise of digital learning, many reputable institutions offer online certification programs that provide flexibility and accessibility. These programs typically include video lectures, interactive modules, and assignments that can be completed remotely, making them ideal for busy professionals.

6.3 Types of Continuing Education Opportunities

Attending workshops and seminars provides hands-on learning experiences and opportunities to interact with experts and peers. These events often cover specific topics in-depth, such as herbal formulation, therapeutic applications, or traditional healing practices.

Online courses and webinars offer convenience and flexibility, allowing herbalists to learn at their own pace. Many institutions and individual practitioners offer high-quality online education covering various topics, from beginner to advanced.

Herbal conferences and symposia bring together practitioners, researchers, and educators to share knowledge and discuss advancements in the field. These events often include lectures, panel discussions, and networking opportunities, providing a comprehensive educational experience.

Engaging in mentorship programs allows herbalists to learn directly from experienced practitioners. Mentorship provides personalized guidance, practical insights, and professional support, fostering growth and development in a collaborative setting.

6.4 Benefits of Continuing Education and Certification

Continuous learning enhances an herbalist's expertise and competence, contributing to professional growth and career advancement. Certification from recognized institutions adds credibility to a practitioner's qualifications, building trust with clients and peers.

Educational programs and events provide opportunities to connect with other herbalists, share experiences, and collaborate on projects.

Advanced knowledge and skills enable herbalists to offer more effective and informed care, improving client health outcomes.

Continuing education and certification programs are vital for herbalists committed to professional excellence and lifelong learning. These programs provide the knowledge, skills, and credentials needed to stay current, enhance practice, and achieve recognition in herbal medicine. By investing in their education, herbalists can ensure they provide the highest quality care to their clients and contribute to the advancement of herbal medicine as a respected and credible health practice.

Here you can access
ADDITIONAL RECIPES

Scan this **QR code** using your phone's camera or click this **LINK** to access your **ADDITIONAL RECIPES** content now:

**SCAN THE QR CODE BELOW AND ENJOY
THE RECIPES FOR YOUR HEALTH:**

**You will access to ADDITIONAL RECIPES Designed
Specifically for Your Healthy Well-Being**

Book 26: Immune-Boosting Recipes

1. Wild Fennel Syrup

Ingredients:

- 1 cup dried wild fennel
- 3 cups water,
- 1 cup honey

Instructions: Simmer wild fennel in water for 30 minutes, then strain. Stir in honey and store in a glass jar.

2. Garlic-Honey Immune Tonic

Ingredients:

- 1 head garlic
- 1 cup raw honey

Instructions: Peel and lightly crush garlic cloves. Add to honey and let sit for at least 3 days.

3. Ginger-Lemon Immune Tea

Ingredients:

- 1-inch fresh ginger root
- 1 lemon
- 1 tbsp honey

Instructions: Grate ginger and steep in hot water for 10 minutes. Add lemon juice and honey.

4. Echinacea Tincture

Ingredients:

- 1 cup dried echinacea root
- 2 cups vodka

Instructions: Place echinacea in a jar and cover with alcohol. Let sit for 4-6 weeks, shaking occasionally.

5. Turmeric-Golden Milk

Ingredients:

- 1 tsp turmeric
- 1 cup coconut milk
- 1 tbsp black pepper

Instructions: Heat all ingredients together in a small pot. Simmer for 5 minutes, then remove from heat and drink warm.

6. Astragalus Root Soup

Ingredients:

- 2-3 slices dried astragalus root
- 4 cups vegetable broth

Instructions: Add astragalus root to broth and simmer for 20 minutes. Remove the root before consuming the soup.

7. Thyme-Infused Honey

Ingredients:

- 1/2 cup fresh thyme
- 1 cup raw honey

Instructions: Gently crush thyme leaves and add them to honey. Let sit for 1-2 weeks. Take 1 tsp as needed.

8. Cinnamon-Clove Immune Tea

Ingredients:

- 1 cinnamon stick
- 4 whole cloves
- 2 cups water

Instructions: Simmer cinnamon and cloves in water for 10 minutes. Strain and drink warm.

9. Lemon-Balm Immune Support Tincture

Ingredients:

- 1 cup fresh lemon balm leaves
- 2 cups vodka

Instructions: Place lemon balm in a jar and cover with vodka. Let it sit for 4 weeks, shaking occasionally. Strain and store.

10. Oregano Oil Capsules

Ingredients:

- Oregano essential oil
- olive oil,
- empty capsules

Instructions: Mix 1 drop of oregano essential oil with a carrier oil like olive oil. Fill capsules and take 1 per day to support the immune system.

11. Rosehip and Hibiscus Tea

Ingredients:

- 1 tbsp dried rosehips
- 1 tbsp dried hibiscus
- 2 cups water

Instructions: Steep rosehips and hibiscus in hot water for 10 minutes. Strain and drink daily to boost vitamin C and support immune health.

12. Garlic and Olive Oil Immune Elixir

Ingredients:

- 3 cloves garlic
- 1/4 cup extra virgin olive oil

Instructions: Mince garlic and mix with olive oil. Let it sit for 1 hour. Drizzle on salads or take 1 tsp daily for a potent immune boost.

13. Ginseng Immune Tonic

Ingredients:

- 1 tsp powdered ginseng
- 1 cup hot water

Instructions: Stir powdered ginseng into hot water and drink once daily to support overall vitality and immune health.

14. Reishi Mushroom Tea

Ingredients:

- 2 slices dried reishi mushroom
- 4 cups water

Instructions: Simmer reishi mushroom slices in water for 30 minutes. Strain and drink 1 cup daily to enhance immune function.

15. Nettle Infusion

Ingredients:

- 1/4 cup dried nettle leaves
- 4 cups water

Instructions: Place nettle leaves in a jar and cover with boiling water. Let steep for 4-6 hours, then strain and drink throughout the day to nourish and support the immune system.

16. Lemon-Ginger Immunity Shots

Ingredients:

- 1 tbsp grated ginger
- juice of 1 lemon

Instructions: Mix all ingredients and take as a shot once per day for a powerful immune boost.

17. Licorice Root and Marshmallow Root Tea

Ingredients:

- 1 tsp dried licorice root
- 1 tsp dried marshmallow root
- 2 cups water

Instructions: Simmer licorice and marshmallow roots in water for 10 minutes.

18. Andrographis Capsules

Ingredients:

- Andrographis powder
- empty capsules

Instructions: Fill empty capsules with Andrographis powder and take 1 capsule daily to enhance immune defense.

19. Probiotic-Infused Kefir Smoothie

Ingredients:

- 1 cup kefir
- 1 banana
- 1 tbsp flaxseed

Instructions: Blend all ingredients and drink daily to support gut health, boosting the immune system.

20. Tulsi (Holy Basil) Tea

Ingredients:

- 1 tbsp dried tulsi leaves
- 2 cups water

Instructions: Steep tulsi leaves in hot water for 10 minutes. Strain and drink 1-2 cups daily to reduce stress and improve immune function.

Book 27: Energy-Boosting Recipes

1. Astragalus and Goji Berry Soup

Ingredients:

- 1 tbsp dried astragalus root
- 1/4 cup goji berries
- 4 cups vegetable broth

Instructions: Simmer astragalus and goji berries in broth for 20 minutes.

2. Thyme and Honey Syrup

Ingredients:

- 1/2 cup fresh thyme
- 1 cup honey
- 1/2 cup water

Instructions: Simmer thyme in water for 10 minutes, strain, and mix with honey.

3. Turmeric Golden Milk

Ingredients:

- 1 tsp turmeric powder
- 1/2 tsp cinnamon
- 1 cup warm almond milk

Instructions: Mix all ingredients into warm almond milk and drink before bed to reduce inflammation and support the immune system.

4. Elderflower and Mint Cold Infusion

Ingredients:

- 1 tbsp dried elderflower
- 1 tbsp dried mint
- 4 cups cold water

Instructions: Steep herbs in cold water for 4 hours. Strain and drink chilled to prevent colds and support immune defense.

5. Shiitake Mushroom Stir-Fry

Ingredients:

- 1 cup sliced shiitake mushrooms
- 2 cloves garlic
- 1 tbsp olive oil
- 1 tbsp soy sauce

Instructions: Sauté shiitake mushrooms and garlic in olive oil, add soy sauce, and serve over rice for a meal rich in immune-boosting beta-glucans.

6. Garlic Fermented Honey

Ingredients:

- 10 garlic cloves
- 1 cup raw honey

Instructions: Crush garlic cloves and cover with honey in a jar. Let sit for 1 week, stirring daily.

7. Echinacea and Ginger Herbal Gummies

Ingredients:

- 1 cup echinacea tea
- 1 tbsp grated ginger
- 2 tbsp gelatin
- 2 tbsp honey

Instructions: Heat tea and ginger, stir in gelatin and honey. Pour into molds and refrigerate. Take 1-2 gummies daily to support the immune system.

8. Pine Needle Tea

Ingredients:

- 1 tbsp fresh pine needles
- 2 cups boiling water

Instructions: Steep pine needles in boiling water for 10 minutes, strain, and drink to boost immune function with its high vitamin C content.

9. Camu Camu Smoothie

Ingredients:

- 1 tsp camu camu powder
- 1/2 cup orange juice

Instructions: Blend all ingredients and drink to get a high dose of vitamin C, which supports immune health.

10. Mullein Steam Inhalation

Ingredients:

- 1 tbsp dried mullein leaves
- 4 cups boiling water

Instructions: Add mullein to boiling water and inhale the steam with a towel over your head to support respiratory health and enhance immune function.

11. Hawthorn berries and Hibiscus Tea

Ingredients:

- 1 tbsp dried hawthorn berries
- 1 tbsp dried hibiscus
- 2 cups boiling water

Instructions: Steep rosehips and hibiscus in boiling water for 10 minutes.

12. Holy Basil and Lemon Balm Infusion

Ingredients:

- 1 tbsp dried holy basil (tulsi)
- 1 tbsp dried lemon balm
- 2 cups hot water

Instructions: Steep holy basil and lemon balm in hot water for 10 minutes. Strain and drink to reduce stress and support immune health.

13. Immunity-Boosting Herbal Oil

Ingredients:

- 1/2 cup olive oil
- 1 tbsp dried oregano
- 1 tbsp thyme

Instructions: Infuse dried herbs in olive oil by warming gently for 30 minutes, strain, and use for cooking.

14. Lemon and Ginger Immune Shots

Ingredients:

- 1/4 cup fresh lemon juice
- 1 tbsp grated ginger

Instructions: Mix all ingredients and take 1 shot in the morning for a burst of vitamin C and anti-inflammatory benefits.

15. Garlic and Cayenne Pepper Tonic

Ingredients:

- 1 garlic clove
- 1/4 tsp cayenne pepper
- 1 cup warm water

Instructions: Mince garlic and stir into warm water with cayenne pepper. Drink daily to stimulate the immune system and improve circulation.

16. Elderberry and Cinnamon Syrup

Ingredients:

- 1/2 cup dried elderberries
- 1 cinnamon stick
- 1 cup honey
- 2 cups water

Instructions: Simmer elderberries and cinnamon in water for 30 minutes, strain, and mix in honey. Take 1 tsp daily to prevent colds and flu.

17. Ashwagandha and Turmeric Latte

Ingredients:

- 1/2 tsp ashwagandha powder
- 1/2 tsp turmeric powder
- 1 cup almond milk
- 1 teaspoon honey

Instructions: Warm almond milk and stir in ashwagandha, turmeric, and honey. Drink in the evening to reduce stress and enhance immune function.

18. Calendula Salve for Immune Support

Ingredients:

- 1/2 cup dried calendula flowers
- 1/2 cup coconut oil
- 1 tbsp beeswax

Instructions: Infuse calendula in coconut oil for 1 hour on low heat, strain, and mix in melted beeswax.

19. Lemon Balm and Ginger Lozenges

Ingredients:

- 1 tbsp dried lemon balm
- 1 tbsp grated ginger
- 1/2 cup honey

Instructions: Simmer lemon balm and ginger in honey for 20 minutes, pour into molds, and let cool to form lozenges.

20. Peppermint and Licorice Root Tea

Ingredients:

- 1 tbsp dried peppermint
- 1 tbsp licorice root
- 2 cups hot water

Instructions: Steep peppermint and licorice root in hot water for 10 minutes. Strain and drink to support respiratory health and boost immune resilience.

21. Astragalus and Ginger Soup

Ingredients:

- 2 slices dried astragalus root
- 1 tbsp grated ginger
- 4 cups vegetable broth

Instructions: Simmer astragalus and ginger in the broth for 30 minutes.

22. Echinacea and Mint Tea

Ingredients:

- 1 tbsp dried echinacea
- 1 tbsp dried mint

- 2 cups boiling water

Instructions: Steep echinacea and mint in boiling water for 10 minutes. Strain and drink to reduce the duration of colds and improve immune function.

23. Clove and Lemon Water

Ingredients:

- 3 cloves
- 1 tbsp fresh lemon juice
- 1 cup hot water

Instructions: Add cloves to hot water and let steep for 10 minutes. Strain and add lemon juice.

24. Sage and Honey Immune Gargle

Ingredients:

- 1 tbsp dried sage
- 1 cup hot water
- 1 tsp honey

Instructions: Steep sage in hot water for 10 minutes, strain, and mix in honey. Gargle with the solution to soothe the throat and reduce inflammation.

25. Elderflower and Chamomile Tea

Ingredients:

- 1 tbsp dried elderflower
- 1 tbsp dried chamomile
- 2 cups boiling water

Instructions: Steep elderflower and chamomile in boiling water for 10 minutes. Strain and drink to reduce stress and enhance immune function.

Book 28: Digestive Health Recipes

1. Ginger Tea

Ingredients:

- 1-inch piece of fresh ginger
- 1 cup boiling water

Instructions: Slice the ginger and steep in boiling water for 10 minutes. Strain and sip slowly to soothe digestion and reduce bloating.

2. Peppermint Infusion

Ingredients:

- 1 tbsp dried peppermint leaves
- 1 cup boiling water

Instructions: Steep peppermint leaves in boiling water for 5-10 minutes. Strain and drink to relieve gas and calm an upset stomach.

3. Fennel Seed Chew

Ingredients:

- 1 tsp fennel seeds

Instructions: Chew on fennel seeds after meals to reduce bloating, gas, and indigestion.

4. Aloe Vera Juice

Ingredients:

- 2 tbsp fresh aloe vera gel
- 1 cup water

Instructions: Blend aloe vera gel with water and drink to soothe inflammation in the gut and support smooth digestion.

5. Apple Cider Vinegar Tonic

Ingredients:

- 1 tbsp apple cider vinegar
- 1 cup warm water

Instructions: Mix apple cider vinegar with water and drink before meals to enhance digestion and reduce acid reflux.

6. Chamomile Tea

Ingredients:

- 1 tbsp dried chamomile flowers
- 1 cup boiling water

Instructions: Steep chamomile flowers in boiling water for 5-10 minutes. Strain and drink to relax the digestive muscles and ease stomach cramps.

7. Turmeric Latte

Ingredients:

- 1/2 tsp turmeric powder
- 1/4 tsp black pepper
- 1 cup almond milk

Instructions: Heat almond milk and mix in turmeric and black pepper.

8. Slippery Elm Water

Ingredients:

- 1 tsp slippery elm powder
- 1 cup warm water

Instructions: Stir slippery elm powder into warm water and drink to coat the digestive tract, relieving irritation and promoting gut healing.

9. Dandelion Root Tea

Ingredients:

- 1 tsp dried dandelion root
- 1 cup boiling water

Instructions: Steep dandelion root in boiling water for 10 minutes. Strain and drink to stimulate digestion and support liver detoxification.

10. Cumin Seed Water

Ingredients:

- 1 tsp cumin seeds
- 1 cup boiling water

Instructions: Boil cumin seeds in water for 5 minutes. Strain and drink to relieve gas, bloating, and indigestion.

11. Lemon and Honey Water

Ingredients:

- Juice of 1/2 lemon
- 1 tsp honey
- 1 cup warm water

Instructions: Mix lemon juice and honey into warm water. Drink first thing in the morning to stimulate digestion and promote bowel movements.

12. Cucumber and Mint Water

Ingredients:

- 1/2 cucumber (sliced)
- a few fresh mint leaves
- 1-liter water

Instructions: Add cucumber slices and mint leaves to water and let it sit for 1-2 hours. Sip throughout the day to hydrate and promote smooth digestion.

13. Caraway Seed Infusion

Ingredients:

- 1 tsp caraway seeds
- 1 cup boiling water

Instructions: Steep caraway seeds in boiling water for 10 minutes. Strain and drink to relieve bloating, gas, and indigestion.

14. Papaya Smoothie

Ingredients:

- 1/2 cup ripe papaya
- 1/2 cup coconut water
- a pinch of cinnamon

Instructions: Blend papaya with coconut water and cinnamon. Drink to aid digestion with papaya's natural enzymes.

15. Ginger and Lemon Digestive Tonic

Ingredients:

- 1-inch piece of ginger
- juice of 1/2 lemon
- 1 cup warm water

Instructions: Grate ginger and squeeze lemon juice into warm water. Drink before meals to enhance digestion and reduce nausea.

16. Pineapple and Ginger Juice

Ingredients:

- 1/2 cup fresh pineapple
- 1-inch piece of ginger
- 1/2 cup water

Instructions: Blend pineapple and ginger with water. Strain and drink to help break down proteins and ease digestion with pineapple's bromelain enzyme.

17. Cabbage Juice

Ingredients:

- 1 cup fresh cabbage
- 1/2 cup water

Instructions: Blend cabbage and water. Strain and drink to support stomach lining health and soothe ulcers.

18. Anise Seed Tea

Ingredients:

- 1 tsp anise seeds
- 1 cup boiling water

Instructions: Steep anise seeds in boiling water for 10 minutes. Strain and drink to reduce gas and bloating.

19. Yogurt and Flaxseed Digestive Mix

Ingredients:

- 1/2 cup plain yogurt
- 1 tbsp ground flaxseed

Instructions: Mix ground flaxseed into yogurt and eat for a probiotic-rich snack that supports gut health and regularity.

20. Cardamom Tea

Ingredients:

- 2-3 crushed cardamom pods
- 1 cup boiling water

Instructions: Steep crushed cardamom pods in boiling water for 5 minutes. Strain and drink to ease indigestion and promote a healthy digestive tract.

Book 29: Liver Health Recipes

1. Fennel and Ginger Digestive Tonic

Ingredients:

- 1 tsp fennel seeds
- 1-inch piece of fresh ginger
- 1 cup boiling water

Instructions: Steep fennel seeds and grated ginger in boiling water for 10 minutes. Strain and drink to soothe indigestion and relieve bloating.

2. Aloe Vera and Coconut Water Smoothie

Ingredients:

- 1 tbsp fresh aloe vera gel
- 1/2 cup coconut water
- 1/4 cup cucumber

Instructions: Blend aloe vera gel with coconut water and cucumber. Drink to hydrate and promote digestive health.

3. Pear and Chia Seed Pudding

Ingredients:

- 1 ripe pear (mashed)
- 1 tbsp chia seeds
- 1/2 cup almond milk

Instructions: Mix mashed pear, chia seeds, and almond milk. Let it sit for 10 minutes to thicken.

4. Peppermint and Chamomile Tea

Ingredients:

- 1 tsp dried peppermint leaves
- 1 tsp dried chamomile flowers
- 1 cup boiling water

Instructions: Steep peppermint and chamomile in boiling water for 5-10 minutes. Strain and drink to relieve indigestion, gas, and cramps.

5. Papaya and Kiwi Salad

Ingredients:

- 1/2 cup ripe papaya
- 1 kiwi (sliced)
- a sprinkle of lime juice

Instructions: Mix papaya and kiwi slices with a splash of lime juice. Enjoy to promote digestive enzyme production and enhance gut health.

6. Cinnamon and Clove Digestive Tea

Ingredients:

- 1 stick cinnamon
- 2-3 cloves
- 1 cup boiling water

Instructions: Simmer cinnamon and cloves in boiling water for 5 minutes. Strain and drink to support digestion and reduce bloating.

7. Apple Cider Vinegar and Honey Drink

Ingredients:

- 1 tbsp apple cider vinegar
- 1 tsp honey
- 1 cup warm water

Instructions: Mix apple cider vinegar and honey into warm water. Drink before meals to stimulate digestive enzymes and aid nutrient absorption.

8. Devil's Claw Tea

Ingredients:

- 1 tsp dried Devil's Claw
- 1 cup boiling water

Instructions: Steep Devil's Claw in boiling water for 10 minutes. Strain and drink to stimulate liver function and support digestion.

9. Beet and Carrot Juice

Ingredients:

- 1/2 beet (peeled)
- 1 carrot
- 1/2 cup water

Instructions: Blend beet and carrot with water. Strain and drink to improve bile flow and aid digestion.

10. Turmeric and Black Pepper Tea

Ingredients:

- 1/2 tsp turmeric powder
- a pinch of black pepper
- 1 cup hot water

Instructions: Stir turmeric and black pepper into hot water. Drink to reduce inflammation and improve digestion.

11. Ginger and Lemon Detox Water

Ingredients:

- 1-inch piece of fresh ginger (sliced)
- 1/2 lemon (sliced)
- 2 cups water

Instructions: Combine ginger and lemon slices with water. Let it infuse for 1-2 hours in the refrigerator.

12. Mint and Cucumber Infused Water

Ingredients:

- 1/2 cucumber (sliced)
- a handful of fresh mint leaves
- 2 cups water

Instructions: Mix cucumber slices and mint leaves with water. Refrigerate for a few hours before drinking to soothe the digestive tract.

13. Oatmeal with Flaxseed and Berries

Ingredients:

- 1/2 cup rolled oats
- 1 tbsp ground flaxseed
- 1/4 cup mixed berries

Instructions: Cook oats as per package instructions. Stir in ground flaxseed and top with berries.

14. Carrot and Ginger Soup

Ingredients:

- 2 carrots (chopped)
- 1-inch piece of fresh ginger (grated)
- 2 cups vegetable broth

Instructions: Simmer carrots and ginger in vegetable broth until carrots are tender.

15. Pomegranate and Mint Smoothie

Ingredients:

- 1/2 cup pomegranate seeds
- a handful of fresh mint leaves
- 1/2 cup Greek yogurt

Instructions: Blend pomegranate seeds, mint leaves, and Greek yogurt until smooth. Drink to benefit from antioxidants and aid digestion.

16. Aloe Vera and Pineapple Juice

Ingredients:

- 1 tbsp fresh aloe vera gel
- 1/2 cup pineapple juice

Instructions: Mix aloe vera gel into pineapple juice. Drink to soothe the digestive system and support hydration.

17. Parsley and Lemon Tea

Ingredients:

- 1 tbsp chopped fresh parsley
- 1/2 lemon (juiced)
- 1 cup boiling water

Instructions: Steep parsley in boiling water for 5 minutes. Add lemon juice before drinking. This tea supports digestion and acts as a natural diuretic.

18. Sweet Potato and Ginger Mash

Ingredients:

- 1 medium sweet potato (peeled and cubed)
- 1-inch piece of fresh ginger (grated)
- a pinch of salt

Instructions: Boil sweet potato until tender. Mash with grated ginger and a pinch of salt.

19. Cinnamon and Apple Infused Tea

Ingredients:

- 1 cinnamon stick
- 1 apple (sliced)
- 1 cup boiling water

Instructions: Steep cinnamon stick and apple slices in boiling water for 10 minutes. Strain and drink to support digestive health and flavor.

20. Cucumber and Lemon Mint Salad

Ingredients:

- 1/2 cucumber (sliced)
- 1/4 cup chopped fresh mint
- 1 tbsp lemon juice

Instructions: Toss cucumber slices with mint and lemon juice. Enjoy this refreshing salad to aid digestion and provide a hydrating boost.

21. Apple Cider Vinegar and Maple syrup

Ingredients:

- 1 tbsp apple cider vinegar
- 1 tsp maple syrup
- 1 cup warm water

Instructions: Mix apple cider vinegar and maple syrup into warm water. Drink before meals to aid digestion and balance stomach acid.

22. Turmeric and Ginger Tea

Ingredients:

- 1/2 tsp ground turmeric
- 1/2 tsp ground ginger

- 1 cup boiling water

Instructions: Combine turmeric and ginger in boiling water. Steep for 5 minutes, then strain. Drink to support digestive health and reduce inflammation.

23. Fennel Seed and Chamomile Tea

Ingredients:

- 1 tsp fennel seeds
- 1 chamomile tea bag
- 1 cup boiling water

Instructions: Steep fennel seeds and chamomile tea bag in boiling water for 10 minutes. Strain and drink to alleviate bloating and gas.

24. Papaya and Pineapple Smoothie

Ingredients:

- 1/2 cup fresh papaya
- 1/2 cup pineapple chunks
- 1/2 cup coconut water

Instructions: Blend papaya, pineapple, and coconut water until smooth. Enjoy this smoothie to aid digestion and boost enzyme intake.

25. Artichoke and Lemon Dip

Ingredients:

- 1 cup cooked artichoke hearts
- 1 tbsp lemon juice
- 1 tbsp olive oil

Instructions: Blend artichoke hearts with lemon juice and olive oil until smooth. Use as a dip or spread to support digestive function.

Book 30: Respiratory Support Recipes

1. Ginger and Lemon Tea

Ingredients:

- 1-inch fresh ginger root
- 1 lemon 1-2 tsp honey
- 2 cups water

Instructions: Boil water and add sliced ginger. Simmer for 10 minutes. Strain into a cup, add lemon juice and honey.

2. Thyme and Eucalyptus Steam Inhalation

Ingredients:

- 1 tbsp dried thyme
- 1-2 drops eucalyptus essential oil
- 4 cups boiling water

Instructions: Place thyme in a bowl, pour boiling, and add eucalyptus oil. Cover your head with a towel and inhale the steam for 5-10 minutes.

3. Ginger Powder Golden Milk

Ingredients:

- 1 cup milk (dairy or plant-based)
- 1 tsp ginger powder
- 1/2 tsp black pepper 1 tsp honey

Instructions: Heat milk in a saucepan and whisk in ginger powder and black pepper. Simmer for 5 minutes, then remove from heat.

4. Peppermint and Lemon Water

Ingredients:

- 1 handful fresh peppermint leaves
- 1 lemon
- 2 cups water

Instructions: Slice lemon and add to a pitcher with peppermint leaves. Fill with water and let infuse in the refrigerator for at least 1 hour before drinking.

5. Garlic and Honey Syrup

Ingredients:

- 4 cloves garlic
- 1/4 cup honey

Instructions: Crush garlic cloves and mix with honey in a jar. Let sit for 24 hours. Take 1 tsp daily to help soothe the respiratory system.

6. Licorice Root Tea

Ingredients:

- 1 tbsp dried licorice root
- 2 cups water

Instructions: Boil water and add licorice root. Simmer for 10-15 minutes. Strain into a cup and drink warm.

7. Oregano Infusion

Ingredients:

- 1 tbsp dried oregano
- 2 cups boiling water

Instructions: Steep oregano in boiling water for 10 minutes. Strain and drink.

8. Cinnamon and Honey Elixir

Ingredients:

- 1/2 tsp cinnamon
- 1 tablespoon honey
- 1 cup warm water

Instructions: Dissolve cinnamon and honey in warm water. Stir well and drink to help soothe the throat and support respiratory health.

9. Rosemary and Sage Tea

Ingredients:

- 1 tsp dried rosemary
- 1 tsp dried sage
- 2 cups water

Instructions: Boil water and add rosemary and sage. Simmer for 10 minutes. Strain and enjoy the tea to help clear respiratory passages.

10. Mullein Leaf Infusion

Ingredients:

- 1 tbsp dried mullein leaves
- 2 cups boiling water

Instructions: Steep mullein leaves in boiling water for 10 minutes. Strain and drink to help with respiratory tract irritation and support lung health.

11. Fennel Seed Tea

Ingredients:

- 1 tbsp fennel seeds
- 2 cups water

Instructions: Crush fennel seeds slightly and add to boiling water. Simmer for 10 minutes. Strain and drink to help alleviate respiratory congestion.

12. Cayenne Pepper and Honey Tonic

Ingredients:

- 1/2 tsp cayenne pepper
- 1 tbsp honey
- 1 cup warm water

Instructions: Stir cayenne pepper and honey into warm water. Drink to help boost circulation and support respiratory function.

13. Elderflower syrup

Ingredients:

- 1 cup dried elderberries
- 3 cups water
- 1 cup honey
- 1 tbsp fresh lemon juice

Instructions: Boil elderberries in water for 30 minutes, then strain. Stir in honey and lemon juice. Let cool before storing.

14. Basil and Mint Infusion

Ingredients:

- 1 tbsp fresh basil leaves
- 1 tbsp fresh mint leaves
- 2 cups boiling water

Instructions: Steep basil and mint leaves in boiling water for 10 minutes. Strain and enjoy the infusion for respiratory support.

15. Ginger and Turmeric Tonic

Ingredients:

- 1-inch fresh ginger root
- 1/2 tsp turmeric powder
- 1 tbsp honey
- 2 cups water

Instructions: Boil water and add sliced ginger and turmeric powder. Simmer for 10 minutes, then strain. Stir in honey and drink warm.

16. Lemon Balm Tea

Ingredients:

- 1 tbsp dried lemon balm leaves
- 2 cups boiling water

Instructions: Steep lemon balm leaves in boiling water for 10 minutes. Strain and drink to support respiratory health and relaxation.

17. Apple Cider Vinegar and Ginger Drink

Ingredients:

- 1 tbsp apple cider vinegar
- 1-inch fresh ginger root
- 1 tbsp honey
- 1 cup water

Instructions: Boil ginger in water for 10 minutes. Strain and stir in apple cider vinegar and honey. Drink warm.

18. Sage and Thyme Tea

Ingredients:

- 1 tsp dried sage
- 1 tsp dried thyme
- 2 cups boiling water

Instructions: Combine sage and thyme in boiling water and steep for 10 minutes. Strain and drink to help soothe the respiratory system.

19. Clove and Cardamom Tea

Ingredients:

- 4-5 whole cloves
- 2-3 cardamom pods
- 2 cups boiling water

Instructions: Crush cloves and cardamom pods slightly. Add to boiling water and steep for 10 minutes. Strain and drink.

20. Juniper Berry Tea

Ingredients:

- 1 tbsp dried juniper berries
- 2 cups boiling water

Instructions: Crush juniper berries slightly and steep in boiling water for 10 minutes. Strain and drink to support respiratory health.

Book 31: Hormone Health Recipes

1. Marshmallow Root Tea

Ingredients:

- 1 tbsp dried marshmallow root
- 2 cups boiling water

Instructions: Steep marshmallow root in boiling water for 15 minutes. Strain and drink to soothe the respiratory tract.

2. Thyme and Lemon Tea

Ingredients:

- 1 tsp dried thyme
- 1 tbsp fresh lemon juice
- 2 cups boiling water

Instructions: Steep thyme in boiling water for 10 minutes. Add lemon juice before drinking to help ease cough and congestion.

3. Onion and Honey Syrup

Ingredients:

- 3 cloves garlic
- 1/4 cup honey

Instructions: Crush Onion and mix with honey. Let sit for at least 4 hours before straining.

4. Rosemary and Eucalyptus Steam

Ingredients:

- 1 tbsp dried rosemary
- 5 drops eucalyptus essential oil
- 2 cups boiling water

Instructions: Add rosemary and eucalyptus oil to boiling water. Lean over the bowl, cover your head with a towel, and inhale the steam for 10 minutes.

5. Peppermint and Echinacea Tea

Ingredients:

- 1 tsp dried peppermint leaves
- 1 tsp dried echinacea
- 2 cups boiling water

Instructions: Steep peppermint and echinacea in boiling water for 10 minutes. Strain and drink to help support immune and respiratory health.

6. Cucumber and Mint Infusion

Ingredients:

- 1/2 cucumber, sliced
- 1 tbsp fresh mint leaves
- 2 cups water

Instructions: Combine cucumber slices and mint leaves in water. Let infuse for 2 hours in the refrigerator.

7. Orange and Ginger Elixir

Ingredients:

- 1 cup fresh orange juice
- 1-inch fresh ginger root
- 1 tbsp honey

Instructions: Juice ginger and mix with orange juice and honey. Drink chilled or at room temperature to support respiratory health.

8. Dill Tea

Ingredients:

- 1 tsp dried Dill
- 2 cups boiling water

Instructions: Steep Dill root in boiling water for 10 minutes. Strain and drink to soothe the throat and support respiratory function.

9. Rooibos Tea

Ingredients:

- 1 tbsp fresh or dried rooibos
- 2 cups boiling water

Instructions: Steep rooibos in boiling water for 10 minutes. Strain and drink to help with respiratory health and boost vitamin C.

10. Dandelion and Ginger Tea

Ingredients:

- 1 tsp dried dandelion root
- 1-inch fresh ginger root
- 2 cups boiling water

Instructions: Boil dandelion root and ginger in water for 15 minutes. Strain and drink to support respiratory health and digestion.

11. Elderberry and Cinnamon Tea

Ingredients:

- 1 tbsp dried elderberries
- 1 cinnamon stick
- 2 cups boiling water

Instructions: Steep elderberries and cinnamon stick in boiling water for 15 minutes. Strain and drink to help with respiratory health and boost immunity.

12. Ginger and Turmeric Lemonade

Ingredients:

- 1-inch fresh ginger root
- 1 tsp ground turmeric
- 1 cup fresh lemon juice
- 2 cups water
- 2 tbsp honey

Instructions: Blend ginger with water, then strain and mix with lemon juice, turmeric, and honey. Chill and drink to support respiratory and overall health.

13. Cardamom and Honey Tea

Ingredients:

- 4 cardamom pods
- 1 tbsp honey
- 2 cups boiling water

Instructions: Crush cardamom pods and steep in boiling water for 10 minutes. Strain, add honey, and drink to help with respiratory discomfort and soothe the throat.

14. Rose and Hibiscus Tea

Ingredients:

- 1 tbsp dried rose petals
- 1 tbsp dried hibiscus flowers
- 2 cups boiling water

Instructions: Steep rose petals and hibiscus flowers in boiling water for 10 minutes. Strain and drink to support respiratory health and provide antioxidants.

15. Fennel Seed and Licorice Tea

Ingredients:

- 1 tsp fennel seeds
- 1 tsp dried licorice root
- 2 cups boiling water

Instructions: Steep fennel seeds and licorice root in boiling water for 10 minutes. Strain and drink to help with respiratory issues and improve digestion.

16. Thyme and Apple Cider Vinegar Tonic

Ingredients:

- 1 tsp dried thyme
- 1 tbsp apple cider vinegar
- 1 cup water

Instructions: Steep thyme in boiling water for 10 minutes. Strain, then add apple cider vinegar. Drink to support respiratory health and overall wellness.

17. Beet and Ginger Juice

Ingredients:

- 1 small beet
- 1-inch fresh ginger root
- 1 cup water

Instructions: Juice beet and ginger, then mix with water. Drink immediately to help clear the respiratory tract and boost vitality.

18. Clove and Honey Infusion

Ingredients:

- 5 whole cloves
- 1 tbsp honey
- 1 cup hot water

Instructions: Steep cloves in hot water for 10 minutes. Strain, then add honey and drink to support respiratory health and soothe the throat.

19. Lemon Balm and Ginger Tea

Ingredients:

- 1 tbsp fresh lemon balm leaves
- 1-inch fresh ginger root
- 2 cups boiling water

Instructions: Steep lemon balm and ginger in boiling water for 10 minutes. Strain and drink to help with respiratory discomfort and provide relaxation.

20. Mullein and Oregano Tea

Ingredients:

- 1 tbsp dried mullein leaves
- 1 tsp dried oregano
- 2 cups boiling water

Instructions: Steep mullein leaves and oregano in boiling water for 10 minutes. Strain and drink to support respiratory health and relieve coughs.

21. Peppermint and Eucalyptus Steam

Ingredients:

- 1 handful fresh peppermint leaves
- 3-4 drops eucalyptus oil
- 2 cups hot water

Instructions: Place peppermint leaves in a bowl and pour hot water over them. Add eucalyptus oil. Drape a towel over your head and the bowl, and inhale the steam for 10 minutes to relieve congestion.

22. Cayenne Pepper and Honey Drink

Ingredients:

- 1/2 tsp cayenne pepper
- 1 tbsp honey
- 1 cup warm water

Instructions: Stir cayenne pepper and honey into warm water. Drink to help clear the airways and provide a warming effect for respiratory support.

23. Rosemary and Thyme Tea

Ingredients:

- 1 tbsp dried rosemary
- 1 tbsp dried thyme
- 2 cups boiling water

Instructions: Steep rosemary and thyme in boiling water for 10 minutes. Strain and drink to help with respiratory congestion and support lung health.

24. Ephedra and Mint Tea

Ingredients:

- 1 tbsp dried Ephedra
- 1 tbsp fresh mint leaves
- 2 cups boiling water

Instructions: Steep echinacea and mint in boiling water for 10 minutes. Strain and drink to support the immune system and respiratory health.

25. Dandelion Root and Ginger Tea

Ingredients:

- 1 tsp dried dandelion root
- 1-inch fresh ginger root
- 2 cups boiling water

Instructions: Steep dandelion root and ginger in boiling water for 10 minutes. Strain and drink to help with respiratory health and detoxification.

Book 32: Stress and Anxiety Relief Recipes

1. Burdock Tea

Ingredients:

- 1 tsp dried burdock
- 1 cup boiling water

Instructions: Steep chamomile in water for 5 mins. Strain and drink to soothe stress and anxiety.

2. Lavender Infused Water

Ingredients:

- 1 tsp dried lavender
- 1 cup water

Instructions: Steep lavender in water for 10 mins. Strain and chill. Sip to relax.

3. Linden Tea

Ingredients:

- 1 tsp dried linden
- 1 cup hot water

Instructions: Steep linden in water for 7 mins. Strain and enjoy to calm nerves.

4. Peppermint Relaxation Smoothie

Ingredients:

- 1 cup spinach
- 1/2 banana
- 1/4 tsp peppermint extract

Instructions: Blend all ingredients until smooth. Drink to relieve stress and anxiety.

5. Valerian Root Tincture

Ingredients:

- 15 drops valerian tincture
- 1/4 cup water

Instructions: Mix valerian tincture with water. Drink before bed to aid relaxation.

6. Passionflower Tea

Ingredients:

- 1 tsp dried passionflower
- 1 cup boiling water

Instructions: Steep passionflower in water for 10 mins. Strain and enjoy to reduce anxiety.

7. Ashwagandha Smoothie

Ingredients:

- 1/2 cup yogurt
- 1/2 banana
- 1/4 tsp ashwagandha powder

Instructions: Blend all ingredients until smooth. Drink to combat stress and enhance mood.

8. Calming Lemonade

Ingredients:

- 1 cup water
- 1 tbsp lemon juice
- 1 tsp honey

Instructions: Mix all ingredients well. Chill and drink to calm the mind.

9. Ginger Honey Tea

Ingredients:

- 1 tsp grated ginger
- 1 cup boiling water
- 1 tsp honey

Instructions: Steep ginger in water for 5 mins. Add honey, stir, and drink to relax.

10. Oatmeal with Cinnamon

Ingredients:

- 1/2 cup oats
- 1 cup water
- 1/4 tsp cinnamon

Instructions: Cook oats in water, stir in cinnamon, and serve warm to promote relaxation.

11. Safflower Golden Milk

Ingredients:

- 1 cup milk
- 1/4 tsp Safflower
- 1/4 tsp honey

Instructions: Heat milk with Safflower. Stir in honey and drink to soothe the mind.

12. Honey Lemon Ginger Tea

Ingredients:

- 1 cup boiling water
- 1 tsp honey
- 1 tbsp lemon juice
- 1 tsp grated ginger

Instructions: Steep ginger in water for 5 mins. Strain, then add honey and lemon juice. Drink to calm nerves.

13. Cinnamon Apple Water

Ingredients:

- 1 apple, sliced
- 1 stick cinnamon
- 1 liter water

Instructions: Combine all ingredients in a pitcher. Let infuse overnight. Drink to relieve stress.

14. Cinnamon Tea

Ingredients:

- 1/2 tsp crushed cinnamon
- 1 cup boiling water

Instructions: Steep cinnamon in water for 5 mins. Strain and drink to reduce anxiety.

15. Peppermint Infused Coconut Water

Ingredients:

- 1 cup coconut water
- 1/4 tsp peppermint extract

Instructions: Mix peppermint extract into coconut water. Chill and sip to ease stress.

16. Sage Tea

Ingredients:

- 1 tsp dried sage
- 1 cup boiling water

Instructions: Steep sage in water for 7 mins. Strain and enjoy to relax.

17. Celery Seed Tea

Ingredients:

- 1 tsp celery seeds
- 1 cup boiling water

Instructions: Steep Celery seeds in water for 5 mins. Strain and drink to ease anxiety.

18. Rhodiola Smoothie

Ingredients:

- 1/2 cup Greek yogurt
- 1/2 cup berries
- 1/4 tsp rhodiola powder

Instructions: Blend all ingredients until smooth. Drink to boost mood and reduce stress.

19. Rosemary Mint Tea

Ingredients:

- 1 sprig rosemary
- 5 fresh mint leaves
- 1 cup boiling water

Instructions: Steep rosemary and mint in water for 5 mins. Strain and enjoy to calm the mind.

20. Apple Cider Vinegar Drink

Ingredients:

- 1 tbsp apple cider vinegar
- 1 cup water
- 1 tsp honey

Instructions: Mix all ingredients well. Drink to help reduce stress and improve digestion.

Book 33: Bone Health Recipes

1. Lavender Lemonade

Ingredients:

- 1 cup water
- 1 tbsp dried lavender
- juice of 1 lemon
- 1 tsp honey

Instructions: Steep lavender in hot water for 5 mins. Strain, then add lemon juice and honey. Chill and drink to relax.

2. Valerian Root Tea

Ingredients:

- 1 tsp dried valerian root
- 1 cup boiling water

Instructions: Steep valerian root in water for 10 mins. Strain and drink to support restful relaxation.

3. Chamomile and Honey Tea

Ingredients:

- 1 tbsp dried chamomile
- 1 cup boiling water
- 1 tsp honey

Instructions: Steep chamomile in water for 5 mins. Strain and stir in honey. Drink to soothe nerves.

4. Ginger and Lemon Infused Water

Ingredients:

- 1 tsp grated ginger
- juice of 1/2 lemon
- 1 liter water

Instructions: Combine ginger and lemon juice in water. Let infuse for 1 hour. Drink to alleviate stress.

5. Ashwagandha Tea

Ingredients:

- 1 tsp ashwagandha powder
- 1 cup boiling water

Instructions: Stir ashwagandha powder into boiling water. Steep for 5 mins, then drink to enhance relaxation.

6. Cucumber Mint Water

Ingredients:

- 1/2 cucumber, sliced
- 5 fresh mint leaves
- 1 liter water

Instructions: Combine cucumber and mint in water. Let infuse for 1 hour. Drink to refresh and reduce anxiety.

7. Warm Almond Milk with Nutmeg

Ingredients:

- 1 cup almond milk
- 1/4 tsp nutmeg

Instructions: Heat almond milk and stir in nutmeg. Drink warm to calm the mind and body.

8. Jamaica Dogwood Tea

Ingredients:

- 1 tsp dried Jamaica Dogwood
- 1 cup boiling water

Instructions: Steep Jamaica Dogwood in water for 5 mins. Strain and drink to support relaxation and reduce anxiety.

9. Peppermint Lavender Tea

Ingredients:

- 1 tsp dried lavender
- 1 tsp peppermint leaves
- 1 cup boiling water

Instructions: Steep lavender and peppermint in water for 5 mins. Strain and enjoy to calm the senses.

10. Orange Blossom Water Drink

Ingredients:

- 1 cup water
- 1 tsp orange blossom water
- 1 tsp honey

Instructions: Mix orange blossom water and honey into water. Drink to help soothe nerves and uplift mood.

11. Lemon-Ginger Herbal Infusion

Ingredients:

- 1 tsp dried ginger
- juice of 1/2 lemon
- 1 cup boiling water

Instructions: Steep ginger in boiling water for 5 mins. Add lemon juice, stir, and drink to relieve stress.

12. Rosewater and Honey Elixir

Ingredients:

- 1 cup water
- 1 tsp rosewater
- 1 tsp honey

Instructions: Mix rosewater and honey into water. Stir well and drink to soothe the mind and body.

13. Holy Basil (Tulsi) Tea

Ingredients:

- 1 tsp dried holy basil
- 1 cup boiling water

Instructions: Steep holy basil in boiling water for 5-7 mins. Strain and drink to support stress reduction.

14. Cinnamon and Apple Cider Vinegar Drink

Ingredients:

- 1 cup water
- 1 tbsp apple cider vinegar
- 1/4 tsp cinnamon

Instructions: Combine apple cider vinegar and cinnamon in water. Stir well and drink to calm and detoxify.

15. Spearmint Lemon Infusion

Ingredients:

- 1 tsp dried spearmint
- juice of 1/2 lemon
- 1 cup water

Instructions: Steep spearmint in boiling water for 5 mins. Add lemon juice, stir, and enjoy to refresh and relax.

16. Warm Coconut Milk with Vanilla

Ingredients:

- 1 cup coconut milk
- 1/2 tsp vanilla extract

Instructions: Heat coconut milk and stir in vanilla extract. Drink warm to promote relaxation.

17. Echinacea Tea

Ingredients:

- 1 tsp dried echinacea
- 1 cup boiling water

Instructions: Steep echinacea in boiling water for 5-7 mins. Strain and drink to support the immune system and reduce stress.

18. Cardamom and Clove Infused Water

Ingredients:

- 1 cardamom pod
- 2 cloves
- 1 liter water

Instructions: Infuse cardamom and cloves in water for 1 hour. Strain and drink to calm nerves and uplift mood.

19. Tumeric and Honey Golden Milk

Ingredients:

- 1 cup milk (dairy or non-dairy)
- 1/2 tsp turmeric,
- 1 tsp honey

Instructions: Heat milk and stir in turmeric and honey. Drink warm to soothe and relax.

20. Apple-Cinnamon Relaxation Tea

Ingredients:

- 1 cup water
- 1/2 apple (sliced)
- 1/2 tsp cinnamon

Instructions: Heat water with apple slices and cinnamon. Simmer for 10 mins, then strain and drink to ease stress.

21. Chamomile and Lavender Tea

Ingredients:

- 1 tsp dried chamomile
- 1 tsp dried lavender
- 1 cup boiling water

Instructions: Steep chamomile and lavender in boiling water for 5-7 mins. Strain and drink to promote relaxation and calm.

22. Peppermint and Lemon Balm Infusion

Ingredients:

- 1 tsp dried peppermint
- 1 tsp dried lemon balm
- 1 cup boiling water

Instructions: Steep peppermint and lemon balm in boiling water for 5-7 mins. Strain and drink to ease tension and stress.

23. Siberian Ginseng Tea

Ingredients:

- 1 tsp dried Siberian Ginseng
- 1 cup boiling water

Instructions: Steep Siberian Ginseng in boiling water for 10 mins. Strain and drink to support restful sleep and reduce anxiety.

24. Ginger and Lime Zinger

Ingredients:

- 1 tsp grated fresh ginger
- juice of 1 lime
- 1 cup water

Instructions: Mix ginger and lime juice into water. Stir well and drink to refresh and alleviate stress.

25. Honey and Cinnamon Relaxation Drink

Ingredients:

- 1 cup warm water
- 1 tsp honey
- 1/4 tsp cinnamon

Instructions: Stir honey and cinnamon into warm water. Drink to soothe nerves and improve mood.

Book 34: Skin and Beauty Recipes

1. Honey and Lemon Face Mask

Ingredients:

- 1 tbsp honey
- 1 tsp lemon juice

Instructions: Mix honey with lemon juice. Apply to face, leave for 10 min, then rinse with warm water.

2. Avocado and Yogurt Face Mask

Ingredients:

- 1/2 avocado
- 2 tbsp yogurt

Instructions: Mash avocado and mix with yogurt. Apply to face, leave for 15 min, then rinse with lukewarm water.

3. Green Tea and Aloe Vera Toner

Ingredients:

- 1 cup brewed green tea
- 2 tbsp aloe vera gel

Instructions: Combine green tea with aloe vera. Apply to face with a cotton pad after cleansing.

4. Oatmeal and Honey Scrub

Ingredients:

- 2 tbsp oatmeal
- 1 tbsp honey

Instructions: Mix oatmeal with honey. Gently massage onto damp face, then rinse off.

5. Cucumber and Mint Eye Soother

Ingredients:

- 1/2 cucumber
- a few mints leaves

Instructions: Blend cucumber and mint. Apply mixture to closed eyes, leave for 10 min, then rinse with cool water.

6. Coconut Oil and Brown Sugar Exfoliant

Ingredients:

- 2 tbsp coconut oil
- 1 tbsp brown sugar

Instructions: Combine coconut oil with brown sugar. Gently massage onto skin, then rinse with warm water.

7. Banana and Honey Face Mask

Ingredients:

- 1 banana
- 1 tbsp honey

Instructions: Mash banana and mix with honey. Apply to face, leave for 10 min, then rinse with lukewarm water.

8. Rosewater and Witch Hazel Toner

Ingredients:

- 1/2 cup rosewater
- 1/2 cup witch hazel

Instructions: Mix rosewater with witch hazel. Apply to face with a cotton pad after cleansing.

9. Aloe Vera and Turmeric Face Mask

Ingredients:

- 2 tbsp aloe vera gel
- 1/2 tsp turmeric powder

Instructions: Mix aloe vera with turmeric. Apply to face, leave for 10 min, then rinse with warm water.

10. Yogurt and Cucumber Face Mask

Ingredients:

- 2 tbsp yogurt
- 1/4 cucumber

Instructions: Blend cucumber and mix with yogurt. Apply to face, leave for 15 min, then rinse with cool water.

11. Almond Oil and Honey Moisturizer

Ingredients:

- 1 tbsp almond oil
- 1 tbsp honey

Instructions: Mix almond oil with honey. Apply to face and neck as a nighttime moisturizer.

12. Lemon and Sugar Lip Scrub

Ingredients:

- 1 tsp lemon juice
- 1 tsp sugar

Instructions: Mix lemon juice with sugar. Gently rub onto lips to exfoliate, then rinse off.

13. Apple Cider Vinegar and Water Toner

Ingredients:

- 1/2 cup apple cider vinegar
- 1/2 cup water

Instructions: Dilute apple cider vinegar with water. Apply to face with a cotton pad after cleansing.

14. Papaya and Honey Face Mask

Ingredients:

- 1/2 cup mashed papaya
- 1 tbsp honey

Instructions: Mix papaya with honey. Apply to face, leave for 10 min, then rinse with warm water.

15. Avocado and Olive Oil Moisturizer

Ingredients:

- 1/2 avocado
- 1 tbsp olive oil

Instructions: Mash avocado and mix with olive oil. Apply to face as a hydrating mask, leave for 15 min, then rinse.

16. Green Tea and Honey Face Mask

Ingredients:

- 1 tbsp green tea (cooled)
- 1 tbsp honey

Instructions: Mix green tea with honey. Apply to face, leave for 10 min, then rinse with lukewarm water.

17. Honey and Cinnamon Spot Treatment

Ingredients:

- 1 tsp honey
- 1/2 tsp cinnamon

Instructions: Mix honey with cinnamon. Apply to blemishes, leave for 10 min, then rinse with warm water.

18. Milk and Honey Bath Soak

Ingredients:

- 1 cup milk
- 1/2 cup honey

Instructions: Mix milk with honey in a warm bath. Soak for 20 min to soothe and soften skin.

19. Sea Salt and Olive Oil Scrub

Ingredients:

- 2 tbsp sea salt
- 2 tbsp olive oil

Instructions: Combine sea salt with olive oil. Gently scrub onto skin, then rinse with warm water.

20. Carrot and Honey Face Mask

Ingredients:

- 1/2 cup grated carrot
- 1 tbsp honey

Instructions: Mix grated carrot with honey. Apply to face, leave for 15 min, then rinse with warm water.

21. Strawberry and Yogurt Face Mask

Ingredients:

- 3 strawberries
- 2 tbsp yogurt

Instructions: Mash strawberries and mix with yogurt. Apply to face, leave for 10 min, then rinse with lukewarm water.

22. Coconut Milk and Honey Facial Cleanser

Ingredients:

- 1/2 cup coconut milk
- 1 tbsp honey

Instructions: Mix coconut milk with honey. Massage onto face, then rinse with warm water.

23. Turmeric and Milk Brightening Mask

Ingredients:

- 1 tbsp milk
- 1/2 tsp turmeric powder

Instructions: Mix milk with turmeric. Apply to face, leave for 10 min, then rinse with warm water.

24. Chamomile and Honey Eye Compress

Ingredients:

- 1 chamomile tea bag
- 1 tbsp honey

Instructions: Brew chamomile tea, let it cool, and mix with honey. Soak cotton pads in the mixture and place them on closed eyes for 10 minutes.

25. Grapefruit and Mint Body Scrub

Ingredients:

- 2 tbsp grapefruit juice
- 2 tbsp sugar
- a few mints leaves

Instructions: Mix grapefruit juice with sugar and crushed mint leaves. Gently scrub onto body, then rinse with warm water.

26. Aloe Vera and Cucumber Gel

Ingredients:

- 2 tbsp aloe vera gel
- 1/2 cucumber (blended)

Instructions: Mix aloe vera gel with blended cucumber. Apply to face and leave for 15 min, then rinse with cool water.

27. Honey and Green Tea Face Mist

Ingredients:

- 1 cup brewed green tea (cooled)
- 1 tbsp honey

Instructions: Combine green tea with honey. Pour into a spray bottle and mist over face for hydration.

28. Papaya and Almond Oil Facial Cream

Ingredients:

- 1/2 cup mashed papaya
- 1 tbsp almond oil

Instructions: Mix papaya with almond oil. Apply to face, leave for 20 min, then rinse with warm water.

29. Yogurt and Mint Face Pack

Ingredients:

- 2 tbsp yogurt
- 1 tsp dried mint

Instructions: Combine yogurt with dried mint. Apply to face, leave for 10 min, then rinse with lukewarm water.

30. Rosewater and Glycerin Toner

Ingredients:

- 1/2 cup rosewater
- 1 tbsp glycerin

Instructions: Mix rosewater with glycerin. Apply to face with a cotton pad after cleansing.

31. Banana and Milk Hydrating Mask

Ingredients:

- 1 banana
- 2 tbsp milk

Instructions: Mash banana and mix with milk. Apply to face, leave for 15 min, then rinse with lukewarm water.

32. Avocado and Honey Hair Treatment

Ingredients:

- 1/2 avocado
- 1 tbsp honey

Instructions: Mash avocado and mix with honey. Apply to hair, leave for 20 min, then rinse with warm water.

33. Lemon and Honey Brightening Mask

Ingredients:

- 1 tbsp honey
- 1 tsp lemon juice

Instructions: Mix honey with lemon juice. Apply to face, leave for 10 min, then rinse with warm water.

34. Cucumber and Aloe Vera Hydrating Mist

Ingredients:

- 1/2 cucumber (blended)
- 2 tbsp aloe vera juice

Instructions: Blend cucumber and mix with aloe vera juice. Pour into a spray bottle and mist over face.

35. Orange Peel and Yogurt Face Mask

Ingredients:

- 2 tbsp dried orange peel powder
- 2 tbsp yogurt

Instructions: Combine orange peel powder with yogurt. Apply to face, leave for 15 min, then rinse with warm water.

36. Coconut Oil and Vitamin E Moisturizer

Ingredients:

- 1 tbsp coconut oil
- 1 tsp vitamin E oil

Instructions: Mix coconut oil with vitamin E oil. Apply to face and neck as a nighttime moisturizer.

37. Green Tea and Aloe Vera Face Spray

Ingredients:

- 1/2 cup brewed green tea (cooled)
- 2 tbsp aloe vera gel

Instructions: Combine green tea with aloe vera gel. Pour into a spray bottle and use as a face refresher.

38. Strawberry and Honey Exfoliant

Ingredients:

- 3 strawberries
- 1 tbsp honey

Instructions: Mash strawberries and mix with honey. Gently rub onto skin, then rinse with warm water.

39. Chamomile and Honey Facial Steam

Ingredients:

- 1 chamomile tea bag
- 1 cup hot water

Instructions: Steep chamomile tea bag in hot water. Place face over steam for 10 min to open pores.

40. Olive Oil and Lemon Scrub

Ingredients:

- 2 tbsp olive oil
- 1 tsp lemon juice
- 1 tbsp sugar

Instructions: Mix olive oil with lemon juice and sugar. Gently scrub onto skin, then rinse with warm water.

41. Beetroot and Yogurt Brightening Mask

Ingredients:

- 1 tbsp beetroot juice
- 2 tbsp yogurt

Instructions: Combine beetroot juice with yogurt. Apply to face, leave for 15 min, then rinse with lukewarm water.

42. Pineapple and Honey Face Mask

Ingredients:

- 2 tbsp pineapple juice
- 1 tbsp honey

Instructions: Mix pineapple juice with honey. Apply to face, leave for 10 min, then rinse with warm water.

43. Milk and Rosewater Soothing Lotion

Ingredients:

- 1/2 cup milk
- 1/4 cup rosewater

Instructions: Mix milk with rosewater. Apply to face and body for a soothing effect.

44. Turmeric and Yogurt Face Mask

Ingredients:

- 2 tbsp yogurt
- 1/2 tsp turmeric powder

Instructions: Combine yogurt with turmeric powder. Apply to face, leave for 10 min, then rinse with warm water.

45. Honey and Almond Scrub

Ingredients:

- 2 tbsp honey
- 1 tbsp ground almonds

Instructions: Mix honey with ground almonds. Gently massage onto skin, then rinse with warm wate

Book 35: Pain Relief and Anti-Inflammatory Recipes

1. Curry Powder Golden Milk

Ingredients:

- 1 cup milk
- 1/2 tsp curry powder
- 1/4 tsp black pepper
- 1 tsp honey

Instructions: Heat milk and whisk in curry powder, black pepper, and honey.

2. Ginger and Cinnamon Tea

Ingredients:

- 1-inch ginger root (sliced)
- 1 stick cinnamon
- 2 cups water

Instructions: Boil ginger and cinnamon in water for 10 minutes. Strain and drink to soothe sore muscles and reduce inflammation.

3. Epsom Salt Foot Soak

Ingredients:

- 1/2 cup Epsom salt
- 2 liters warm water

Instructions: Dissolve Epsom salt in warm water. Soak feet for 15 minutes to relieve muscle pain and inflammation.

4. Chamomile and Peppermint Tea

Ingredients:

- 1 chamomile tea bag
- 1 tsp dried peppermint
- 1 cup boiling water

Instructions: Steep chamomile and peppermint in boiling water for 5 minutes. Drink to help with digestive pain and inflammation.

5. Arnica Infused Oil

Ingredients:

- 1/4 cup dried arnica flowers
- 1/2 cup carrier oil (like coconut or olive)

Instructions: Infuse arnica flowers in carrier oil for 2 weeks. Strain and apply to sore muscles to reduce pain and swelling.

6. Rice Wine Vinegar Drink

Ingredients:

- 1 tbsp rice Wine Vinegar
- 1 cup water
- 1 tsp honey

Instructions: Mix Rice Wine Vinegar, water, and honey. Drink to support joint health and reduce inflammation.

7. Aloe Vera Gel

Ingredients:

- 1/4 cup fresh
- aloe vera gel

Instructions: Apply fresh aloe vera gel directly to inflamed areas to soothe and reduce redness.

8. Clove and Cinnamon Infusion

Ingredients:

- 1/2 tsp ground cloves
- 1 stick cinnamon
- 1 cup water

Instructions: Boil cloves and cinnamon in water for 10 minutes. Strain and drink to ease arthritis pain.

9. Garlic and Ginger Paste

Ingredients:

- 2 cloves garlic
- 1-inch ginger root
- 1 tbsp honey

Instructions: Blend garlic and ginger into a paste and mix with honey. Take a small spoonful daily to reduce inflammation and pain.

10. Green Tea with Honey

Ingredients:

- 1 green tea bag
- 1 tsp honey
- 1 cup boiling water

Instructions: Steep green tea bag in boiling water for 3 minutes. Stir in honey and drink to reduce inflammation and soothe sore throat.

11. Lavender Essential Oil Blend

Ingredients:

- 5 drops lavender essential oil
- 1 tbsp carrier oil

Instructions: Mix lavender oil with carrier oil and apply to sore areas for pain relief and relaxation.

12. Turmeric and Honey Paste

Ingredients:

- 1 tbsp turmeric powder
- 1 tbsp honey

Instructions: Mix turmeric powder with honey to form a paste. Apply it topically to inflamed areas to relieve pain and swelling.

13. Willow Bark Tea

Ingredients:

- 1 tsp dried willow bark
- 1 cup boiling water

Instructions: Steep willow bark in boiling water for 10 minutes. Strain and drink to help alleviate pain and inflammation.

14. Cucumber and Aloe Vera Soothing Mask

Ingredients:

- 1/2 cucumber (blended)
- 2 tbsp aloe vera gel

Instructions: Mix cucumber and aloe vera gel to form a paste. Apply to inflamed skin to reduce redness and swelling.

15. Pineapple and Turmeric Smoothie

Ingredients:

- 1 cup pineapple chunks
- 1/2 tsp turmeric powder
- 1 cup coconut water

Instructions: Blend pineapple, turmeric, and coconut water. Drink to benefit from anti-inflammatory properties.

16. Rosehip Tea

Ingredients:

- 1 tsp dried rosehips
- 1 cup boiling water

Instructions: Steep rosehips in boiling water for 10 minutes. Strain and drink to help with joint pain and inflammation.

17. Calendula Infused Oil

Ingredients:

- 1/4 cup dried calendula flowers
- 1/2 cup carrier oil

Instructions: Infuse calendula flowers in carrier oil for 2 weeks. Strain and apply to inflamed areas to reduce swelling and pain.

18. Fenugreek Seed Tea

Ingredients:

- 1 tsp fenugreek seeds
- 1 cup boiling water

Instructions: Steep fenugreek seeds in boiling water for 10 minutes. Strain and drink to help with inflammation and joint pain.

19. Peppermint and Ginger Tea

Ingredients:

- 1 tsp dried peppermint
- 1-inch ginger root (sliced)
- 1 cup boiling water

Instructions: Steep peppermint and ginger in boiling water for 5 minutes. Strain and drink to alleviate stomach pain and inflammation.

20. Mustard Seed Compress

Ingredients:

- 1/4 cup mustard seeds
- 1/2 cup warm water

Instructions: Grind mustard seeds and mix with warm water to paste. Apply to sore muscles for pain relief.

Book 36: Recipes for Mobility Issues

1. Oregano oil pods

Ingredients:

- 1 oregano oil capsule (standard dosage)

Instructions: Take an oregano oil capsule daily to benefit from its anti-inflammatory properties.

2. Chamomile and Lavender Bath

Ingredients:

- 1/4 cup dried chamomile flowers
- 1/4 cup dried lavender flowers

Instructions: Add chamomile and lavender to a warm bath. Soak for 20 minutes to relax muscles and reduce pain.

3. Ginger and Turmeric Soup

Ingredients:

- 1 cup vegetable broth
- 1-inch ginger root (sliced)
- 1/2 tsp turmeric powder

Instructions: Simmer ginger and turmeric in vegetable broth for 10 minutes. Strain and drink to help with inflammation.

4. Honey and Cinnamon Paste

Ingredients:

- 1 tbsp honey
- 1/2 tsp cinnamon powder

Instructions: Mix honey and cinnamon to form a paste. Apply to inflamed areas for soothing relief.

5. Green Tea Ice Cubes

Ingredients:

- 1 cup brewed green tea
- ice cube trays

Instructions: Pour brewed green tea into ice cube trays and freeze. Rub green tea ice cubes on sore areas to reduce pain and inflammation.

6. Ginger and orange juice

Ingredients:

- 1-inch ginger root (sliced)
- juice of orange
- 1 cup boiling water

Instructions: Steep ginger in boiling water for 10 minutes. Stir in orange juice and drink to help ease pain and inflammation.

7. Clove Oil Massage

Ingredients:

- 2 drops clove essential oil
- 1 tbsp carrier oil

Instructions: Mix clove oil with carrier oil. Massage gently onto sore areas to relieve pain and reduce inflammation.

8. Cabbage Leaf Compress

Ingredients:

- 2 fresh cabbage leaves

Instructions: Warm cabbage leaves in hot water, then apply to inflamed areas for 15 minutes to soothe and reduce swelling.

9. Caraway seeds Tea

Ingredients:

- 1 tsp caraway seeds
- 1 cup boiling water

Instructions: Steep caraway seeds in boiling water for 10 minutes. Strain and drink to alleviate joint pain and inflammation.

10. Basil and Lemon Juice

Ingredients:

- 1/4 cup fresh basil leaves
- juice of 1/2 lemon
- 1 cup water

Instructions: Blend basil leaves with lemon juice and water. Strain and drink to help with inflammation and pain.

11. Turmeric and Ginger Infused Oil

Ingredients:

- 1/4 cup turmeric powder
- 1-inch ginger root (sliced)
- 1/2 cup carrier oil

Instructions: Infuse turmeric and ginger in carrier oil for 2 weeks. Strain and apply to inflamed areas for soothing relief.

12. Hot Pepper and Olive Oil Rub

Ingredients:

- 1/2 tsp cayenne pepper
- 2 tbsp olive oil

Instructions: Mix cayenne pepper with olive oil. Apply gently to sore muscles to help reduce pain and inflammation.

13. Apricots and Ginger Juice

Ingredients:

- 1 cup apricots juice
- 1-inch ginger root (grated)

Instructions: Mix apricots juice with grated ginger. Drink to benefit from the anti-inflammatory properties.

14. Sage and Honey Tea

Ingredients:

- 1 tsp dried sage leaves
- 1 tsp honey
- 1 cup boiling water

Instructions: Steep sage leaves in boiling water for 5 minutes. Stir in honey and drink to soothe inflammation and pain.

15. Green Apple and Ginger Smoothie

Ingredients:

- 1 green apple (chopped)
- 1-inch ginger root
- 1 cup water

Instructions: Blend apple and ginger with water. Drink to support pain relief and reduce inflammation.

16. Turmeric Ground Tea

Ingredients:

- 1 tbsp dried Turmeric Ground
- 1 cup boiling water

Instructions: Steep Turmeric Ground in boiling water for 10 minutes. Strain and drink to help soothe pain and inflammation.

17. Turmeric and Black Pepper Capsules

Ingredients:

- 1 tsp turmeric powder
- 1/4 tsp black pepper
- 1 tbsp coconut oil

Instructions: Mix turmeric and black pepper with coconut oil. Pour into empty capsules and take daily to reduce inflammation.

18. Thyme and Lemon Infusion

Ingredients:

- 1 tsp dried thyme
- juice of 1/2 lemon
- 1 cup boiling water

Instructions: Steep thyme in boiling water for 5 minutes. Stir in lemon juice and drink to ease pain and reduce inflammation.

19. Summer Savory and Eucalyptus Steam

Ingredients:

- 1 tbsp dried summer savory
- 1 tbsp eucalyptus leaves
- 1-liter hot water

Instructions: Steep summer savory and eucalyptus in hot water. Place your face over the bowl, cover with a towel, and inhale steam to relieve pain and inflammation.

20. Black Pepper and Ginger Tea

Ingredients:

- 1/2 tsp black pepper
- 1-inch ginger root (sliced)
- 1 cup boiling water

Instructions: Steep black pepper and ginger in boiling water for 10 minutes. Strain and drink to reduce pain and inflammation.

21. Oatmeal and Chamomile Bath

Ingredients:

- 1 cup oatmeal
- 1/2 cup dried chamomile flowers

Instructions: Add oatmeal and chamomile to a warm bath. Soak for 20 minutes to soothe inflammation and relax muscles.

22. Sweet Potato and Turmeric Mash

Ingredients:

- 1 medium sweet potato (cooked and mashed)
- 1/2 tsp turmeric powder

Instructions: Mix turmeric powder into mashed sweet potato. Eat to benefit from its anti-inflammatory properties.

23. Hibiscus Tea

Ingredients:

- 1 tbsp dried hibiscus flowers
- 1 cup boiling water

Instructions: Steep hibiscus flowers in boiling water for 10 minutes. Strain and drink to help with inflammation and pain.

24. Papaya and Ginger Smoothie

Ingredients:

- 1 cup papaya chunks
- 1-inch ginger root
- 1 cup water

Instructions: Blend papaya and ginger with water. Drink to support anti-inflammatory effects.

25. Moringa Leaf Tea

Ingredients:

- 1 tsp dried moringa leaves
- 1 cup boiling water

Instructions: Steep moringa leaves in boiling water for 10 minutes. Strain and drink to reduce inflammation and pain.

Book 37: Detoxification Recipes

1. Lemon and Ginger Water

Ingredients:

- 1 lemon (sliced)
- 1 tsp grated ginger
- 1 liter water

Instructions: Infuse lemon slices and ginger in water for 1 hour. Strain and drink to support digestion and detoxification.

2. Cucumber and Lemon Detox Water

Ingredients:

- 1/2 cucumber (sliced),
- lemon (sliced)
- 1 liter water

Instructions: Combine cucumber and lemon slices in water. Let sit for 1 hour before drinking to refresh and detoxify.

3. Beet and Daikon radish

Ingredients:

- 1 beet (peeled)
- 2 Daikon radish
- 1 apple,1
- 1/2 cup water

Instructions: Juice all ingredients and drink to boost liver function and detoxify the body.

4. Green Apple and Spinach Smoothie

Ingredients:

- 1 green apple
- 1 cup spinach
- 1/2 cucumber
- 1 cup water

Instructions: Blend all ingredients until smooth. Drink to support detoxification and provide essential nutrients.

5. Turmeric and Honey Tea

Ingredients:

- 1 tsp turmeric powder
- 1 tbsp honey
- 1 cup hot water

Instructions: Stir turmeric and honey into hot water. Drink to reduce inflammation and support detoxification.

6. Celery and Apple Juice

Ingredients:

- 2 stalks celery
- 1 apple
- 1/2 cup water.

Instructions: Juice all ingredients and drink to aid in digestion and detoxification.

7. Pineapple and Mint Smoothie

Ingredients:

- 1 cup pineapple chunks
- 1/4 cup fresh mint leaves
- 1/2 cup water

Instructions: Blend pineapple and mint leaves with water. Drink to refresh and cleanse your system.

8. Grapefruit and Rosemary Infusion

Ingredients:

- 1 grapefruit (sliced)
- 1 sprig rosemary
- 1 liter water

Instructions: Infuse grapefruit and rosemary in water for 1 hour. Strain and drink to support liver function.

9. Feverfew Tea

Ingredients:

- 1 tsp dried Feverfew
- 1 cup hot water

Instructions: Steep Feverfew in hot water for 10 minutes. Strain and drink to aid in liver detoxification.

10. Apple Cider Vinegar Detox Drink

Ingredients:

- 1 tbsp apple cider vinegar
- 1 tsp honey
- 1 cup water

Instructions: Mix apple cider vinegar and honey in water. Drink to support metabolism and detoxification.

11. Aloe Vera and Lemon Juice

Ingredients:

- 2 tbsp aloe vera gel
- juice of 1 lemon
- 1 cup water

Instructions: Blend aloe vera gel and lemon juice with water. Drink to soothe and detoxify the digestive system.

12. Watermelon and Basil Infusion

Ingredients:

- 1 cup watermelon (cubed)
- 1/4 cup fresh basil leaves
- 1 liter water

Instructions: Infuse watermelon and basil in water for 1 hour. Strain and drink to refresh and detoxify.

13. Matcha Green Tea

Ingredients:

- 1 tsp matcha powder
- 1 cup hot water

Instructions: Whisk matcha powder into hot water. Drink to provide antioxidants and support detoxification.

14. Curcuma longa and Lemon Tea

Ingredients:

- 1 tsp grated curcuma longa
- juice of 1/2 lemon
- 1 cup hot water

Instructions: Steep curcuma longa in hot water, add lemon juice. Strain and drink to boost digestion and detoxify.

15. Cucumber and Ginger Juice

Ingredients:

- 1 cucumber (peeled)
- 1 inch ginger
- 1/2 lemon (juiced)
- 1/2 cup water

Instructions: Juice cucumber and ginger, add lemon juice. Drink to help cleanse and revitalize.

16. Mint and Lime Water

Ingredients:

- 1/4 cup fresh mint leaves
- juice of 1 lime
- 1 liter water

Instructions: Infuse mint and lime juice in water for 1 hour. Strain and drink to refresh and detoxify.

17. Carrot and Orange Juice

Ingredients:

- 2 carrots
- 1 orange
- 1/2 cup water

Instructions: Juice carrots and orange together. Drink to provide vitamins and aid in detoxification.

18. Parsley and Lemon Infusion

Ingredients:

- 1/4 cup fresh parsley
- juice of 1 lemon
- 1 liter water

Instructions: Infuse parsley and lemon juice in water for 1 hour. Strain and drink to support liver health.

19. Cilantro and Lime Smoothie

Ingredients:

- 1/4 cup fresh cilantro
- juice of 1 lime
- 1 cup water

Instructions: Blend cilantro and lime juice with water. Drink to help cleanse and detoxify your body.

20. Strawberry and Basil Infusion

Ingredients:

- 1/2 cup strawberries (sliced)
- 1/4 cup fresh basil leaves
- 1 liter water

Instructions: Infuse strawberries and basil in water for 1 hour. Strain and drink to refresh and detoxify.

21. Papaya and Lime Smoothie

Ingredients:

- 1 cup papaya chunks
- juice of 1 lime
- 1/2 cup water

Instructions: Blend papaya and lime juice with water. Drink to support digestion and detoxification.

22. Cranberry and Ginger Juice

Ingredients:

- 1 cup cranberry juice
- 1 inch ginger

- 1/2 cup water

Instructions: Juice ginger, mix with cranberry juice. Drink to support urinary tract health and detoxify.

23. Green Tea and Lemon Infusion

Ingredients:

- 1 green tea bag
- juice of 1/2 lemon
- 1 cup hot water

Instructions: Steep green tea bag, add lemon juice. Drink to provide antioxidants and aid in detoxification.

24. Blueberry and Mint Infusion

Ingredients:

- 1/2 cup blueberries
- 1/4 cup fresh mint leaves
- 1 liter water

Instructions: Infuse blueberries and mint in water for 1 hour. Strain and drink to refresh and support detoxification.

25. Pomegranate and Ginger Juice

Ingredients:

- 1 cup pomegranate juice
- 1 inch ginger
- 1/2 cup water

Instructions: Juice ginger, mix with pomegranate juice. Drink to support detoxification and provide antioxidants.

26. Lemon and Cucumber Juice

Ingredients:

- 1 lemon (juiced)
- 1/2 cucumber (sliced)
- 1 cup water

Instructions: Mix lemon juice and cucumber slices in water. Drink to refresh and support detoxification.

27. Raspberry and Mint Infusion

Ingredients:

- 1/2 cup raspberries
- 1/4 cup fresh mint leaves
- 1 liter water

Instructions: Infuse raspberries and mint in water for 1 hour. Strain and drink to support hydration and detoxification.

28. Pear and Ginger Smoothie

Ingredients:

- 1 pear
- 1 inch ginger
- 1/2 cup water

Instructions: Blend pear and ginger with water. Drink to aid digestion and support detoxification.

29. Artichoke and Lemon Tea

Ingredients:

- 1 artichoke heart (steamed)
- juice of 1/2 lemon

- 1 cup hot water

Instructions: Steep artichoke heart in hot water, add lemon juice. Strain and drink to support liver health.

30. Pineapple and Turmeric Juice

Ingredients:

- 1 cup pineapple chunks
- 1/2 tsp turmeric powder
- 1/2 cup water

Instructions: Juice pineapple and mix with turmeric powder. Drink to support digestion and detoxification.

31. Apple and Cinnamon Infusion

Ingredients:

- 1 apple (sliced)
- 1 stick cinnamon
- 1 liter water

Instructions: Infuse apple slices and cinnamon in water for 1 hour. Strain and drink to support digestion and detoxification.

32. Grapefruit and Mint Water

Ingredients:

- 1 grapefruit (sliced)
- 1/4 cup fresh mint leaves
- 1 liter water

Instructions: Infuse grapefruit and mint in water for 1 hour. Strain and drink to refresh and aid detoxification.

33. Ginger and Turmeric Tea

Ingredients:

- 1 inch ginger
- 1/2 tsp turmeric powder
- 1 cup hot water

Instructions: Steep ginger and turmeric in hot water. Strain and drink to reduce inflammation and support detoxification.

34. Mango and Lime Smoothie

Ingredients:

- 1 cup mango chunks
- juice of 1 lime
- 1/2 cup water

Instructions: Blend mango and lime juice with water. Drink to support digestion and detoxification.

35. Kiwi and Cucumber Juice

Ingredients:

- 2 kiwis
- 1/2 cucumber (peeled)
- 1/2 cup water

Instructions: Juice kiwis and cucumber together. Drink to hydrate and aid detoxification.

36. Agave and Pineapple Juice

Ingredients:

- 2 tbsp agave gel
- 1 cup pineapple chunks
- 1/2 cup water

Instructions: Blend agave gel and pineapple with water. Drink to support digestion and detoxify.

37. Cranberry and Lemon Infusion

Ingredients:

- 1/2 cup cranberry juice
- juice of 1 lemon
- 1 liter water

Instructions: Mix cranberry juice and lemon juice in water. Drink to support kidney health and detoxification.

38. Pear and Cinnamon Infusion

Ingredients:

- 1 pear (sliced)
- 1 stick cinnamon
- 1 liter water

Instructions: Infuse pear slices and cinnamon in water for 1 hour. Strain and drink to aid digestion and detoxify.

39. Blueberry and Lime Smoothie

Ingredients:

- 1/2 cup blueberries
- juice of 1 lime
- 1/2 cup water

Instructions: Blend blueberries and lime juice with water. Drink to provide antioxidants and support detoxification.

40. Artichoke and Mint Tea

Ingredients:

- 1 artichoke heart (steamed)
- 1/4 cup fresh mint leaves
- 1 cup hot water

Instructions: Steep artichoke heart and mint in hot water. Strain and drink to support liver health and detoxify.

41. Beet and Lemon Juice

Ingredients:

- 1 beet (peeled)
- juice of 1 lemon
- 1/2 cup water

Instructions: Juice beet and lemon together. Drink to boost liver function and detoxify.

42. Pineapple and Ginger Smoothie

Ingredients:

- 1 cup pineapple chunks
- 1 inch ginger
- 1/2 cup water

Instructions: Blend pineapple and ginger with water. Drink to aid digestion and support detoxification.

43. Strawberry and Cucumber Infusion

Ingredients:

- 1/2 cup strawberries (sliced)
- 1/2 cucumber (sliced)
- 1 liter water

Instructions: Infuse strawberries and cucumber in water for 1 hour. Strain and drink to refresh and detoxify.

44. Green Tea and Ginger Infusion

Ingredients:

- 1 green tea bag
- 1 inch ginger
- 1 cup hot water

Instructions: Steep green tea bag and ginger in hot water. Strain and drink to support metabolism and detoxification.

45. Raspberry and Lemon Juice

Ingredients:

- 1/2 cup raspberries
- juice of 1/2 lemon
- 1/2 cup water

Instructions: Juice raspberries and mix with lemon juice. Drink to support detoxification and provide antioxidants.

Book 38: Sleep and Relaxation Recipes

1. Chamomile Lavender Tea

Ingredients:

- 1 tsp dried chamomile
- 1 tsp dried lavender
- 1 cup boiling water

Instructions: Steep chamomile and lavender in boiling water for 5 minutes. Strain and sip before bed to calm the mind and promote restful sleep.

2. American Ginseng Tincture

Ingredients:

- 1 tsp American Ginseng extract
- 1 cup water

Instructions: Mix American Ginseng extract with water. Drink 30 minutes before bedtime to aid in falling asleep.

3. Warm Milk and Honey

Ingredients:

- 1 cup milk
- 1 tsp honey

Instructions: Heat milk and stir in honey. Drink warm before bed to soothe and relax.

4. Lemon Balm Infusion

Ingredients:

- 1 tsp dried lemon balm
- 1 cup hot water

Instructions: Steep lemon balm in hot water for 5 minutes. Strain and drink to help reduce anxiety and improve sleep.

5. Galangal and Turmeric Tea

Ingredients:

- 1 tsp galangal
- 1/2 tsp turmeric powder
- 1 cup hot water

Instructions: Steep galangal and turmeric in hot water for 5 minutes. Strain and sip to relax muscles and calm the mind.

6. Peppermint and Sage Tea

Ingredients:

- 1 tsp dried peppermint
- 1 tsp dried sage
- 1 cup boiling water

Instructions: Steep peppermint and sage in boiling water for 5 minutes. Strain and drink to ease tension and promote relaxation.

7. Almond and Oat Smoothie

Ingredients:

- 1/2 cup almond milk
- 1/4 cup oats
- 1 banana

Instructions: Blend almond milk, oats, and banana until smooth. Drink in the evening to help relax and unwind.

8. Lavender Essential Oil Diffuser Blend

Ingredients:

- 3 drops lavender essential oil
- 1 cup water

Instructions: Add lavender oil to water in a diffuser. Run the diffuser in your bedroom to promote relaxation and better sleep.

9. Cinnamon and Apple Infusion

Ingredients:

- 1 cinnamon stick
- 1 apple (sliced)
- 1 cup hot water

Instructions: Infuse cinnamon stick and apple slices in hot water for 10 minutes. Strain and sip to enjoy a calming drink.

10. Dong Quai Tea

Ingredients:

- 1 tsp dried Dong Quai
- 1 cup boiling water

Instructions: Steep Dong Quai in boiling water for 5 minutes. Strain and drink to alleviate stress and improve sleep quality.

11. Turmeric and Honey Milk

Ingredients:

- 1 cup milk
- 1/2 tsp turmeric
- 1 tsp honey

Instructions: Heat milk, stir in turmeric and honey. Drink warm before bed to help relax and reduce inflammation.

12. Relaxation Bath Soak

Ingredients:

- 1 cup Epsom salt
- 1/2 cup baking soda
- 5 drops lavender essential oil

Instructions: Dissolve Epsom salt and baking soda in a warm bath. Add lavender oil and soak for 20 minutes to relax muscles.

13. Celery Mint Water

Ingredients:

- 1/2 Celery (sliced)
- 5 mint leaves
- 1 liter water

Instructions: Infuse Celery and mint in water for 1 hour. Strain and drink throughout the day for a calming effect.

14. Rose Water and Chamomile Spray

Ingredients:

- 2 tbsp rose water
- 1 tbsp chamomile tea
- 1 cup water

Instructions: Mix ingredients in a spray bottle. Lightly mist your room or pillow to promote relaxation.

15. Herbal Sleep Sachet

Ingredients:

- 1 tbsp dried lavender

- 1 tbsp dried chamomile
- 1 small cloth bag

Instructions: Combine herbs in the cloth bag. Place under your pillow to help with relaxation and sleep.

16. Melatonin-Boosting Cherry Juice

Ingredients:

- 1/2 cup cherry juice

Instructions: Drink cherry juice in the evening to help boost natural melatonin levels and promote sleep.

17. Warm Lemon Ginger Drink

Ingredients:

- 1 tsp grated ginger
- juice of 1 lemon
- 1 cup warm water

Instructions: Mix ginger and lemon juice in warm water. Sip before bed to help soothe and relax.

18. Blueberry Lavender Smoothie

Ingredients:

- 1/2 cup blueberries
- 1/2 cup almond milk
- 1 tsp dried lavender

Instructions: Blend blueberries, almond milk, and lavender until smooth. Drink to relax before bed.

19. Oatmeal with Cinnamon and Honey

Ingredients:

- 1/2 cup oats
- 1 cup milk
- 1/2 tsp cinnamon
- 1 tsp honey

Instructions: Cook oats in milk, then stir in cinnamon and honey. Enjoy this soothing dish in the evening to promote relaxation.

20. Valerian and Peppermint Tea

Ingredients:

- 1 tsp valerian root
- 1 tsp dried peppermint
- 1 cup boiling water

Instructions: Steep valerian and peppermint in boiling water for 5 minutes. Strain and drink to aid sleep.

21. Coconut Water and Lime Drink

Ingredients:

- 1 cup coconut water
- juice of 1 lime

Instructions: Mix coconut water and lime juice. Drink to stay hydrated and relaxed.

22. Herbal Relaxation Infusion

Ingredients:

- 1 tsp dried rose petals
- 1 tsp dried chamomile

- 1 cup boiling water

Instructions: Steep rose petals and chamomile in boiling water for 5 minutes. Strain and enjoy to ease tension.

23. Almond Butter Banana Smoothie

Ingredients:

- 1 banana
- 1 tbsp almond butter
- 1/2 cup almond milk

Instructions: Blend banana, almond butter, and almond milk until smooth. Drink before bed to promote relaxation.

24. Calendula and Echinacea Tea

Ingredients:

- 1 tsp dried calendula
- 1 tsp dried echinacea
- 1 cup hot water

Instructions: Steep calendula and echinacea in hot water for 5 minutes. Strain and sip to calm and relax.

25. Apple Cider Vinegar and Corn syrup Drink

Ingredients:

- 1 tbsp apple cider vinegar
- 1 tsp corn syrup
- 1 cup warm water

Instructions: Mix vinegar and Corn syrup in warm water. Drink to help relax before bed.

26. Ginger and Nutmeg Tea

Ingredients:

- 1 tsp grated ginger
- 1/2 tsp nutmeg
- 1 cup boiling water

Instructions: Steep ginger and nutmeg in boiling water for 5 minutes. Strain and drink to help unwind.

27. Peppermint and Fennel Infusion

Ingredients:

- 1 tsp dried peppermint
- 1 tsp dried fennel seeds, 1 cup hot water

Instructions: Steep peppermint and fennel in hot water for 5 minutes. Strain and enjoy to soothe and relax.

28. Lavender and Chamomile Pillow Spray

Ingredients:

- 2 tbsp lavender water
- 2 tbsp chamomile tea
- 1 cup water

Instructions: Mix ingredients in a spray bottle. Lightly spray on your pillow before bed for calming effects.

29. Banana and Mint Smoothie

Ingredients:

- 1 banana, 5 mint leaves
- 1/2 cup coconut water

Instructions: Blend banana, mint, and coconut water until smooth. Drink to relax and hydrate.

30. Honey Lemon mace Tea

Ingredients:

- 1 tsp grated mace
- juice of 1/2 lemon
- 1 tsp honey
- 1 cup hot water

Instructions: Steep mace in hot water, then stir in lemon juice and honey. Drink to calm and prepare for restful sleep.

31. Chamomile Mint Tea

Ingredients:

- 1 tsp dried chamomile
- 1 tsp dried mint
- 1 cup boiling water

Instructions: Steep chamomile and mint in boiling water for 5 minutes. Strain and drink to relax.

32. Warm Almond Milk and Allspice

Ingredients:

- 1 cup almond milk, 1/4 tsp allspice

Instructions: Heat almond milk and stir in allspice. Drink warm before bed to calm the senses.

33. Vanilla and Lavender Infused Water

Ingredients:

- 1/2 tsp vanilla extract
- 1 tsp dried lavender
- 1 liter water

Instructions: Infuse vanilla extract and lavender in water for 1 hour. Strain and drink for a soothing effect.

34. Ginger Lemonade

Ingredients:

- 1 tsp grated ginger
- juice of 1 lemon
- 1 cup cold water

Instructions: Mix ginger and lemon juice with water. Stir well and drink to refresh and unwind.

35. Cinnamon and Clove Tea

Ingredients:

- 1 cinnamon stick
- 2 cloves
- 1 cup boiling water

Instructions: Steep cinnamon and cloves in boiling water for 5 minutes. Strain and enjoy for relaxation.

36. Blueberry Lavender Infusion

Ingredients:

- 1/2 cup blueberries
- 1 tsp dried lavender

Instructions: Infuse blueberries and lavender in boiling water for 10 minutes. Strain and sip to unwind.

37. Pineapple and Mint Juice

Ingredients:

- 1/2 cup pineapple juice
- 5 mint leaves

Instructions: Mix pineapple juice with mint leaves. Drink to refresh and soothe before bed.

38. Coconut Milk and Honey Blend

Ingredients:

- 1 cup coconut milk
- 1 tsp honey

Instructions: Warm coconut milk and stir in honey. Drink before bedtime to relax.

39. Rose and Chamomile Tea

Ingredients:

- 1 tsp dried rose petals
- 1 tsp dried chamomile
- 1 cup boiling water

Instructions: Steep rose petals and chamomile in boiling water for 5 minutes. Strain and enjoy to relax.

40. Pear and cinnamon Smoothie

Ingredients:

- 1 pear
- 1 tsp grated cinnamon
- 1/2 cup almond milk

Instructions: Blend pear, cinnamon, and almond milk until smooth. Drink to unwind and relax.

41. Passionfruit and Lemon Water

Ingredients:

- 1/2 passionfruit
- juice of 1 lemon
- 1 liter water

Instructions: Mix passionfruit and lemon juice in water. Infuse for 1 hour and drink to calm the mind.

42. Apple Cinnamon Water

Ingredients:

- 1 apple (sliced)
- 1 cinnamon stick
- 1 liter water

Instructions: Infuse apple slices and cinnamon stick in water for 2 hours. Strain and drink for a soothing effect.

43. Lemon Balm and mace Tea

Ingredients:

- 1 tsp dried mace
- 1 tsp grated ginger
- 1 cup hot water

Instructions: Steep mace and ginger in hot water for 5 minutes. Strain and enjoy to ease tension.

44. Blackberry and Sage Infusion

Ingredients:

- 1/2 cup blackberries
- 1 tsp dried sage
- 1 cup boiling water

Instructions: Infuse blackberries and sage in boiling water for 10 minutes. Strain and sip to relax.

Book 39: Women's Health Recipes

1. Red Clover Tea

Ingredients:

- 1 tbsp dried red clover

Instructions: Steep red clover in boiling water for 10 minutes. Strain and drink to support hormonal balance.

2. Ginger and Turmeric Elixir

Ingredients:

- 1 tsp grated ginger
- 1 tsp turmeric powder

Instructions: Mix ginger and turmeric in hot water. Let steep for 5 minutes and drink to reduce inflammation.

3. Raspberry Leaf Infusion

Ingredients:

- 1 tbsp dried raspberry leaves

Instructions: Steep raspberry leaves in boiling water for 10 minutes. Strain and drink to ease menstrual discomfort.

4. Chamomile and Spearmint Tea

Ingredients:

- 1 tsp dried chamomile
- 1 tsp dried spearmint

Instructions: Steep chamomile and spearmint in boiling water for 5 minutes. Strain and drink for relaxation and digestive support.

5. Flaxseed and Almond Smoothie

Ingredients:

- 1 tbsp ground flaxseed
- 1/4 cup almonds
- 1 cup almond milk

Instructions: Blend flaxseed, almonds, and almond milk until smooth. Drink to support hormonal health.

6. Aloe Vera and Cucumber Juice

Ingredients:

- 1/2 cup aloe vera gel
- 1/2 cucumber
- 1 cup water

Instructions: Blend aloe vera gel, cucumber, and water until smooth. Strain and drink to promote skin health.

7. Marjoram and Honey Tea

Ingredients:

- 1 tsp dried marjoram
- 1 tsp honey
- 1 cup boiling water

Instructions: Steep marjoram in boiling water for 5 minutes. Add honey and drink to soothe the throat and support digestive health.

8. Oat and Berries Smoothie

Ingredients:

- 1/2 cup oats

- 1/2 cup mixed berries
- 1 cup yogurt

Instructions: Blend oats, berries, and yogurt until smooth. Drink to support energy levels and overall health.

9. Roman Chamomile Tea

Ingredients:

- 1 tbsp dried Roman Chamomile
- 1 cup boiling water

Instructions: Steep Roman Chamomile in boiling water for 10 minutes. Strain and drink to support liver function.

10. Lemon and Ginger Infusion

Ingredients:

- Juice of 1 lemon
- 1 tsp grated ginger
- 1 cup hot water

Instructions: Mix lemon juice and ginger in hot water. Steep for 5 minutes and drink to boost immunity.

11. Allspice and Apple Cider Vinegar Drink

Ingredients:

- 1 tsp allspice
- 1 tbsp apple cider vinegar

Instructions: Mix allspice and apple cider vinegar in water. Stir and drink to support metabolic health.

12. Nettle Leaf Tea

Ingredients:

- 1 tbsp dried nettle leaves

Instructions: Steep nettle leaves in boiling water for 10 minutes. Strain and drink to support energy levels and detoxification.

13. Lavender and Chamomile Tea

Ingredients:

- 1 tsp dried lavender
- 1 tsp dried chamomile

Instructions: Steep lavender and chamomile in boiling water for 5 minutes. Strain and drink to relax and promote sleep.

14. Pomegranate and Beet Juice

Ingredients:

- 1/2 cup pomegranate juice
- 1/2 cup beet juice

Instructions: Mix pomegranate and beet juices with water. Stir and drink to support cardiovascular health.

15. Ginkgo Biloba Tea

Ingredients:

- 1 tsp dried ginkgo biloba leaves
- 1 cup boiling water

Instructions: Steep ginkgo biloba leaves in boiling water for 10 minutes. Strain and drink to support cognitive function.

16. Avocado and Spinach Smoothie

Ingredients:

- 1/2 avocado
- 1 cup spinach

Instructions: Blend avocado, spinach, and water until smooth. Drink to support overall health and energy.

17. Echinacea and Honey Tea

Ingredients:

- 1 tsp dried echinacea
- 1 tsp honey

Instructions: Steep echinacea in boiling water for 5 minutes. Add honey and drink to boost the immune system.

18. Squash and Celery Juice

Ingredients:

- 1 cup squash juice
- 1/2 cup celery juice

Instructions: Mix carrot and celery juices with water. Stir and drink to support skin health and digestion.

19. Basil and Lemon Balm Tea

Ingredients:

- 1 tsp dried basil
- 1 tsp dried lemon balm

Instructions: Steep basil and lemon balm in boiling water for 5 minutes. Strain and drink for relaxation and digestive support.

20. Rosehip and althea Tea

Ingredients:

- 1 tbsp dried rosehips
- 1 tbsp dried althea

Instructions: Steep rosehips and hibiscus in boiling water for 10 minutes. Strain and drink to support skin health.

21. Persian Cucumber and Mint Infusion

Ingredients:

- 1/2 Persian Cucumber (sliced)
- 1 tsp dried mint

Instructions: Infuse Persian Cucumber slices and mint in water for 1 hour. Strain and drink to soothe and refresh.

22. Garlic and Lemon Drink

Ingredients:

- 1 clove garlic (minced)
- juice of 1 lemon

Instructions: Mix garlic and lemon juice in water. Stir and drink to support immune health.

23. Peppermint and Fennel Tea

Ingredients:

- 1 tsp dried peppermint
- 1 tsp fennel seeds
- 1 cup boiling water

Instructions: Steep peppermint and fennel in boiling water for 5 minutes. Strain and drink to support digestion.

24. Aloe Vera and Ginger Smoothie

Ingredients:

- 1/4 cup aloe vera gel
- 1 tsp grated ginger
- 1 cup coconut water

Instructions: Blend aloe vera gel, ginger, and coconut water until smooth.

25. Ground allspice and Lemon Tea

Ingredients:

- 1 tsp ground allspice
- juice of 1/2 lemon

Instructions: Steep ground allspice in boiling water for 5 minutes. Add lemon juice and drink to aid digestion and boost immunity.

26. Apple Cider Vinegar and Turmeric Drink

Ingredients:

- 1 tbsp apple cider vinegar
- 1/2 tsp turmeric powder
- 1 cup water

Instructions: Mix apple cider vinegar and turmeric in water. Stir and drink to support anti-inflammatory processes.

27. Sour Cherries and Ginger Juice

Ingredients:

- 1/2 cup Sour Cherries juice
- 1 tsp grated ginger

Instructions: Mix Sour Cherries juice and ginger in water. Stir and drink to support urinary health.

28. Dill and Lemon Tea

Ingredients:

- 1 tsp dried dill
- juice of 1/2 lemon
- 1 cup boiling water

Instructions: Steep dill in boiling water for 5 minutes. Add lemon juice and drink to support digestive health.

29. Turmeric and Coconut Milk Latte

Ingredients:

- 1 tsp turmeric powder
- 1 cup coconut milk
- 1 tsp honey

Instructions: Warm coconut milk and stir in turmeric powder and honey. Drink to support joint health.

30. Mint and Ginger Infused Water

Ingredients:

- 1/2 cup fresh mint leaves
- 1 tsp grated ginger

Instructions: Infuse mint leaves and ginger in water for 2 hours. Strain and drink to refresh and aid digestion.

31. Hibiscus and Lemon Tea

Ingredients:

- 1 tbsp dried hibiscus flowers

- juice of 1 lemon

Instructions: Steep hibiscus flowers in boiling water for 10 minutes. Add lemon juice and drink to support cardiovascular health.

32. Parsley and Honey Infusion

Ingredients:

- 1 tsp dried parsley
- 1 tsp honey

Instructions: Steep parsley in boiling water for 5 minutes. Add honey and drink to soothe coughs and support respiratory health.

33. Chia and Berries Smoothie

Ingredients:

- 1 tbsp chia seeds
- 1/2 cup mixed berries
- 1 cup almond milk

Instructions: Blend chia seeds, berries, and almond milk until smooth. Drink to support hormone balance and skin health.

34. Beetroot and Carrot Juice

Ingredients:

- 1/2 cup beet juice
- 1/2 cup carrot juice

Instructions: Mix beet and carrot juices with water. Stir and drink to support liver health and energy levels.

35. Pomegranate and Green Tea Blend

Ingredients:

- 1/2 cup pomegranate juice
- 1 cup brewed green tea
- 1 tsp honey

Instructions: Mix pomegranate juice with green tea and honey. Stir and drink to support antioxidant levels.

36. Lemon Balm and Chamomile Tea

Ingredients:

- 1 tsp dried lemon balm
- 1 tsp dried chamomile
- 1 cup boiling water

Instructions: Steep lemon balm and chamomile in boiling water for 5 minutes. Strain and drink to promote relaxation and reduce stress.

37. Apple and Cinnamon Water

Ingredients:

- 1/2 apple (sliced)
- 1 cinnamon stick

Instructions: Infuse apple slices and cinnamon stick in water for 1 hour. Strain and drink to support digestion and metabolism.

38. Cranberry and Ginger Tea

Ingredients:

- 1/2 cup cranberry juice
- 1 tsp grated ginger

- 1 cup hot water

Instructions: Mix cranberry juice and ginger in hot water. Steep for 5 minutes and drink to support urinary tract health.

39. Rosemary and Lemon Infusion

Ingredients:

- 1 tsp dried rosemary
- juice of 1 lemon
- 1 cup boiling water

Instructions: Steep rosemary in boiling water for 5 minutes. Add lemon juice and drink to aid digestion and improve concentration.

40. Avocado and Kale Smoothie

Ingredients:

- 1/2 avocado
- 1 cup kale
- 1 cup coconut water

Instructions: Blend avocado, kale, and coconut water until smooth. Drink to support overall wellness and skin health.

41. Goji Berry and Mint Tea

Ingredients:

- 1 tbsp dried goji berries
- 1 tsp dried mint

Instructions: Steep goji berries and mint in boiling water for 10 minutes. Strain and drink to support immune function.

42. Cinnamon and Ginger Tea

Ingredients:

- 1 tsp cinnamon
- 1 tsp grated ginger
- 1 cup boiling water

Instructions: Steep cinnamon and ginger in boiling water for 5 minutes. Strain and drink to support metabolic health.

43. Celery and Cucumber Juice

Ingredients:

- 1/2 cup celery juice
- 1/2 cup cucumber juice

Instructions: Mix celery and cucumber juices with water. Stir and drink to support hydration and digestion.

44. Dandelion and Lemon Tea

Ingredients:

- 1 tbsp dried dandelion leaves
- juice of 1/2 lemon

Instructions: Steep dandelion leaves in boiling water for 10 minutes. Add lemon juice and drink to support liver health

Book 40: Cold and Flu Recipes

1. Ginger and Honey Tea

Ingredients:

- 1 tbsp fresh ginger (grated)
- 1 tbsp honey
- 1 cup hot water

Instructions: Steep ginger in hot water for 5 minutes. Strain, add honey, and drink to soothe sore throat and reduce inflammation.

2. Lemon and Echinacea Drink

Ingredients:

- Juice of 1 lemon
- 1 tsp echinacea powder

Instructions: Mix lemon juice and echinacea powder in water. Stir well and drink to support immune function.

3. Garlic and Lemon Infusion

Ingredients:

- 2 cloves garlic (crushed)
- juice of 1 lemon
- 1 cup hot water

Instructions: Steep garlic in hot water for 10 minutes. Strain, add lemon juice, and drink to combat cold symptoms.

4. Turmeric and Ginger chai tea

Ingredients:

- 1 tsp turmeric powder
- 1 tsp fresh ginger (grated)
- 1 cup hot water

Instructions: Mix turmeric and ginger in hot water. Steep for 5 minutes, strain, and drink to reduce inflammation and ease discomfort.

5. Apple Cider Vinegar and Honey Tonic

Ingredients:

- 1 tbsp apple cider vinegar
- 1 tbsp honey

Instructions: Stir apple cider vinegar and honey into water. Drink to help boost immunity and soothe a sore throat.

6. Peppermint and Lemon Tea

Ingredients:

- 1 tsp dried peppermint
- juice of 1/2 lemon

Instructions: Steep peppermint in hot water for 5 minutes. Strain, add lemon juice, and drink to relieve congestion.

7. Cinnamon and Honey Mix

Ingredients:

- 1/2 tsp cinnamon powder
- 1 tbsp honey

Instructions: Mix cinnamon and honey in warm water. Stir well and drink to help reduce cold symptoms.

8. Tarragon and Lemon Infusion

Ingredients:

- 1 tsp dried tarragon
- juice of 1/2 lemon
- 1 cup hot water

Instructions: Steep tarragon in hot water for 5 minutes. Strain, add lemon juice, and drink to ease cough and sore throat.

9. Warm Ginger and Lemon Elixir

Ingredients:

- 1 tbsp fresh ginger (sliced)
- juice of 1 lemon
- 1 cup warm water

Instructions: Steep ginger in warm water for 5 minutes. Strain, add lemon juice, and drink to support digestion and immune health.

10. Arnica and Honey Tea

Ingredients:

- 1 tsp dried Arnica flowers
- 1 tbsp honey
- 1 cup hot water

Instructions: Steep Arnica in hot water for 5 minutes. Strain, add honey, and drink to relax and soothe throat irritation.

11. Orange and Ginger Drink

Ingredients:

- Juice of 1 orange
- 1 tsp fresh ginger (grated)

Instructions: Mix orange juice and ginger in water. Stir well and drink to boost vitamin C and reduce cold symptoms.

12. Clove and Cinnamon Tea

Ingredients:

- 2 cloves
- 1/2 tsp cinnamon powder
- 1 cup hot water

Instructions: Steep cloves and cinnamon in hot water for 10 minutes. Strain and drink to relieve congestion and improve circulation.

13. Honey and Ginger Tonic

Ingredients:

- 1 tbsp honey
- 1 tsp fresh ginger (grated)

Instructions: Mix honey and ginger in hot water. Stir well and drink to reduce coughing and soothe throat.

14. Elderberry and Lemon Drink

Ingredients:

- 1 tbsp elderberry syrup
- juice of 1/2 lemon

Instructions: Mix elderberry syrup and lemon juice in water. Stir well and drink to support immune health and fight off colds.

15. Ginger and Mint Tea

Ingredients:

- 1 tbsp fresh ginger (sliced)
- 1 tsp dried mint
- 1 cup hot water

Instructions: Steep ginger and mint in hot water for 5 minutes. Strain and drink to alleviate nausea and congestion.

16. Green apple and Turmeric Juice

Ingredients:

- 1 cup green apple juice
- 1/2 tsp turmeric powder
- 1 cup water

Instructions: Mix green apple juice and turmeric in water. Stir well and drink to boost immunity and reduce inflammation.

17. Rosemary and Lemon Tea

Ingredients:

- 1 tsp dried rosemary
- juice of 1/2 lemon
- 1 cup hot water

Instructions: Steep rosemary in hot water for 5 minutes. Strain, add lemon juice, and drink to ease respiratory symptoms.

18. Green Tea and Honey Blend

Ingredients:

- 1 green tea bag
- 1 tbsp honey
- 1 cup hot water

Instructions: Steep green tea bag in hot water for 3 minutes. Remove tea bag, add honey, and drink to support overall health.

19. Sage and Ginger Infusion

Ingredients:

- 1 tsp dried sage
- 1 tsp fresh ginger (grated)
- 1 cup hot water

Instructions: Steep sage and ginger in hot water for 5 minutes. Strain and drink to relieve throat irritation and improve digestion.

20. Lemon and Turmeric Water

Ingredients:

- Juice of 1 lemon
- 1/2 tsp turmeric powder

Instructions: Mix lemon juice and turmeric in water. Stir well and drink to support immune function and reduce inflammation.

21. Echinacea and Ginger Tea

Ingredients:

- 1 tsp echinacea powder
- 1 tsp fresh ginger (grated)
- 1 cup hot water

Instructions: Steep echinacea and ginger in hot water for 5 minutes. Strain and drink to help fight off colds and flu.

22. Carrot and Green bell pepper Juice

Ingredients:

- 1 carrot (chopped)
- 1 green bell pepper (chopped)
- 1 cup water

Instructions: Blend carrot and green bell pepper with water. Strain and drink to support overall health and boost immunity.

23. Apple and ginger Infusion

Ingredients:

- 1 apple (sliced)
- 1/2 tsp ginger

Instructions: Steep apple slices and ginger in hot water for 10 minutes. Strain and drink to soothe throat and reduce inflammation.

24. Peppermint and Eucalyptus Tea

Ingredients:

- 1 tsp dried peppermint
- 1 tsp dried eucalyptus leaves
- 1 cup hot water

Instructions: Steep peppermint and eucalyptus in hot water for 5 minutes. Strain and drink to alleviate congestion and support respiratory health.

25. Lime and Honey Drink

Ingredients:

- Juice of 1 lime
- 1 tbsp honey

Instructions: Mix lime juice and honey in water. Stir well and drink to ease throat discomfort and support immune function.

26. Honey and Cinnamon Tea

Ingredients:

- 1 tbsp honey
- 1/2 tsp cinnamon powder
- 1 cup hot water

Instructions: Mix honey and cinnamon in hot water. Stir well and drink to reduce cold symptoms and soothe throat.

27. Rose Tea and Ginger

Ingredients:

- 1 rose tea bag
- 1 tsp fresh ginger (sliced)

Instructions: Steep rose tea bag and ginger in hot water for 5 minutes. Remove tea bag, strain, and drink to support immune health.

28. Lemon and Ginger Syrup

Ingredients:

- Juice of 1 lemon
- 1 tbsp fresh ginger (grated)
- 2 tbsp honey

Instructions: Mix lemon juice, ginger, and honey. Take 1 tsp every few hours to soothe throat and boost immunity.

29. Zucchini and Mint Water

Ingredients:

- 1/2 Zucchini (sliced)
- 1 tsp dried mint
- 1 liter water

Instructions: Infuse Zucchini slices and mint in water for 1 hour. Strain and drink to refresh and hydrate.

30. Apple and ground allspice

Ingredients:

- 1 apple (sliced)
- 1 tsp ground allspice

Instructions: Steep apple slices and ground allspice in hot water for 5 minutes. Strain and drink to support digestion and boost immunity.

31. Ginger and Lemon

Ingredients:

- 1 tbsp fresh ginger (sliced)
- juice of 1 lemon

Instructions: Steep ginger in warm water for 5 minutes. Strain, add lemon juice, and drink to soothe and energize.

32. Turmeric and Honey Drink

Ingredients:

- 1/2 tsp turmeric powder
- 1 tbsp honey

Instructions: Mix turmeric and honey in hot water. Stir well and drink to reduce inflammation and support overall health.

33. Clove and Ginger Tea

Ingredients:

- 2 cloves
- 1 tsp fresh ginger (grated)
- 1 cup hot water

Instructions: Steep cloves and ginger in hot water for 10 minutes. Strain and drink to alleviate cold symptoms and support digestion.

34. Peppermint and Echinacea Infusion

Ingredients:

- 1 tsp dried peppermint
- 1 tsp echinacea powder

Instructions: Steep peppermint and echinacea in hot water for 5 minutes. Strain and drink to support immune function and soothe respiratory issues.

35. Honey and Lemon Gargle

Ingredients:

- Juice of 1 lemon
- 1 tbsp honey
- 1 cup warm water

Instructions: Mix lemon juice and honey in warm water. Gargle to relieve sore throat and reduce inflammation.

36. Goji Berries and Ginger Juice

Ingredients:

- 1/2 cup Goji Berries juice
- 1 tsp fresh ginger (grated)
- 1 cup water

Instructions: Mix Goji Berries juice and ginger in water. Stir well and drink to boost immune health and support digestion.

37. Garlic and Lemon Tonic

Ingredients:

- 2 cloves garlic (crushed)
- juice of 1/2 lemon

Instructions: Mix garlic and lemon juice in water. Stir well and drink to help fight off colds and support immune health.

38. Kale and Ginger Smoothie

Ingredients:

- 1 cup kale
- 1 tsp fresh ginger (grated)
- 1/2 cup water

Instructions: Blend kale and ginger with water. Drink to boost immunity and aid digestion.

39. Oregano and Lemon Infusion

Ingredients:

- 1 tsp dried oregano
- juice of 1/2 lemon
- 1 cup hot water

Instructions: Steep oregano in hot water for 5 minutes. Strain, add lemon juice, and drink to relieve cough and congestion.

40. Green Tea and Mint Cooler

Ingredients:

- 1 green tea bag
- 1 tsp dried mint

Instructions: Steep green tea and mint in hot water for 3 minutes. Remove tea bag, strain, and chill. Drink to refresh and soothe.

41. Elderberry and Ginger Drink

Ingredients:

- 1 tbsp elderberry syrup
- 1 tsp fresh ginger (grated)
- 1 cup water

Instructions: Mix elderberry syrup and ginger in water. Stir well and drink to boost immunity and ease cold symptoms.

42. Cinnamon and Apple Cider Vinegar Tonic

Ingredients:

- 1 tsp cinnamon powder
- 1 tbsp apple cider vinegar

Instructions: Mix cinnamon and apple cider vinegar in water. Stir well and drink to help balance blood sugar and boost immune health.

43. Lemon and Peppermint Tea

Ingredients:

- Juice of 1/2 lemon
- 1 tsp dried peppermint

Instructions: Steep peppermint in hot water for 5 minutes. Strain, add lemon juice, and drink to soothe and refresh.

Conclusion

Barbara O'Neill's holistic approach invites us to explore the intricate connections between our physical, emotional, and mental health, empowering us to take charge of our health naturally and sustainably.

The significance of the topics we've explored cannot be overstated. In an era where quick fixes and pharmaceutical interventions often dominate the healthcare landscape, the principles of natural healing stand out as beacons of hope.

Through this guide, we've delved into various aspects of natural health, each underscoring the power of holistic healing. From detoxification to nutrition, from herbal remedies to essential oils, the evidence and insights presented reinforce the efficacy of these approaches. This dual foundation of ancient wisdom and modern science ensures that the strategies offered are not just reliable but also effective, giving readers the confidence and tools they need to improve their health.

Detoxification, a critical practice in maintaining health, has been highlighted for its role in eliminating toxins and revitalizing the body. The practical steps and protocols shared in this guide, such as fasting, consuming specific foods, and avoiding certain substances, make detoxification accessible and achievable, allowing readers to support their body's natural cleansing processes.

Nutrition, another critical element of Barbara O'Neill's philosophy, emphasizes the transformative power of whole, natural foods. A diet rich in nutrient-dense foods not only fuels the body and guards against disease but also enhances mental clarity, opening the door to a new level of health and well-being. The nutritional advice equips readers with the knowledge to make healthy, informed dietary choices that promote long-term vitality.

Herbal remedies and essential oils, known for their potent therapeutic properties, offer natural alternatives to conventional treatments. Their versatility and effectiveness make them indispensable tools in any health regimen.

Managing chronic illness and pain through natural methods highlights the potential of holistic strategies to offer relief where conventional medicine often falls short. Focusing on lifestyle changes, dietary adjustments, and natural therapies provides comprehensive solutions to persistent health challenges, underscoring the body's remarkable ability to heal when given the proper support.

Emotional and mental health, which is deeply connected to physical well-being, is addressed through holistic practices that foster resilience and balance. Techniques for stress reduction, mindfulness, and emotional support are integral to overall health.

Beyond the immediate benefits of natural remedies, this guide also touches on broader aspects of holistic living. Preventive care and lifestyle modifications extend to creating a healthy living environment and nurturing supportive social networks. These elements emphasize the all-encompassing nature of true wellness, which includes every aspect of our lives.

Embracing the teachings of Barbara O'Neill offers a transformative journey toward self-discovery and empowerment. It's about reclaiming control over our health through natural, sustainable practices that honor the body's innate wisdom. Let this journey inspire you to explore, experiment, and fully embrace the path to natural health and holistic living.

Made in United States
Cleveland, OH
15 November 2024

10564633R20299